CLINICAL REASONING

COACHING THE STRUGGLING MEDICAL LEARNER

CLINICAL REASONING

COACHING THE STRUGGLING MEDICAL LEARNER

Andrew S. Parsons, MD, MPH
Karen M. Warburton, MD

AHME | ASSOCIATION FOR HOSPITAL MEDICAL EDUCATION

The objective of this book is to provide knowledge and practical guidance to medical education professionals in accordance with the mission of AHME to promote improvement in medical education to meet health care needs, serve as a forum and resource for medical education information, develop professionals in the field of medical education, and support medical education in health care.

Association for Hospital Medical Education
109 Brush Creek Road
Irwin, PA 15642
724-864-7321 phone
724-864-6153 fax
info@ahme.org email
www.ahme.org

The text of this book is set in Minion
Book designed by Michael Sayre

Printed in United States of America
1 3 5 7 9 10 8 6 4 2

Clinical Reasoning: Coaching the Struggling Medical Learner /
by Andrew S. Parsons, MD, MPH and Karen M. Warburton, MD

Library of Congress Control Number: 2025945137

ISBN 979-8-218-70169-7

Cover design by Michael Sayre

CONTENTS

FOREWORD

Above all its other valuable features, this book is an example of how theory and practice should work together. The first several chapters introduce the theoretical foundations of clinical reasoning while the rest of the chapters emphasize the pragmatics of coaching. However, throughout the book, theory and application are woven together continuously. The theory-practice pairings may address large and complex phenomena, like self-regulated learning, or focused practices and underlying theory for micro skills of coaching, but throughout, a thoughtful balance characterizes the richness of this volume. In many cases, the authors use theory as a way to understand a phenomenon and extend that understanding to practice. In other cases, established practice gets linked to theoretical mechanisms to better understand and improve educational tools. The mastery of so many methods and theories is truly remarkable and the book is worth acquiring if only for its comprehensive bibliographies for each chapter.

Clinical reasoning is the primary focus of this book, and the authors provide a rich and diverse set of viewpoints on this complex professional competency. In these chapters, the reader will find comprehensive reviews of key phenomena and thoughtful analysis of both established and novel conceptual frameworks. For example, the authors argue that reasoning combines both diagnostic reasoning and management reasoning but also propose that we consider prognosis as a third facet. This novel proposal demonstrates the creativity with which the authors think creatively about complex constructs.

A key theme in the book is that clinical reasoning is highly situated, dependent on the content and the context of the problem. At the same time, teaching the struggling learner requires very individualized diagnosis and teaching methods, both for the teacher and the learner. Finding the balance between the idiosyncratic and the generalizable is a tension that the authors recognize does not have a simple, definitive answer. Instead, methods for "diagnosing" and "treating" these learning problems are left to the reader's judgment and application of the guidelines and tools the authors offer.

The struggling learner is the focus of the second part of the book and builds on the broader framework of self-regulated learning. Although the goal of medical education is to produce professionals who can independently identify gaps in their knowledge, plan activities to address these gaps, put that plan into action, and evaluate its efficacy, such self-regulated learning is never perfect. The authors excel in translating the theory of self-regulated learning into coaching practice though educational principles, teaching methods and specific tools and mnemonics, which help coaches more effectively diagnosis and remedy self-regulated learning problems.

The coaching methods addressed in the second half of the book are essential for coaching individuals who struggle. These struggles are grouped into a series of "phenotypes" or common learning problems that are linked to specific coaching methods. This is where the marriage of clinical reasoning and coaching practice produces a wealth of teaching strategies and coaching tools. These tools can be customized to both common and unique struggles that students may be having.

The richness and scope of the literature examined in this book may leave some readers with additional questions, but the concepts and dynamics of thinking, learning, and medical practice are far too complex to allow for a single explanatory framework. The multiplicity of teaching mnemonics and scenarios is extensive. This is not a book that can be used once; it will prove to be a valuable resource for many years and in many, many situations. This is a book that should be in the library of any faculty member concerned with teaching clinical reasoning or coaching learners – and parts of it will be valuable to learners seeking to develop their self-regulated learning skills.

Larry Gruppen, PhD
Professor, University of Michigan

PREFACE

We begin by acknowledging the pioneers of remediation in medical education who have influenced our work. In a seminal paper from 2009, Dr. Karen Hauer and colleagues proposed a model for remediation of the struggling learner that begins with a comprehensive assessment using multiple tools, followed by determination of the primary deficit and development of an individualized learning plan.[1] In their model, remediation itself consists of a cycle of deliberate practice followed by real-time feedback and time for reflection, concluding ultimately with reassessment and determination of competence. In addition to introducing a framework that has inspired most existing centralized remediation programs in the US, this publication served as a call to action for educators to engage in multi-institutional, outcomes-based research to develop best practice guidelines for remediation of training clinicians with long-term follow-up data.

Drs. Calvin Chou and Adina Kalet have also profoundly shaped the discussion around remediation over the last decade. Their book *Remediation in Medical Education: A Mid-Course Correction*,[2] now in its second edition,[3] provides a wealth of practical and theoretical evidence-based guidance. Drawing on the collective expertise of clinicians and medical educators across the world, they define remediation in medical education as the act of facilitating a correction for learners who began the journey toward becoming competent physicians and have moved off course. In a subsequent article entitled "The dos, don'ts and don't knows of remediation in medical education," Drs. Chou and Kalet and colleagues offer practical guidelines for remediation that clarify evidence-based best practices and pitfalls.[4]

Dr. Jeannette Guerrasio, in her extensive body of published work which includes two books and numerous scholarly articles published over a similar time period, has laid the groundwork for medical educators who work with struggling medical learners across the continuum of their training. Her book *Remediation of the Struggling Medical Learner*,[5] now in its second edition,[6] presents a case-based, practical approach to the identification, diagnosis, and remediation of the struggling medical learner that has greatly informed our program development. In her more recent companion volume, *Remediation Case Studies: Helping Struggling Medical Learners*,[7] educators (including us) contribute 24 real-life cases, discuss remediation approaches and pitfalls, and benefit from the wisdom of Dr. Guerrasio's commentary.

Dr. Guerrasio has been incredibly generous and giving of her time and expertise over the last 10 years, and we owe her a tremendous debt of gratitude. We enthusiastically recommend her books.

Finally, Dr. Marie-Claude Audétat and colleagues have been a leading voice in the study and remediation of clinical reasoning for more than a decade. In their 2013 study, her group published a taxonomy that categorizes common clinical reasoning difficulties based on real-world clinical teaching experiences.[8] A follow-up publication in 2017 proposed specific remediation strategies for each step of the clinical reasoning process.[9] Their research underscores the need for early identification of and structured support for the struggling learner, encouraging clinical teachers to integrate remediation strategies within everyday supervision practices.

I, Dr. Karen Warburton, am a Professor of Medicine and Associate Designated Institutional Official at the University of Virginia School of Medicine. I built and direct a centralized remediation program known as COACH (Committee on Achieving Competency Through Help) that provides support for approximately 850 graduate medical learners and 200 program leaders in over 100 different programs at our institution.

I, Dr. Andrew Parsons, am an Associate Professor of Medicine and Associate Dean for Clinical Competency at the University of Virginia School of Medicine. I designed and direct an evidence-based approach to clinical reasoning coaching for struggling learners across the medical educational continuum.

We jointly lead faculty development efforts focused on the teaching and assessment of clinical reasoning for practicing clinicians at the University of Virginia and provide support for educators at other academic institutions who are interested in building similar programs. Together, we have worked with hundreds of struggling medical students, residents (physician and nonphysician), and fellows. Our work has been presented at national and international educational and scientific conferences and published in high-impact journals.

In this book, we draw upon the methods of Dr. Guerrasio and her mentor, Dr. Eva Aagaard, as we focus on the learner struggling with clinical reasoning. Our understanding of clinical reasoning has grown in recent years and, with it, our sophistication in teaching and assessment. Despite this, there are currently no best-practice guidelines for the individualized remediation of medical learners who struggle with clinical reasoning. We aim to provide educators with a standardized approach to clinical reasoning assessment and a library of coaching tools that are accessible to all educators and do not require specialized expertise in remediation. In doing so, we hope ultimately to facilitate earlier detection of and intervention for struggling learners and improve assessment and teaching of clinical reasoning for all learners.

We have chosen to use the term medical learner to encompass all levels of training, from student through practitioner, in allopathic and osteopathic medicine, among advanced practice practitioners, and in select physical therapy, pharmacy, podiatry, and dentistry programs. This book is meant to serve as a resource for educators at all levels, in any specialty providing clinical care, who are working with learners across the continuum as they care for patients.

References

1. Hauer KE, Ciccone A, Henzel TR, et al. Remediation of the Deficiencies of Physicians Across the Continuum From Medical School to Practice: A Thematic Review of the Literature: *Acad Med.* 2009;84(12):1822-1832. doi:10.1097/ACM.0b013e3181bf3170

2. Kalet A. *Remediation in Medical Education: A Mid-Course Correction.* 2014 edition. (Chou CL, ed.). Springer; 2013.

3. Kalet A, Chou CL, eds. *Remediation in Medical Education: A Mid-Course Correction.* Springer International Publishing; 2023. doi:10.1007/978-3-031-32404-8

4. Chou CL, Kalet A, Costa MJ, Cleland J, Winston K. Guidelines: The dos, don'ts and don't knows of remediation in medical education. *Perspect Med Educ.* 2019;8(6):322-338. doi:10.1007/s40037-019-00544-5

5. Guerrasio J. *Remediation of the Struggling Medical Learner.* 1 edition. Association for Hospital Medical Education; 2013.

6. Guerrasio J. *Remediation of the Struggling Medical Learner.* 2nd Edition. Association for Hospital Medical Education; 2018.

7. Guerrasio J. *Remediation Case Studies: Helping Struggling Medical Learners.* 2nd Edition. Association for Hospital Medical Education; 2021.

8. Audétat MC, Laurin S, Sanche G, et al. Clinical reasoning difficulties: A taxonomy for clinical teachers. *Med Teach.* 2013;35(3):e984-e989. doi:10.3109/0142159X.2012.733041

9. Audétat MC, Laurin S, Dory V, Charlin B, Nendaz MR. Diagnosis and management of clinical reasoning difficulties: Part II. Clinical reasoning difficulties: Management and remediation strategies. *Med Teach.* 2017;39(8):797-801. doi:10.1080/0142159X.2017.1331034

ACKNOWLEDGEMENTS

WE CONTRIBUTED EQUALLY to this book and are appreciative of the generous support and encouragement we received along the way. Thank you to our contributors for sharing cases and coaching exercises and to our peer reviewers who provided thoughtful guidance on every chapter. This publication continues a tradition of successful works dedicated to remediation in medical education under the auspices of the Association for Hospital Medical Education (AHME). We owe special thanks to this remarkable organization, its executive director Tia O. Drake, and literary agent Joan Parker of Parker Literary Agency, LLC, for the opportunity to author this book and for your steadfast guidance. Your partnership and support made this project a reality. Our personal acknowledgements are below.

Sincerely,
Karen and Andrew

Karen M. Warburton, MD:

My journey working with struggling learners began more than two decades ago during my time as a chief resident. I came to this work unexpectedly and without formal preparation. Since then, most of my learning has taken place in real time, shaped by the needs of learners and the lessons they have taught me along the way. It has been my good fortune to have trained at a rigorous program in which clinical reasoning was both a spoken value of patient care and woven deliberately into our education.

Thank you to Dr. Lisa Bellini, my mentor and confidante, who led the Penn Internal Medicine Residency Program for twenty years. A transformational leader, Lisa sets a high bar for excellence and is deeply committed to advancing the careers of her mentees. In 2014, she entrusted me with a formal role in working with struggling learners, a role that would ultimately define my career. I am forever grateful for this gift and to Lisa for her support over the years.

My own clinical reasoning took shape under the leadership of a spectacular line of chief residents, Drs. Alison Loren, Todd Barton, Vin Lo Re, and Joe Rencic, to name a few. At Penn, I learned from these and other master clinicians and educators how to think critically, methodically, and creatively when approaching a clinical problem. As residents, we were routinely encouraged, in the context of patient care and in teaching conferences, to think aloud, to think on our feet, and to justify our decisions—practices which eventually became ingrained.

Their training influenced every aspect of how I teach and practice medicine and has greatly informed the lessons in this book.

I am profoundly grateful to Drs. Mitchell Rosner and John Schorling, my mentors at the University of Virginia, whose guidance, wisdom, and unwavering support have shaped my career in ways I could not have imagined. Thank you for your advocacy and for the doors you have opened for me in different but equally impactful ways.

Dr. Eric Goren, my former colleague and collaborator, deserves much recognition for his work with struggling learners and his creative ideas about coaching and program development. Eric is an exceptionally gifted educator, and his contributions to this book have been invaluable. Thank you to Dr. Andrew Parsons for your partnership on this project and for being the type of mentee who reminds mentors why we mentor. The epitome of a self-starter, Andrew's enthusiasm and dedication continue to inspire and motivate me daily.

To the hundreds of residents and fellows with whom I have had the privilege of working over the last twenty years, thank you for your bravery and your willingness to put in the work. You have taught me more than I could ever teach you.

With infinite gratitude, I acknowledge JS, MA, and ER, my team without whom there would be no book. Thank you for believing in me and trusting me and teaching me, through your example, to lead with curiosity rather than judgment. Thank you for your kindness and equanimity. And thank you especially to ER for reminding me that there is so much more to life than getting to a diagnosis.

And, finally, a huge thank you to my husband, Dr. Alden Doyle, and my remarkable, thoughtful, creative, curious, and hilarious 11-year old daughter, Harper, for your patience and encouragement as this book has taken me away from my roles at home.

It truly takes a village, and I am so fortunate to have this village.

Andrew S. Parsons, MD, MPH:

This journey has only been possible because of the love and support of my family. To my wife, Dr. Laura Parsons, you are so strong and steady. Thank you for being with me every step of the way. To my daughter, Grayce: your independence, confidence, enthusiasm, and sense of humor are inspiring; you make the world a better place for so many. I am grateful to my mom for helping me to truly see, hear, and know people; to my dad for giving me strength, an innate ability to teach, and an enjoyment of writing that I found later in life. Thank you to my sister for giving me all my good ideas, my brother-in-law for being the quintessential professional, and to "the twins" for your curiosity and joyful presence.

Numerous individuals have shaped my professional path. Thank you to Dr. George Hoke for igniting my early interest in high-value care that eventually became a fascination with decision-making. Your sponsorship laid the foundation for everything that followed—and continues to this day. To Dr. Joe Rencic for encouraging me to look beyond the field of medicine to grow my understanding of clinical reasoning—you are an aspirational clinician educator; to Dr. Michelle Daniel for keeping me grounded in theory and pushing me to think outside the box; to Dr. Andrew Olson for setting the standard for hard work; and to Dr. Steven Durning for your mentorship and encouragement to dive headfirst into a PhD program.

To Drs. Jess Dreicer, Glenn Moulder, MJ Sacco, and Greg Young: I am appreciative of your friendship and camaraderie. Special thanks to Dr. Maryellen Gusic, who taught me how to formulate research questions and produce scholarship that matters, and to Drs. Michael Ryan and Jim Martindale, who have carried that torch as both friend and mentor. To Dr. Paul Helgerson: thank you for the opportunity to become a hospitalist and for providing such thoughtful advice. To Dr. Amber Inofuentes: thank you for your leadership and unwavering belief in doing what's right. To Dr. Peggy Plews-Ogan: I appreciate your early guidance and wisdom. Thank you to Drs. Megan Bray, Mohan Nadkarni, Brian Uthlaut, and Meg Keeley for always opening doors, and to Drs. Emily Abdoler and Thilan Wijesekera for proving how enriching collaboration can be.

To my co-author, Dr. Karen Warburton, who entrusted a new faculty member with the opportunity to support struggling learners and the freedom to innovate: I have learned so much from you and am truly thankful for your partnership.

Finally, to the learners I've had the privilege to teach and learn alongside: your commitment to growth makes this work fulfilling. It's always been about the journey, and I'm grateful to those of you who have shared it with me.

CONTRIBUTORS AND PEER REVIEWERS

Stephanie Bajo, PsyD
Assistant Professor of Psychiatry and Neurobehavioral Sciences
University of Virginia School of Medicine
sdb7q@uvahealth.org

Cara A. Cipriano, MD, MSc
Associate Professor of Orthopaedic Surgery
Perelman School of Medicine at the University of Pennsylvania
cara.cipriano@pennmedicine.upenn.edu

Ian Crane, MD
Assistant Professor of Medicine
University of Virginia School of Medicine
ian.crane@uvahealth.org

Michelle Daniel, MD, MHPE
Professor of Emergency Medicine
University of California, San Diego School of Medicine
midaniel@health.ucsd.edu

Jessica J. Dreicer, MD
Associate Professor of Medicine
University of Virginia School of Medicine
jessica.dreicer@uvahealth.org

Katherine T. Forkin, MD
Associate Professor of Anesthesiology
University of Virginia School of Medicine
ket2a@uvahealth.org

Eric N. Goren, MD
Professor of Clinical Medicine
Perelman School of Medicine at the University of Pennsylvania
eric.goren@gmail.com

Sook Chan Hoang, MD
Associate Professor of Surgery
University of Virginia School of Medicine
sh7je@uvahealth.org

Matthew Kelleher, MD, MEd
Associate Professor of Pediatrics and Internal Medicine
University of Cincinnati College of Medicine
kellehmw@ucmail.uc.edu

Casey N. McQuade, MD, MSEd
Assistant Professor of Medicine
University of Pittsburgh School of Medicine
mcquadec@upmc.edu

Joseph J. Rencic, MD
Professor of Medicine
Boston University Chobanian & Avedisian School of Medicine
jrencic@bu.edu

Adam Rodman, MD, MPH
Assistant Professor of Medicine
Harvard Medical School
arodman@bidmc.harvard.edu

Melissa J. Sacco, MD, MS
Associate Professor of Pediatrics
University of Virginia School of Medicine
ms4xe@uvahealth.org

John B. Schorling, MD, MPH
Professor of Medicine
University of Virginia School of Medicine
jbs7f@uvahealth.org

Jessica Sheeran, MD
Associate Professor of Anesthesiology
University of Virginia School of Medicine
js5cu@uvahealth.org

Sarah E. Vick, MD
Associate Professor of Medicine
University of Kentucky College of Medicine
sarah.vick@uky.edu

Kevin M. Watson, MSc
Learning Specialist
University of Virginia School of Medicine
ryj5xz@virginia.edu

Thilan Wijesekera, MD, MHS
Assistant Professor of Medicine
Yale School of Medicine
thilan.wijesekera@yale.edu

Gregory Young, MD
Associate Professor of Medicine
University of Virginia School of Medicine
gregory.young@uvahealth.org

CLINICAL REASONING

COACHING THE STRUGGLING MEDICAL LEARNER

Section 1

General Principles: The Struggling Medical Learner

While learner struggle is an inevitable part of medical education, it is often not adequately addressed. As educators, we have a vital responsibility to move beyond simply identifying performance gaps and must also work to create learning environments that embrace challenges as opportunities for growth.

In chapter 1, "Normalizing Struggle and Promoting Learner Buy-In," we highlight the importance of redefining how educators and learners perceive challenges.

We introduce a developmental perspective to frame the varied factors that may hinder learner progress in chapter 2, "Global Assessment of the Struggling Medical Learner."

CHAPTER 1

Normalizing Struggle and Promoting Learner Buy-In

THE LAST 25 years have been characterized by a fundamental shift in the way we teach and assess learners in the health professions. Medical education has evolved toward a competency-based model which places a greater emphasis on assessing what learners can do in practice rather than simply what they know.[1,2] This shift reflects the recognition that clinical competence is multi-dimensional, involving not only knowledge but also skills and the ability to integrate these elements in real-world contexts.[3] A key tenet of competency-based education (CBE) is that each learner's developmental trajectory is unique; curricula, assessment strategies, and remediation efforts must be individualized to meet learners where they are.[4,5] Rather than progressing on a fixed timeline, learners are expected to demonstrate competency before advancing, allowing for greater flexibility in both pace and pathways of learning.

Implicit in this framework is the recognition that struggling learners are an expected part of any CBE program. Struggle is not only normal but inevitable in a system designed to challenge learners to meet the high standards of clinical competence. The reported prevalence of struggling learners, however, varies widely depending on how struggle is characterized and the willingness to acknowledge it. In graduate medical education, reports from specialty-specific surveys of program directors and single-center retrospective reviews suggest that the prevalence of "problem residents" or fellows requiring formal remediation ranges from 3.5% to 22%.[6–13] These numbers reflect both the wide range of specialties and the varying criteria used to define underperformance. For example, some programs define struggle narrowly (e.g., failure to pass licensing exams) while others adopt a broader perspective that includes concerns about mental well-being or deficiencies in clinical reasoning, professionalism, and teamwork.

In undergraduate medical education and other health professions, the prevalence of struggling learners is less well defined due to the lack of standardized criteria and an almost exclusive focus of remedial efforts on test-taking rather than clinical skill development. An estimated 5 to 15% of medical students will face academic difficulties requiring remediation, characterized most commonly as flaws in clinical reasoning.[14–16] For the majority of these students, struggles are not identified until clinical rotations.[17,18] Later identification is associated with learner discouragement and disengagement.[19]

While this represents a minority of learners throughout the continuum and across specialties, struggling learners consume a disproportionate share of time and resources, requiring intensive effort from clinicians, administrators, and remediation coaches.[20,21] Effectively addressing the needs of these learners is not only a matter of fairness but also a critical component of maintaining the integrity of training programs and institutions and ensuring patient safety.

THE IMPORTANCE OF ACKNOWLEDGING LEARNER DEFICIENCY

The early recognition of struggling learners is vital for successful intervention because it allows sufficient time for coaching and eventual demonstration of competence.[22,23] However, learners are often identified late in their struggle, if at all. Deficits are rarely self-reported.[24] The Dunning-Kruger effect occurs when an individual's lack of knowledge or skill in a certain area leads them to overestimate their performance.[25] A systematic review of more than 700 articles concluded that, similar to other professions, clinicians have a limited ability to accurately self-assess.[26] Underperforming learners often overestimate—whereas more competent learners tend to underestimate—their abilities;

the latter is particularly true for women.[27] Lack of insight, whether due to overconfidence or underestimation, creates a significant barrier to timely intervention. Later in this chapter we will discuss strategies for enhancing learner insight and fostering openness to feedback.

Learner buy-in, critical for the success of remediation efforts, is contingent on educator buy-in.[28] Educators must recognize and accept their role in identifying and supporting struggling learners, yet this process is often hindered by flawed assessment tools and cognitive biases.[29] Clinical evaluations, for instance, are frequently submitted or shared late, lack specificity, and suffer from various rating errors.[30–32] Written feedback is often too vague or focuses on irrelevant aspects of performance.[33] In our experience, evaluators tend to make global inferences about clinical competence based on work ethic and interpersonal skills. "They are working so hard." "They are wonderful with patients and a real team player." In the busy clinical environment where there is limited time or opportunity to directly observe learners throughout the workday, clinicians may fail to look past these qualities and consequently may overlook significant problems with clinical reasoning, leading to missed opportunities for early intervention.

Additionally, cognitive biases such as the halo effect can obscure the recognition of deficits. Coined by psychologist Dr. Edward Thorndike, the halo error (or effect) refers to the tendency to let one positive attribute, such as a learner's likability or dedication, influence judgments about unrelated areas of performance.[34,35] For example, a learner who is well-liked by patients and supervisors may receive favorable evaluations that overlook significant struggles with other aspects of performance. Recognizing and addressing these barriers is essential for creating a culture that normalizes struggle while ensuring early identification and support for those who need it most.

CASE

Dr. Smith is a first-year resident who struggles to triage clinical tasks. At the conclusion of rounds on the inpatient wards, for example, he is not sure which item on his to-do list to tackle first. When presenting patients, his management plans are cursory, and he prefers to focus on reporting the objective data and let his supervisors develop a plan. Dr. Smith also struggles to identify "sick versus not sick." These issues are most prominent on busy days, when he is covering the team by himself, or when patient census and complexity is high. Recently, Dr. Smith's failure to recognize a patient's acute change in clinical status resulted in a delay in transfer of this patient to the intensive care unit. Upon review of his file, the program director finds that Dr. Smith's numeric end-of-rotation evaluations are average. He is noted by his supervisors and fellow residents to be kind, compassionate, and extremely hardworking. They vaguely acknowledge that he can improve in certain areas but are reluctant to express their true concerns directly to him or in his evaluations.

Learners like Dr. Smith, who struggles with multiple aspects of clinical reasoning and is unable to manage a full census of patients independently, commonly fly under the radar for extended periods of time in an educational or training program. Peers and supervisors may minimize concerns and avoid bringing them to anyone's attention out of concern that they will offend the learner or negatively impact their career advancement.[29,36] Issues often come to light when the learner is covering their team on a supervisor's day off or following a medical error. When written evaluations are unrevealing, leaders rely on hallway chatter and confidential comments communicated over email to formulate an accurate assessment of the struggling learner. These practices result in delays in intervention and may hinder learner buy-in.

In a series of seminal articles over the last 20 years, educational scholars have explored the complex psychological and systemic contributors to the common practices of "failure to fail" or "kicking the can down the road" in medical education.[37–39] Denial and avoidance are strategies employed by many of us to cope with the discomfort we experience when faced with an underperforming medical learner. In our experience, most learners who present with performance issues in residency or fellowship also struggled with similar issues in medical school or residency, respectively. In most cases, we come to this conclusion by reading between the lines of the medical school or residency file and talking directly with the learner. The objective is not more failures but rather the prevention of failures with earlier recognition and appropriate deployment of resources. In our experience, we are far more likely to help than hurt someone's career by acknowledging difficulty and providing dedicated help. Struggle is a normal and expected component of medical training and should be treated as such. It is critical to intervene before the learner enters clinical practice, where supervision is less predictable and patient safety is at greater risk.

BARRIERS TO RECOGNITION OF THE STRUGGLING MEDICAL LEARNER

These observations reflect the many barriers to recognition and acknowledgement of the struggling medical learner. Sometimes we are unaware of a learner's deficiency because we are not directly observing closely enough or in the correct settings. In other cases, we do see the problem but are reluctant to acknowledge it officially. Time is a major barrier for all of us who work in busy academic and clinical settings. We may lack comfort with how to remediate someone. Our institutions may not have well-defined or easily accessible resources for remediation. Many of us are worried about the impact of stigma on the learner's feelings or on their career.[40,41] In certain cases, we may even fear retaliation. And while we, as authors, acknowledge the legitimacy of all these concerns, they must be weighed against the consequences of ignoring the struggle, which in most cases will not improve without targeted intervention. Earlier recognition of the struggling medical learner often requires a programmatic, or even institutional, culture change (Table 1.1). Such culture change necessitates faculty development, particularly around the importance of giving corrective feedback and providing skills to do this effectively.

Table 1.1. Changing the Culture Around Remediation: Faculty and Institutional Goals

1. Admit that learners struggle
2. Help learners expect and embrace both reinforcing and corrective feedback as part of the progression toward competence
3. Gain comfort giving corrective feedback and being honest in written evaluations
4. Implement widespread faculty development focused on coaching
5. Embed remediation programs at high levels within the institution or program
6. Celebrate remediation success stories

WORD CHOICE MAKES A DIFFERENCE

So how do we help learners feel more comfortable with the idea that they need additional support to meet competency standards? For starters, the language we use carries weight. Remediation itself is a charged word, and some places avoid the term altogether. The meanings and implications of the word remediation vary between programs and institutions. Differences center around the threshold for putting a learner on remediation, the level of formality and specifics of the process, the type of documentation, and the consequences to the learner within the program and beyond. In US graduate medical education programs, remediation is usually a pre-disciplinary step that is not reportable to licensing boards or other regulatory entities unless associated with an extension of training or significant modification in scope of practice. The literature describing remediation in medical students or non-physician health care professionals is scant and primarily focuses on test performance. Typically, remediation implies something in writing. Formal remediation is a path that one might consider if there is a lack of learner buy-in, if initial efforts to coach the learner in deficient skills have been unsuccessful, and/or if struggles involve misconduct or are significant enough to impact patient care.

Dr. Carol Dweck's research in educational psychology underscores the importance of a growth mindset, a perspective that reframes challenges and setbacks as valuable opportunities for personal development.[42] This approach is particularly relevant in medical education, for which the stakes are high and the learning curve is steep. Adopting a growth mindset encourages learners to perceive struggle not as a sign of failure but as an expected and essential aspect of their journey toward clinical competence. By normalizing the inevitability of challenges, educators can help learners embrace feedback, persist through difficulties, and approach remediation with a sense of purpose rather than shame. This shift in perspective is not only beneficial for individual growth but also paramount for creating a supportive learning environment that prioritizes continuous improvement.

In alignment with this approach, for most medical learners we prefer the term *clinical coaching* to *remediation.* This terminology reflects less righting a wrong and more the developmental approach of modern medical education.

In other words, remediation often implies correcting deficits, while coaching focuses on helping learners to refine their skills in a supportive environment. In this book we use the word *remediation* when referencing the work of others and when speaking generally about our program and programmatic processes. We use the word *coaching* when describing the one-on-one work with learners. Effective clinical coaching relies on the creation of a supportive and neutral space for learners to engage in deliberate practice of unmastered skills under direct observation by a coach. Implicit in the concept of deliberate practice is the belief that, with proper coaching, performance can improve with dedicated effort.[43] The concept and roles of a *coach* in a remediation setting, which remain complex and at times controversial, are discussed in more detail in chapter 6.

Table 1.2 includes a list of strategies to promote learner buy-in with an evidence-based rationale for each.

Table 1.2. Strategies to Promote Learner Buy-in for Effective Remediation

Strategy	Description	Rationale
Establish psychological safety	Create an environment in which learners feel safe to acknowledge challenges and participate in coaching without fear of judgment or repercussions	Psychological safety supports openness to feedback and engagement in growth-focused interventions[44]
Clarify expectations	Use explicit, competency-based objectives to define areas requiring improvement and the definition of success	Clear goals align with the principles of competency-based education, improving learner understanding and motivation
Set goals collaboratively	Involve learners in developing their coaching plan to enhance ownership and investment in the process	Collaboration fosters autonomy, a key driver of motivation, as outlined in self-determination theory[45]

(continued)

Table 1.2. Strategies to Promote Learner Buy-in for Effective Remediation *(continued)*

Strategy	Description	Rationale
Provide timely, specific feedback	Deliver actionable feedback focusing on observed behaviors and their impact, avoiding vague or overly general statements that make assumptions about intent	Timely, specific feedback promotes insight and mitigates overconfidence[33,46]
Use data to foster insight	Share objective performance data such as assessment scores or observed clinical behaviors to help learners understand their areas of struggle	Data-driven discussions reduce defensiveness and increase learner self-awareness[24,47]
Normalize struggle	Frame remediation as a routine and expected part of professional development, reducing stigma around the process	Emphasizing the normalcy of struggle aligns with the principles of growth mindset and improves acceptance[42]
Highlight long-term benefits	Emphasize how addressing deficiencies now contributes to future success and patient safety, characterizing remediation as a professional investment	Linking remediation to professional growth fosters motivation and reduces learner resistance[48]

THE CENTRAL ROLE OF INSIGHT AND INTRINSIC MOTIVATION

Many underperforming medical learners have trouble identifying and actualizing feedback, and some may appear to be resistant to feedback. Insight and ability to self-reflect are two of the most important predictors of effective coaching.[49–51] Similarly, successful coaching hinges on actively engaging the learner and adopting the principles of self-regulated learning (SRL) as the learners participate in the intervention.[52,53] SRL and its critical relationship to coaching clinical reasoning is discussed in chapters 6 and 7. Learners should be encouraged to set specific goals, participate in the development of the coaching plan, and continuously self-monitor and self-evaluate.[54] Successful involvement in this process requires motivation. Motivation is ideally intrinsic, though in our experience the threat of remediation can serve as a powerful extrinsic motivator as coaches work to uncover and/or develop intrinsic motivation. Those who present with apparent lack of insight or motivation should be approached with curiosity rather than judgment. Encouraging self-reflection and goal setting can help learners take ownership of their learning process. In most cases, the barriers to insight or motivation relate to fear of failing, learned responses to perceived criticism, burnout, and/or concomitant mental health conditions such as depression or anxiety. Many struggling medical learners arrive with a fixed mindset in which their primary goal is avoiding failure. As a result, they are intolerant of their own imperfections and resistant to feedback. Creating a supportive space to understand and address these fears and barriers is crucial to overcoming them. The importance of this supportive space is discussed in more detail in chapter 2.

SEPARATION OF COACHING AND ASSESSMENT

For all medical learners, we recommend establishing a clear boundary between coaching and formal assessment, including reassessment following the coaching intervention (Table 1.3). Learners tend to be more engaged in coaching and more likely to ask for help or clarification if they feel that they can make mistakes and say "I don't know" without fear of repercussions.[55,56] Furthermore, learners engaged in coaching interventions are often scrutinized to a degree that is not the standard for their peers. For many reasons, this sets up an unlevel playing field from the standpoint of assessment. Therefore, we feel strongly that, for the purposes of summative feedback and decisions regarding advancement, the learner's progress in coaching should be measured using the standard, programmatic evaluation system and based solely on their performance in the clinical environment. Feedback provided by the coach to the learner during coaching sessions should not be included in the learner's summative assessment.

Table 1.3. Separation of Coaching and Assessment

Roles of program or institutional leader
• Communicates expectations to the learner and provides notification if expectations are not being met • Ensures that supervising clinicians are giving frequent, formative feedback • Documents concerns in writing • Assesses and reassesses learner using standard evaluation methods
Roles of coach
• Processes feedback with the learner • Promotes skill development, observes learner performing skills, gives formative feedback about performance of skills • Examines barriers to insight, motivation, actualization of feedback, and/or improvement

SUMMARY

Normalizing struggle and promoting learner buy-in are critical elements in the success of remediation programs for medical learners. Recognizing the uniqueness of each learner's trajectory allows educators to provide timely and effective support, helping learners overcome challenges and achieve competency. By fostering a culture that values growth, resilience, and honest feedback, we can promote an environment in which learners feel safe to acknowledge their difficulties and engage fully in their development. Encouraging the separation of coaching from assessment further supports this process, ensuring that remediation is seen as an opportunity for development rather than as a punishment. By investing in early recognition, targeted coaching, and a supportive learning environment, we can help all medical learners reach their full potential.

References

1. Frank JR, Mungroo R, Ahmad Y, Wang M, De Rossi S, Horsley T. Toward a definition of competency-based education in medicine: a systematic review of published definitions. *Med Teach.* 2010;32(8):631-637. doi:10.3109/0142159X.2010.500898
2. Ross S, Hauer KE, van Melle E. Outcomes are what matter: Competency-based medical education gets us to our goal. *MedEdPublish.* 2018;7:85. doi:10.15694/mep.2018.0000085.1
3. ten Cate O, Khursigara-Slattery N, Cruess RL, Hamstra SJ, Steinert Y, Sternszus R. Medical competence as a multilayered construct. *Med Educ.* 2024;58(1):93-104. doi:10.1111/medu.15162
4. Carraccio C, Englander R, Van Melle E, et al. Advancing Competency-Based Medical Education: A Charter for Clinician–Educators. *Acad Med.* 2016;91(5):645. doi:10.1097/ACM.0000000000001048
5. Frank JR, Snell L, Englander R, Holmboe ES, ICBME Collaborators. Implementing competency-based medical education: Moving forward. *Med Teach.* 2017;39(6):568-573. doi:10.1080/0142159X.2017.1315069
6. Yao DC, Wright SM. National Survey of Internal Medicine Residency Program Directors Regarding Problem Residents. *JAMA.* 2000;284(9):1099-1104. doi:10.1001/jama.284.9.1099
7. Riebschleger MP, Haftel HM. Remediation in the Context of the Competencies: A Survey of Pediatrics Residency Program Directors. *J Grad Med Educ.* 2013;5(1):60-63. doi:10.4300/JGME-D-12-00024.1
8. Roback HB, Crowder MK. Psychiatric resident dismissal: A national survey of training programs. *Am J Psychiatry.* 1989;146(1):96-98. doi:10.1176/ajp.146.1.96
9. Williams RG, Roberts NK, Schwind CJ, Dunnington GL. The nature of general surgery resident performance problems. *Surgery.* 2009;145(6):651-658. doi:10.1016/j.surg.2009.01.019
10. Reamy BV, Harman JH. Residents in Trouble: An In-depth Assessment of the 25- year Experience of a Single Family Medicine Residency. *Fam Med.* 38(4):6.
11. Warburton KM, Goren E, Dine CJ. Comprehensive Assessment of Struggling Learners Referred to a Graduate Medical Education Remediation Program. *J Grad Med Educ.* 2017;9(6):763-767. doi:10.4300/JGME-D-17-00175.1
12. Warburton KM, Shahane AA. Mental Health Conditions Among Struggling GME Learners: Results From a Single Center Remediation Program. *J Grad Med Educ.* 2020;12(6):773-777. doi:10.4300/JGME-D-20-00007.1
13. Tabby DS, Majeed MH, Schwartzman RJ. Problem neurology residents: a national survey. *Neurology.* 2011;76(24):2119-2123. doi:10.1212/WNL.0b013e31821f4636
14. Hunt RG, Krzystofiak FJ, Meindl JR, Yousry AM. Cognitive style and decision making. *Organ Behav Hum Decis Process.* 1989;44(3):436-453. doi:10.1016/0749-5978(89)90018-6
15. Audétat MC, Laurin S, Sanche G, et al. Clinical reasoning difficulties: A taxonomy for clinical teachers. *Med Teach.* 2013;35(3):e984-e989. doi:10.3109/0142159X.2012.733041

16. Yates J, James D. Risk factors for poor performance on the undergraduate medical course: cohort study at Nottingham University. *Med Educ.* 2007;41(1):65-73. doi:10.1111/j.1365-2929.2006.02648.x

17. Hauer KE, Ciccone A, Henzel TR, et al. Remediation of the Deficiencies of Physicians Across the Continuum From Medical School to Practice: A Thematic Review of the Literature: *Acad Med.* 2009;84(12):1822-1832. doi:10.1097/ACM.0b013e3181bf3170

18. Boileau E, St-Onge C, Audétat MC. Is there a way for clinical teachers to assist struggling learners? A synthetic review of the literature. *Adv Med Educ Pract.* 2017;8:89-97. doi:10.2147/AMEP.S123410

19. Kalet A, Chou CL, Ellaway RH. To fail is human: remediating remediation in medical education. *Perspect Med Educ.* 2017;6(6). doi:10.1007/S40037-017-0385-6

20. Parsons AS, Warburton KM, Martindale JR, Rosenberg IL. Characterization of Clinical Skills Remediation: A National Survey of Medical Schools. *South Med J.* 2022;115(3):202-207. doi:10.14423/SMJ.0000000000001361

21. Parsons AS, Dreicer JJ, Martindale JR, Young G, Warburton KM. A Targeted Clinical Reasoning Remediation Program for Residents and Fellows in Need. *J Grad Med Educ.* 2024;16(4):469. doi:10.4300/JGME-D-23-00822.1

22. Bennion LD, Torre D, Durning SJ, et al. Early identification of struggling learners: using prematriculation and early academic performance data. *Perspect Med Educ.* 2019;8(5). doi:10.1007/S40037-019-00539-2

23. Landoll RR, Bennion LD, Maranich AM, et al. Extending growth curves: a trajectory monitoring approach to identification and interventions in struggling medical student learners. *Adv Health Sci Educ.* 2022;27(3):645-658. doi:10.1007/s10459-022-10109-7

24. Eva KW, Cunnington JPW, Reiter HI, Keane DR, Norman GR. How can I know what I don't know? Poor self assessment in a well-defined domain. *Adv Health Sci Educ Theory Pract.* 2004;9(3):211-224. doi:10.1023/B:AHSE.0000038209.65714.d4

25. Kruger J, Dunning D. Unskilled and unaware of it: how difficulties in recognizing one's own incompetence lead to inflated self-assessments. *J Pers Soc Psychol.* 1999;77(6):1121-1134. doi:10.1037//0022-3514.77.6.1121

26. Davis DA, Mazmanian PE, Fordis M, Van Harrison R, Thorpe KE, Perrier L. Accuracy of physician self-assessment compared with observed measures of competence: a systematic review. *JAMA.* 2006;296(9):1094-1102. doi:10.1001/jama.296.9.1094

27. Rahmani M. Medical Trainees and the Dunning–Kruger Effect: When They Don't Know What They Don't Know. *J Grad Med Educ.* 2020;12(5):532-534. doi:10.4300/JGME-D-20-00134.1

28. Krzyzaniak SM, Wolf SJ, Byyny R, et al. A qualitative study of medical educators' perspectives on remediation: Adopting a holistic approach to struggling residents. *Med Teach.* 2017;39(9):967-974. doi:10.1080/0142159X.2017.1332362

29. Castanelli DJ, Molloy E, Bearman M. The stigma of underperformance in assessment and remediation. *Adv Health Sci Educ Theory Pract.* Published online October 16, 2024. doi:10.1007/s10459-024-10382-8

30. McQueen SA, Petrisor B, Bhandari M, Fahim C, McKinnon V, Sonnadara RR. Examining the barriers to meaningful assessment and feedback in medical training. *Am J Surg.* 2016;211(2):464-475. doi:10.1016/j.amjsurg.2015.10.002

31. Cleland JA, Knight LV, Rees CE, Tracey S, Bond CM. Is it me or is it them? Factors that influence the passing of underperforming students. *Med Educ.* 2008;42(8):800-809. doi:10.1111/j.1365-2923.2008.03113.x

32. Dolan BM, Arnold J, Green MM. Establishing Trust When Assessing Learners: Barriers and Opportunities. *Acad Med.* 2019;94(12):1851. doi:10.1097/ACM.0000000000002982

33. Veloski J, Boex JR, Grasberger MJ, Evans A, Wolfson DB. Systematic review of the literature on assessment, feedback and physicians' clinical performance: BEME Guide No. 7. *Med Teach.* 2006;28(2):117-128. doi:10.1080/01421590600622665

34. Nisbett RE, Wilson TD. The halo effect: Evidence for unconscious alteration of judgments. *J Pers Soc Psychol.* 1977;35(4):250-256. doi:10.1037/0022-3514.35.4.250

35. Thorndike EL. A constant error in psychological ratings. *J Appl Psychol.* 1920;4(1):25-29. doi:10.1037/h0071663

36. Scarff CE, Bearman M, Chiavaroli N, Trumble S. Assessor discomfort and failure to fail in clinical performance assessments. *BMC Med Educ.* 2023;23(1):901. doi:10.1186/s12909-023-04688-1

37. Dudek NL, Marks MB, Regehr G. Failure to Fail: The Perspectives of Clinical Supervisors. *Acad Med.* 2005;80(10):S84.

38. Guerrasio J, Furfari KA, Rosenthal LD, Nogar CL, Wray KW, Aagaard EM. Failure to fail: the institutional perspective. *Med Teach.* 2014;36(9):799-803. doi:10.3109/0142159X.2014.910295

39. Santen SA, Christner J, Mejicano G, Hemphill RR. Kicking the Can Down the Road - When Medical Schools Fail to Self-Regulate. *N Engl J Med.* 2019;381(24):2287-2289. doi:10.1056/NEJMp1908940

40. Mills LM, Stenfors T, Duffy M, et al. "When You're in It, It Feels Like It's Everything": Medical Students' Experience of Failure and Remediation in the United States and the Netherlands. *Acad Med.* 2024;99(11):1254. doi:10.1097/ACM.0000000000005845

41. Shaker L, Amilcar C, Kothari N, Murano T. KNOWLEDGE, ATTITUDES AND PERCEPTIONS OF REMEDIATION AMONG TRAINEES IN GRADUATE MEDICAL EDUCATION PROGRAMS. *J Emerg Med.* 2023;65(1):e41-e49. doi:10.1016/j.jemermed.2023.04.008

42. Dweck CS. *Mindset: The New Psychology of Success.* Random House; 2006:x, 276.

43. Ericsson KA. Deliberate Practice and the Acquisition and Maintenance of Expert Performance in Medicine and Related Domains. *Acad Med.* 2004;79(10):S70.

44. Edmondson A. Psychological safety and learning behavior in work teams. *Adm Sci Q.* 1999;44(2):350-383. doi:10.2307/2666999

45. Ryan RM, Deci EL. Self-determination theory and the facilitation of intrinsic motivation, social development, and well-being. *Am Psychol.* 2000;55(1):68-78. doi:10.1037//0003-066x.55.1.68

46. Sargeant J, Mann K, Sinclair D, Van der Vleuten C, Metsemakers J. Understanding the influence of emotions and reflection upon multi-source feedback acceptance and use. *Adv Health Sci Educ Theory Pract.* 2008;13(3):275-288. doi:10.1007/s10459-006-9039-x

47. Sargeant J. Toward a common understanding of self-assessment. *J Contin Educ Health Prof.* 2008;28(1):1-4. doi:10.1002/chp.148

48. Winston KA, Vleuten CPMVD, Scherpbier AJJA. The role of the teacher in remediating at-risk medical students. *Med Teach.* 2012;34(11):e732-e742. doi:10.3109/0142159X.2012.689447

49. White CB, Ross PT, Gruppen LD. Remediating Students' Failed OSCE Performances at One School: The Effects of Self-Assessment, Reflection, and Feedback. *Acad Med.* 2009;84(5):651. doi:10.1097/ACM.0b013e31819fb9de

50. Price T, Wong G, Withers L, et al. Optimising the delivery of remediation programmes for doctors: A realist review. *Med Educ.* 2021;55(9):995-1010. doi:10.1111/medu.14528

51. Ng IKS, Lin NHY, Goh WGW, Teo DB, Tan LF, Ban KHK. "Insight" in medical training: what, why, and how? *Postgrad Med J.* 2024;100(1181):196-202. doi:10.1093/postmj/qgad115

52. Durning SJ, Cleary TJ, Sandars J, Hemmer P, Kokotailo P, Artino AR. Perspective: Viewing "Strugglers" Through a Different Lens: How a Self-Regulated Learning Perspective Can Help Medical Educators With Assessment and Remediation. *Acad Med.* 2011;86(4):488. doi:10.1097/ACM.0b013e31820dc384

53. Patel R, Tarrant C, Bonas S, Yates J, Sandars J. The struggling student: a thematic analysis from the self-regulated learning perspective. *Med Educ.* 2015;49(4):417-426. doi:10.1111/medu.12651

54. Zimmerman BJ. Attaining self-regulation: A social cognitive perspective. In: *Handbook of Self-Regulation.* Academic Press; 2000:13-39. doi:10.1016/B978-012109890-2/50031-7

55. Dyre Rasmussen L, Grierson L, Morcke AM, Rasmussen K, Ringsted C, Tolsgaard M. A change of mind: Error motivation is shaped by error perceptions in different learning environments. *Med Teach.* Published online October 15, 2024:1-9. doi:10.1080/0142159X.2024.2412783

56. Bakke BM, Sheu L, Hauer KE. Fostering a Feedback Mindset: A Qualitative Exploration of Medical Students' Feedback Experiences With Longitudinal Coaches. *Acad Med.* 2020;95(7):1057. doi:10.1097/ACM.0000000000003012

CHAPTER 2

Global Assessment of the Struggling Medical Learner

Assessment of the struggling medical learner begins with confirmation that the learner is actually struggling. With the advent of standardized methods for determining competence, medical educators now have a more objective lens through which to identify when a learner has strayed off course or exhibited a change in their trajectory. However, even when operating within a competency-based framework as discussed in chapter 1, accurate detection of performance concerns can be difficult due to inadequate direct observation, imprecise standards, and lack of formal reporting by supervisors.[1,2] Dr. Janae Heath, an expert in medical education assessment at the University of Pennsylvania, highlights the importance of supervisor intuition and hallway chatter as common first hints of learner struggle. Dr. Heath advises us to pay attention to these informal mechanisms and design evaluation systems for which these are not the main source of information about a learner's performance. We must also recognize the potential for bias (i.e., our understandings and assumptions about learners that are unrelated to their actual ability) at all stages of assessment. In an excellent article, Dr. Hauer and colleagues offer strategies for creating assessment systems to mitigate bias and preserve fairness and evidence of validity.[3]

For more than 20 years combined, we have participated in the assessment and remediation of struggling medical learners as program leader, director of centralized remediation programs, and focused clinical reasoning coach. This work spans the continuum of medical education and training. The current chapter is a compilation of lessons learned from our work with hundreds of students, residents, and fellows and is a testament to the importance of an accurate, holistic assessment as a critical first step in any remediation effort. A clarification on the term assessment in this context: in this chapter we are referring to a specialized type of assessment that is meant to understand the learner's struggle in the broader context of their life experience, inspire the dynamic and often longitudinal process of coaching for purposes of remediation, and support ongoing self-appraisal and reflection as the learner advances. To facilitate this developmental process, we encourage educators and institutional leaders to create a space for struggling learners to explore these factors that is separate from the programmatic evaluation and summative reassessment following remediation.

IMPORTANCE OF THE BIOPSYCHOSOCIAL CONTEXT IN WHICH LEARNER DEFICITS OCCUR

The biopsychosocial approach to medical practice was developed in 1977 by Dr. George Engel at the University of Rochester.[4] Dr. Engel proposed the integration of the objective scientific facts of a patient's disease with the more subjective human experiences of patients and their families as they faced the disease. He believed that considering health and illness in a broader context affords clinicians a deeper understanding of their complexities and a more meaningful relationship with patients. Similarly, we cannot view any aspect of a medical learner's performance in a vacuum. Nor can we assume that we intuitively understand a learner's perspective or that all learners will respond to the challenges of medical training in an identical, or even predictable, fashion. A learner's success, or lack thereof, in training is impacted by numerous biological, psychological, and social factors that are summarized in Figure 2.1.

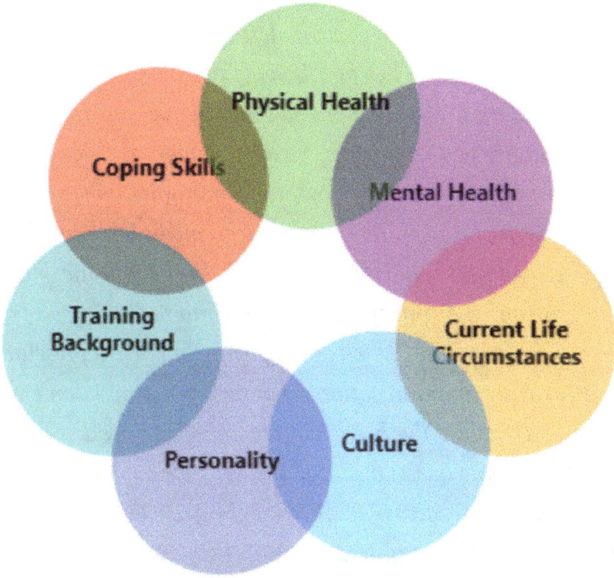

Figure 2.1. Biopsychosocial Factors Associated with Learner Performance

Consequently, there is no one-size-fits-all approach to remediation. Part of what makes this field so interesting is that every case is unique. Effective remediation plans are individualized and consider not only the specific deficit being remediated, but the context in which the deficit occurs.

CASE 1

Dr. Ortiz is an intern who is referred by her program director to our remediation program with concerns about clinical reasoning. Specific observations include patient presentations with missing information, a tendency to anchor, and difficulties justifying her diagnoses and plans. The program has tried informal coaching, but the perception is that Dr. Ortiz is resistant to feedback. All of Dr. Ortiz' written evaluations comment on her excellent work ethic and natural rapport with patients and their families. Some members of the interprofessional team offer superlative comments about her advocacy for patients; others note that she is occasionally argumentative.

Dr. Ortiz grew up in a densely populated urban area. Her parents divorced when she was young, and her mother has struggled with depression

throughout Dr. Ortiz' life. Dr. Ortiz describes herself as a "strong-willed child." She was the first of her family to go to college and plans to practice primary care in an underserved area. She attended medical school in her home city, and her performance in medical school was average. Evaluators praised her work ethic, compassion, and community advocacy efforts. Her father died in the spring of her fourth year of medical school. She describes pushing back against authority occasionally throughout life, but only if she had "good reason" (i.e., refusing to go alone into the room of a patient who made her uncomfortable). When asked about her patient presentations, she replies, "People say communication is not my strength…I don't feel the need to explain myself a lot…I've been this way since I was a kid." She admits that she doesn't like being questioned and pushes back or shuts down when she perceives feedback as criticism. Dr. Ortiz volunteers that she doesn't feel that she belongs in her current program, which is in a small town in a different part of the country from where she grew up. She has been struggling with insomnia for many months.

To help Dr. Ortiz become more open to feedback and begin to work on her clinical reasoning deficiencies, it is important to understand both her background and her current experiences in the residency program. The approach to a learner with observed resistance to feedback should begin with an exploration of that resistance. In this case, Dr. Ortiz is triggered by a longstanding distrust for certain authority figures. Our mentor, Dr. Betsy Williams, teaches that people who have experienced difficulties with authority figures early in life may struggle with feedback in medical training. Dr. Ortiz is also experiencing symptoms of depression and social isolation and has not fully processed her father's death. Assignment of a remediation coach in this case must be undertaken thoughtfully. Remediation programs should have a confidential, expedited referral process for mental health support.

Dr. Ortiz establishes care with a primary care clinician and is referred to a therapist with a similar ethnic and cultural background. She is also given the opportunity to select a mentor in the program whom she trusts. Only after establishing these supportive relationships and beginning treatment for her insomnia and depression is the clinical reasoning coaching program undertaken.

CASE 2

Sid Banner is referred by a sub-internship director to our remediation program late in their fourth year of medical school with a suspected clinical reasoning deficiency. Evaluations note that their "presentations are all over the place" and they rarely seem to understand "the big picture" with their patients. Recently, a cross-cover patient became acutely hypoxic in the middle of the night, and Sid appeared to lack an organized approach to evaluating and managing the patient, leading to a delay in appropriate care. Sid has always performed well on standardized tests. Their clinical grades in clerkship, however, were consistently below average. They are universally viewed as a hard worker, enthusiastic learner, and team player.

Sid discloses that they are under a great deal of stress. They have a new baby at home, and their significant other is struggling with postpartum depression. They feel tremendous guilt that they are away from the family for long hours at work. Sid reports carrying a maximum census of three patients during their prior clinical rotations and lacks frameworks for patient presentations and management of urgent clinical situations. They describe increasing symptoms of anxiety when on call and when presenting patients on rounds. Acutely, their heart races, their palms become sweaty, and they "freeze." "I could tell you right now how to begin caring for that hypoxic patient, but in the moment my mind went blank."

Given what we know about their early medical school experience and performance (e.g., relative inexperience with high patient volume and acuity, lack of clinical reasoning frameworks, and below-average clinical grades), Sid's struggles in residency are expected. Coaching and broader remediation efforts should consider the impact of personal stressors and what is likely performance anxiety on their clinical reasoning performance.

Sid is referred, confidentially, to a psychologist for cognitive behavioral therapy and encouraged to establish care with a primary care provider. Simultaneously, they are matched with a coach to begin targeted clinical reasoning coaching in a low-pressure, simulated environment during which they can develop effective frameworks for presenting patients and managing urgent situations.

CONDITIONS THAT UNDERLIE CLINICAL PERFORMANCE DEFICITS

As we have seen in these two cases, struggling medical learners often have a lot going on beneath the surface. Figure 2.2 summarizes the conditions that, in our experience, commonly underlie performance issues among learners. These factors are complex and interrelated.

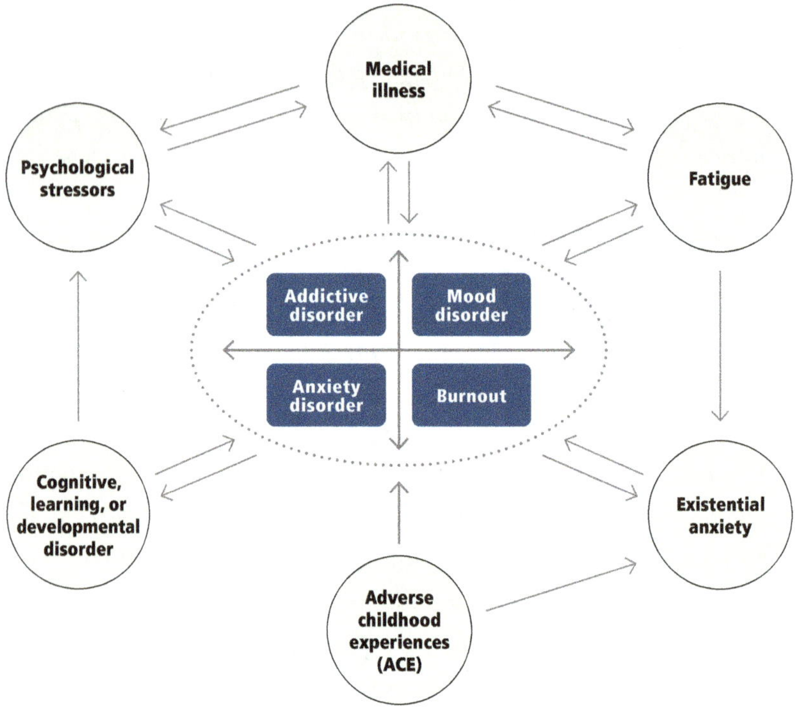

Figure 2.2. Conditions that May Underlie Medical Learner Performance Deficits[5]

According to program director surveys and single-center reviews, underlying mental health conditions are present in between 18% to 40% of struggling medical learners.[6–11] Our experience directing remediation programs that screen all referrals for depression, anxiety, psychological stressors, cognitive and learning disorders, and adverse childhood experiences suggests that this number is even higher. Approximately 50% of residents and fellows referred to our program with performance deficits also disclose or are diagnosed with mental health conditions.[7,12] Nearly all these data come from the graduate medical education population. Statistics reflecting the coexistence of similar issues among medical students and non-physician health care trainees are not available to report. Anxiety disorders, including performance anxiety, generalized anxiety disorder, panic disorder, and obsessive-compulsive disorder, are the most common types of mental health conditions diagnosed in struggling medical learners. Many learners experience existential anxiety related to their career choice that impacts performance. Family stressors associated with partner or parental conflict, estrangement or difficulties with extended family, and changes to the family composition are common. Addictive disorders include substance use disorders and other behavioral addictions such as gambling. An increasing body of literature connects adverse childhood experiences with performance issues, especially professionalism, among training and practicing clinicians.[13,14]

Sometimes the presence of an underlying issue, as well as the type of issue, is obvious. Other times, even significant problems remain hidden for some time. Clinicians are usually extremely skilled at concealing their symptoms, until they are not. And work tends to be the last area of life to fold. It is important to maintain a high index of suspicion any time a learner deviates from the expected course during training, especially if there are inconsistencies in behavior and/or otherwise unexplained changes in trajectory of performance. Deficits across multiple competencies can also point to an underlying mental health concern.

Table 2.1. Common Descriptors of Medical Learners with Underlying Mental Health Conditions*

- Emotional dysregulation, erratic behavior or moods
- Frequent interpersonal conflict
- Disheveled appearance or change in appearance
- Poor performance on standardized tests
- Lack of engagement
  - Delay in completing work, missed deadlines
  - Inappropriate delegation of tasks to colleagues
  - Absent or late to required activities

(continued)

Table 2.1. Common Descriptors of Medical Learners with Underlying Mental Health Conditions* *(continued)*

- – Lack of attention to detail
- – "Checked out" on rounds
- Repeated duty-hour violations
- Pervasive cynicism and negativity
- Dishonest behavior, rule-breaking
- Lack of appropriate response in urgent clinical situations
- Frequent errors in documentation or orders
- Poor clinical judgment
- General disorganization
- Resistance to feedback

*especially if out of character

When given space, some learners come forward and admit that they are depressed, anxious, burned out, or under stress. Others remain reluctant to do so. Unfortunately, the pervasive stigma around learners and clinicians with mental illness remains, for many, a barrier to seeking help.[15,16] Many learners avoid disclosing their symptoms for fear that doing so will put their career in jeopardy. In our experience, not seeking treatment when it is warranted is more likely to damage a career than seeking treatment proactively. As educators, we should model vulnerability for our learners to normalize the experience of admitting and asking for help when we need it. Later in this chapter, we will review the structure of our program, which includes an integrated pathway for mental health referral. To be optimally effective, it is critical that those overseeing remediation efforts are familiar with their own institutional and community resources supporting the mental health of medical learners.

ATTENTION DEFICIT HYPERACTIVITY DISORDER IN STRUGGLING MEDICAL LEARNERS

CASE 3

Dr. Mouawad is referred to our remediation program by her program director in the fall of intern year with concerns about clinical reasoning and time management. Evaluators routinely comment on her positive attitude, "high EQ," and openness to feedback. She works longer hours than her peers and never complains. While she has many strengths, Dr. Mouawad struggles to collect and synthesize data efficiently, and she has trouble building and prioritizing her differential diagnosis, especially for complex patients. As a result, her presentations and written notes are disorganized, often with missing and/or extraneous information. She requires a great deal of oversight to triage tasks and develop management plans on all but the most straightforward patients. Dr. Mouawad has received specific feedback about these concerns, and while she is very receptive to the feedback, she is often unable to put it to use. These concerns have been present since the beginning of the year.

Dr. Mouawad denies any difficulties with learning or performance in school growing up, and she did well in college. A review of her medical school performance reveals an overall ranking in the bottom 20% of her graduating class. She failed USMLE Step 1 on first attempt and took a leave of absence to prepare for her second attempt, which she passed. She passed her Step 2 exam on the first attempt after completing an in-person course. She has good insight into the fact that she is struggling in residency and generally feels very overwhelmed. She is working with a peer coach on effective strategies for pre-rounding and approaching new admissions. She has been trying to read more but has had trouble sticking to a schedule. She admits that she has struggled with symptoms of anxiety since medical school but has never sought treatment.

Cognitive, learning, and neurodevelopmental disorders are not well-studied in struggling medical learners. It is important to identify these conditions, many of which are considered disabilities under the Americans with Disabilities Act (ADA) and can be accommodated. According to the ADA of 1990, a disability is a physical or mental impairment that significantly limits one or more "major life activities."[17] A reasonable accommodation is a modification to the job or the work environment that enables the individual with the disability to perform the essential functions of the job. For example, medical learners with cognitive or learning disorders may require more time for test preparation or test-taking.

In our program, 20% of graduate medical learners referred for remediation have attention deficit hyperactivity disorder (ADHD).[12] Many were unaware of their diagnosis until residency or fellowship. Based on past research and general understanding about executive functioning, it is posited that individuals with high IQ and/or other significant cognitive strengths (e.g., strong memory retention) could effectively compensate for symptoms related to ADHD during the developmental period, especially when their life and academic demands are less intense. However, when demands increase, either due to more challenging academic courses or a more intensive occupational role, the longstanding compensatory strategies used by adults with high IQ become much less effective. At this point, performance problems can become more noticeable and begin to interfere with functioning. Therefore, adults with high IQ may in fact meet criteria for ADHD but have previously gone undiagnosed due to masking of their underlying developmental weakness by other intellectual and/or cognitive strengths. In our experience, learners with ADHD may struggle across multiple areas of performance, including medical knowledge and test-taking, clinical reasoning, organization and time management, and professionalism. Clinical reasoning deficits in this group commonly manifest as difficulty triaging tasks, disorganized presentations, and "missing the forest for the trees."

Dr. Mouawad is confidentially referred to the neuropsychologist on our team for neuropsychological testing. She is also assigned a clinical reasoning coach.

Our program's written consent process allows, with learner written release, the members of our team to communicate. This has allowed the coach and clinicians on our team to work together to create a synergistic, multidisciplinary intervention that is effective in the majority of cases. When possible, this coordination between team members both shortens the duration of remediation and increases its likelihood of success.

RECOGNIZING WHEN A MEDICAL LEARNER NEEDS TO BE REMOVED FROM CLINICAL PRACTICE

In a landmark article published in 1973, the American Medical Association (AMA) defined *impairment* as the inability to perform professional and personal responsibilities due to psychiatric illness, alcoholism, or drug dependency.[18] The term impairment is often used to indicate the presence of a substance use disorder, but really any mental or medical health condition can lead to impairment, as can fatigue. There is no one phenotype of impairment. This is a situation in which one must trust one's gut instinct. If there are concerns about learner or patient safety, the learner should be removed from the work environment until they can be evaluated. Because a learner's imminent risk to patient safety is often difficult to determine, supervisors should consider the behaviors and circumstances outlined in Table 2.1 when contemplating whether a learner can safely perform their duties. As discussed in more detail later in this chapter, it is important to know and follow one's institutional policy and to be familiar with one's state laws around mandated reporting.

ESTABLISHING THE CORRECT "DIAGNOSIS"

The term *diagnosis* is in quotation marks here as a reminder that we are not our learners' clinicians and should resist the urge, no matter how compelling, to play diagnostician when they veer off course. That said, successful remediation hinges on accurate identification of the clinical performance deficit(s). Approaching a struggling learner often feels overwhelming.[19] A framework for characterizing learner deficits can alleviate the overwhelm and is necessary to ensure validity. The ACGME/ABMS[20] competencies and the new AAMC Foundational Competencies[21] provide a natural scaffold from which to approach the struggling medical learner. Unfortunately, incorrect "diagnosis" occurs frequently, highlighting some of the flaws in our current practice.

The competency of patient care is broad and has been subdivided by Dr. Guerrasio as follows: clinical skills, clinical reasoning and judgement, and time management and organization (Table 2.2).[19] In addition, she splits interpersonal skills and communication into two competencies and adds mental well-being—defined as psychiatric diagnosis, substance abuse, learning disorder, or psychosocial stressors—as its own competency. The result is ten discrete areas of struggle that she has termed Competencies Plus. In our experience, these adaptations to the original ACGME/ABMS competencies greatly improve accuracy in establishing the correct problem. Over time, we have continued to build on Dr. Guerrasio's framework, expanding some areas and consolidating others.

Table 2.2. Competencies and Competencies "Plus"

ACGME/AGMS* Competencies	Guerrasio Competencies "Plus"
Medical knowledge	• Medical knowledge
Patient care	• Patient care – Clinical skills – Clinical reasoning and judgment – Time management and organization
Interpersonal skills and communication	• Interpersonal skills • Communication
Professionalism	Professionalism
Practice-based learning and improvement	• Practice-based learning and improvement
Systems-based practice	• Systems-based practice • Mental well-being

*the AAMC Foundational Competencies align with the ACGME competencies but add Procedural Skills to Patient Care

Adapted with permission from ACGME.

Through our work with hundreds of struggling learners, we have come to view mental well-being not as a distinct competency or deficit but rather as a contributing factor that potentially impacts all aspects of learner performance. In keeping with consideration of the biopsychosocial context, our program screens all referrals for mental health conditions. Figure 2.3 depicts our process for learner referral and categorization of deficits in graduate medical education (GME).[8] This framework, which we have adapted for work in undergraduate medical education (UME),[22] can be applied to any medical learner working in the clinical environment.

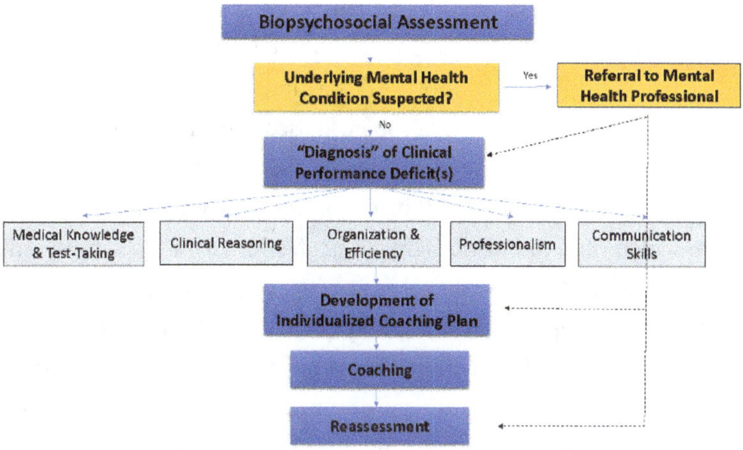

Figure 2.3. Our Process for Learner Referral and Categorization of Performance Deficits[5] (Adapted with permission from ACGME.)

We have retained Dr. Guerrasio's patient care sub-competencies of clinical reasoning and time management and organization, which we call *organization and efficiency.* As discussed in more detail in chapter 4, there is an art to distinguishing between the two, and the "disorganized learner" may struggle in either or both areas. In our framework, the organization and efficiency category addresses the effectiveness and efficiency of a learner's systems for completing their daily work. Common areas of struggle in this domain include admitting a new patient (or approaching a new consult or a new patient in clinic), pre-rounding, note-writing, managing a task list, and preparing for an operative procedure. *Organization and efficiency* maps to multiple ACGME/ABMS/AAMC[20,21] competencies, including patient care, interpersonal and communication skills, professionalism, and systems-based practice. *Clinical reasoning,* on the other hand, refers to data gathering, interpretation, and synthesis to obtain a diagnosis, create a management plan, consider a prognosis, and more broadly to the interactions between the clinician, patient, and their dynamic practice environment. We have adopted Mak-van der Vossen and colleagues' classification of *professionalism* as four domains (Table 2.3) which correspond to the following behavioral themes, respectively: failure to engage, dishonest behavior, disrespectful behavior, and poor self-awareness.[23] *Communication* refers to a learner's ability to effectively communicate with patients, patients' families, and other members of the health care team.

Our remediation team includes domain experts in each of the five areas of concern outlined in Table 2.3. To consolidate resources and simplify the creation of direct observation tools and coaching exercises, we have merged systems-based practice (SBP) and problem-based learning and improvement (PBLI) with other areas. These competencies are often difficult to define and typically overlap with others. SBP incorporates self-awareness and systems thinking, which map to our domains of professionalism (specifically introspection, Table 2.3, 4d) and clinical reasoning, respectively. Chapters 8 and 12 will discuss the approach to the learner who struggles with management reasoning, which like SBP involves risk-benefit analysis, considerations of cost awareness, and effective utilization of resources. Embedded in PBLI is the commitment to lifelong learning, the ability to self-monitor, and the acceptance and actualization of feedback into practice. Fundamentally, we view these as analogous to the involvement and introspection components of professionalism (Table 2.3, 4a and 4d).

Finally, our program is not currently resourced to remediate procedural skills, so these issues are handled within the learner's training program. However, in our experience, most learners who struggle in procedural settings are deficient in the non-technical areas of operative performance. Operative reasoning is discussed in chapter 15.

Table 2.3. Categorization of Medical Learner Performance Deficits

1. Medical knowledge and test-taking
2. Clinical reasoning
3. Organization and efficiency
4. Professionalism
    - A. Involvement
    - B. Integrity
    - C. Interaction
    - D. Introspection
5. Communication

DISCORDANCE BETWEEN STANDARDIZED TEST SCORES AND CLINICAL PERFORMANCE

There are many potential reasons why a medical learner performs well clinically and yet struggles with standardized tests.[24] Anxiety on test day—or while preparing for the test—is common, and learners with test-related anxiety are typically conscious of their symptoms and readily able to describe them.[25,26] Learners with ADHD or other cognitive or learning disorders often do not study effectively for standardized tests and may have trouble finishing tests on time.[12] Learners without any of these conditions may have sufficient knowledge but are unable to apply this knowledge in a testing situation due to poor test-taking strategies such as second-guessing, overthinking, and changing answers.[27] Many learners describe significant distractions or stressors that limit their ability to prepare for standardized tests but do not seem to impact their performance in the clinical setting.

Conversely, learners may excel in a standardized examination setting and struggle in the clinical environment. This is the crux of most clinical reasoning struggles, which are explored in the chapters to come.[28,29] Some learners feel comfortable applying their knowledge in a testing situation but experience anxiety when face to face with a supervisor and while being asked to reason off the cuff. Even without the subjective experience of anxiety, some learners need additional time to process and integrate information and do not do well thinking on their feet in a patient care setting. Cognitive load theory, described by Dr. John Sweller in 1988, asserts that our working memory has limited capacity to process information; when a task overwhelms the capacity of the working memory, performance and learning are negatively impacted.[30,31] Components of cognitive load include intrinsic load (associated with the task itself), extraneous load (related to how material is presented), and germane load (imposed by the development of patterns recognized by our brain to help us learn complex material).[32] Standardized tests are designed to minimize extraneous cognitive load and optimize germane cognitive load to accurately assess a learner's knowledge of the material. On a test, the learner encounters only a finite amount of information, and the test provides prompts in the form of answer choices. Learners in the clinical environment are confronted with seemingly endless amounts of clinical information. Prompts are largely unavailable, making it challenging to integrate and synthesize the relevant information. The prompts afforded by standardized tests also allow the learner to bypass the hypothesis generation step of clinical reasoning, which is discussed in more detail in Section 3.

A SYSTEMATIC APPROACH TO FORMATIVE ASSESSMENT OF THE STRUGGLING MEDICAL LEARNER

Once the struggling medical learner has been identified, effective remediation necessitates a systematic assessment process that incorporates all these principles. In her book *Remediation of the Struggling Medical Learner*, Dr. Guerrasio provides valuable guidance on accessing information about the struggling learner's performance as well as detailed strategies for recognizing different types of performance deficits with many practical examples.[19,33] Table 2.4 presents the components of our formative, global assessment process that is greatly informed by her work.

Table 2.4. Components of the Global Assessment of the Struggling Medical Learner

1. Reconnaissance

- a. Review
  - i. Performance in the current program
  - ii. Performance in prior programs
- b. Assess preparedness for current program
- c. Identify changes in trajectory
- d. Recognize disconnect between standardized test scores and clinical performance

2. Interview

- a. Assess insight, perspective, and characterization of the problem
- b. Investigate for underlying causes, understand the biopsychosocial context
- c. Review of systems[19] for each type of deficit

The reconnaissance component begins with an in-depth review of the learner's performance in the current program. It is important to draw on multiple sources of data, as each deficit is captured in different assessment domains. Conventional sources of information such as test scores, narrative evaluations, global ratings, and multi-source feedback are important. Equally important, in our experience, are the less-traditional sources of data such as confidential comments to the program director and critical incident reviews. Learner self-evaluation can be helpful in assessing insight, if nothing else.

Built into our program is the expectation that our coaches will speak directly to a learner's evaluators. Without exception, these interactions enhance our understanding of the nature of the performance concerns, which are often ill-defined in the clinical evaluations, if mentioned at all. When possible, we advocate for targeted direct observation of the skills in question—either in the learning environment or in a lower-stakes, simulated environment—to help fully characterize the issues. We introduce direct observation strategies for commonly observed clinical reasoning deficits in chapters 9 to 15. We address the question of who should be gathering this information and doing the observing, which will depend on one's program's size and resources, in more detail later in this and subsequent chapters. For learners with significant struggles, or for whom the "diagnosis" is less clear, we arrange a formative clinical rotation (often 1 to 2 weeks in duration) in which the learner is paired with a faculty member who can directly observe them in all aspects of daily work and provide real-time feedback. In chapter 6 specific guidance is offered on how to set up a dedicated coaching rotation.

We review all available information concerning performance in prior training programs to assess trajectory and preparedness for the current program and to identify any disconnect in standardized test scores and clinical performance.

The interview is arguably the most important part of the formative assessment process. There are always at least two sides to every story, and in the interview the coach will hear the learner's perspective and learn a great deal about their insight and motivations. In her book and related publications, Dr. Guerrasio has provided scripts to guide discussions with the learner about their performance.[11,19] We borrow from her the concept of conducting a "review of systems" for each learner deficit. It is important to consider who conducts the interview; this will depend on the size and resources of one's remediation program.

ON STAYING IN THE CORRECT LANE WHEN "ASSESSING" THE STRUGGLING LEARNER

In chapter 1 we advocated for the creation of a supportive and neutral space for learners to explore their resistance to constructive feedback or their reluctance to engage in coaching interventions. Similarly, struggling learners deserve a protected environment in which to reflect upon the performance concerns and the issues that potentially underlie them without fear of retaliation, bias, or conflict of interest.[34,35] Institutional and program leaders, by definition, serve a dual role and therefore should maintain some distance from the details of the learner's mental and physical health and current life circumstances.[36] This is not to say that leaders should withhold emotional support or refrain from sharing concerns if they believe that something more than meets the eye is going on. We encourage all program leaders to familiarize themselves with the conditions that commonly underlie performance struggles. We urge all programs to establish a defined mechanism by which learners can receive confidential evaluation and treatment for mental and physical health conditions that might be contributing to performance issues.

Accordingly, we recommend that someone other than the program or institutional leader direct the formative global assessment of the struggling learner. This role can be undertaken by any faculty member who is trained in the process and is not directly involved in the learner's programmatic assessment. For graduate medical education programs without a centralized remediation program, the Clinical Competency Committee (CCC) structure allows for early recognition and correct "diagnosis" of the struggling medical learner.[37–39] Medical schools may rely on the infrastructure of their Department of Student Affairs or may develop specialized academic enhancement teams that function like a CCC to identify, assess, and remediate struggling students.[40] A number of medical schools have competency-specific advancement committees such as an entrustment committee, and the number of UME CCCs is growing.[41–43] It is possible to participate in the coaching and formative assessment of a struggling learner as a member of the CCC (or equivalent entity) and remove oneself from decisions relating to Milestone scores (or equivalent) and advancement, thus preventing any conflict of interest. For programs which have neither a centralized remediation program nor a CCC equivalent, any invested faculty member can be trained in the formative assessment process.

OUR PROGRAM'S FORMATIVE, GLOBAL ASSESSMENT PROCESS FOR THE STRUGGLING MEDICAL LEARNER

Learner referral to our program can be voluntary or mandated by our institutional policy as part of a formal remediation plan. Following written informed consent, a physician remediation specialist performs a biopsychosocial evaluation to identify specific performance deficits and facilitate the creation of an individualized coaching plan. If concerns arise during the initial assessment for a concomitant mental health issue, confidential referral to a mental health provider is offered. Unless there is concern for impairment, learners are under no obligation to follow through with this referral, nor are they required to share information pertaining to evaluation and/or treatment of mental or medical health issues with the assessor on our team. Most of the learners in our program who screen positive for mental health concerns do follow through with our referrals. Neither the answers to the questions on the formative assessment tool nor any of the information concerning the diagnosis and/or treatment of medical or mental health conditions is shared with the learner's supervisor. Our program created and uses the tool below (Figure 2.4) to structure our formative assessment process. These records are stored on a secure, HIPAA-compliant shared drive accessible only to our faculty and are never shared with the learner's supervisor.

BIOPSYCHOSOCIAL FORMATIVE ASSESSMENT TOOL

Component 1: Reconnaissance

A. INITIAL ASSESSMENT FORM FOR PROGRAM LEADER (IF PROGRAM-LED REFERRAL):

1. *Why are you referring this learner to COACH? Please indicate all that apply. Please provide narrative comments to support your choice(s).*

☐ Medical knowledge	☐ Lack of engagement or ownership
☐ Presentation skills	☐ Dishonest behavior
☐ Understanding "the big picture"	☐ Disruptive or disrespectful behavior
☐ Anchoring/premature closure	☐ Lack of confidence
☐ Data collection or data synthesis	☐ Inadequate response to feedback

(continued)

(continued)

- ☐ Building a differential diagnosis
- ☐ Prioritizing tasks
- ☐ Response in urgent situations
- ☐ Therapeutic decision-making
- ☐ Time management/ organizational skills
- ☐ Poor self-awareness
- ☐ Communication skills
- ☐ Procedural or physical exam skills
- ☐ Concern for mental well-being
- ☐ Other

2. How long have these issues been present?

3. Has the learner received feedback from the program leadership about these concerns? If so, what was the learner's response to feedback? If not, why not?

4. What coaching or remediation strategies have already been tried? Please elaborate and address any prior concerns about the learner and how they have been addressed.

5. What are the consequences if these concerns persist? Has the learner been informed of these consequences?

B. REVIEW OF THE LEARNER'S FILE

Undergraduate Medical Program(s)

- ☐ Preclinical performance (grades, course failures)
- ☐ Performance on OSCEs, miniCEX or EPAs*
- ☐ Clinical performance (grades, course failures, comments in clinical rotations)
- ☐ Standardized test scores (end-of-rotation exams, USMLE, COMLEX)
- ☐ Medical Student Performance Evaluation (MSPE) letter, including class rank if available, letters of recommendation, need for remediation or extension of training

Graduate Medical Program(s)

- ☐ Written evaluations, Milestone ratings
- ☐ Standardized test scores (USMLE, in-training exams, specialty board exams)
- ☐ Program director file, confidential comments, email correspondence
- ☐ Critical incident reviews
- ☐ Multi-source feedback

*OSCE (Objective Structured Clinical Exam); mini-CEX (Clinical Evaluation Exercise); EPA (Entrustable Professional Activity)

Component 2: Interview

1. **Background, reason for referral, awareness and understanding**
    a. Family history, social history
    b. Why did you choose this program?
    c. Insight/awareness of problem(s)
    d. Understanding of consequences of the problem(s)
    e. Career goals
2. **Educational history**
    a. Performance in school
    b. Test result history
3. **Program learning climate**
    a. Mentorship and support
4. **Psychosocial contributors**
    a. Stress (family, social, financial, career)
    b. Adjustment (program, learning climate, new location, living situation)
5. **Mental health (personal and family history)**
    a. Mood or anxiety disorder, symptoms
    b. Trauma, bereavement
    c. Cognitive or learning disorder (including ADHD)
    d. Addictive disorders (current and past use of substances)
6. **Self-care and social support**
    a. Sleep, diet, exercise, hobbies
    b. Social support and important relationships
    c. Coping skills and strategies
7. **Relevant medical history**
8. **Legal history**
    a. Contact with legal system (history of arrests, convictions, protective orders)
9. **Mental status and behavioral observations during the interview**
10. **Clinical performance**
    a. Medical knowledge
        i. Study plan and habits: How much? How effective?

(continued)

(continued)

ii. Global versus specific areas of deficit
iii. Trajectory of test performance, assess preparation for prior tests
iv. Does test performance reflect knowledge?
v. Performance anxiety? Poor self-confidence?

b. Clinical reasoning
   i. Presentations, handoffs of care
   ii. Summarize complex patients in one line
   iii. Ability to triage tasks, respond appropriately in urgent situations
   iv. Situational awareness, ability to troubleshoot

c. Organization/Efficiency
   i. Global organization and time management skills
   ii. Systems for completion of daily work
      aa. Approach to a new patient (admission, clinic)
      bb. Pre-rounding
      cc. Note-writing
      dd. Completion of a task list
      ee. Comfort level in current system, with electronic health record

d. Professionalism
   i. Review any incidents of unprofessional behavior to assess learner perspective
   ii. Assess knowledge of professional norms, cultural and training background

e. Communication
   i. Review any concerns related to communication to assess learner perspective
   ii. Assess performance anxiety, global issues with communication

Figure 2.4. Biopsychosocial Assessment Tool[8] (Adapted from Reference 8.)

COACHING THE LEARNER WITH CONCOMITANT PERFORMANCE AND MENTAL HEALTH CONCERNS

We have presented three learners in this chapter with concomitant struggles involving mental health and clinical performance. The co-existence of these issues, as discussed, is quite common and presents several potential challenges for institutional and program leaders. In some situations, treatment of the mental health condition corrects the performance problem and obviates the need for coaching. In others, the learner benefits from simultaneous clinical treatment and coaching or, in the case of Dr. Ortiz, interventions in close succession. Only a minority of learners must delay the coaching work significantly. In these cases, we usually recommend a leave of absence during which they can focus on their clinical recovery.

Figure 2.5 summarizes a programmatic approach to the struggling learner, starting with this question: Is the learner impaired, and/or is patient safety at risk? If the answer is "yes," as discussed earlier in this chapter, we recommend removing the learner from the clinical environment and proceeding with a mandated independent evaluation of their physical and mental health. All programs that train learners who provide direct patient care should have a *fitness for duty* policy (or equivalent), and programs are encouraged to adhere to their institutional policy.[44–46] Fitness for duty evaluations should be performed by an independent entity with experience in working with health care providers.

In the absence of concern about a learner's ability to safely perform the functions of the job, we do not believe it is ethical to mandate evaluation or treatment for mental or physical health conditions. Policies may differ, however, at other institutions, so it is important to be familiar with yours. We provide all struggling learners with referral options and have partnered with area clinicians to establish a network of providers who are committed to working with medical learners and accommodating their schedules. That we do not mandate evaluation or treatment for underlying conditions is true even in cases of misconduct, which typically refers to serious departures from professionalism standards, law breaking, and/or intentional wrongdoing, unless the decision is made to invoke the fitness for duty policy and related procedure. At some institutions, misconduct in and of itself triggers a fitness for duty evaluation. Regardless of the type or the egregiousness of the conduct violation, all learners deserve a chance to undergo evaluation and treatment for underlying causes. Identification of an underlying mental or physical health condition does not change the fact that learners must still demonstrate competence to advance and may face disciplinary consequences for prior behaviors or performance concerns. If a remediation plan or disciplinary action is indicated based on institutional policy, the learner must abide by this policy, regardless of the underlying contributors.

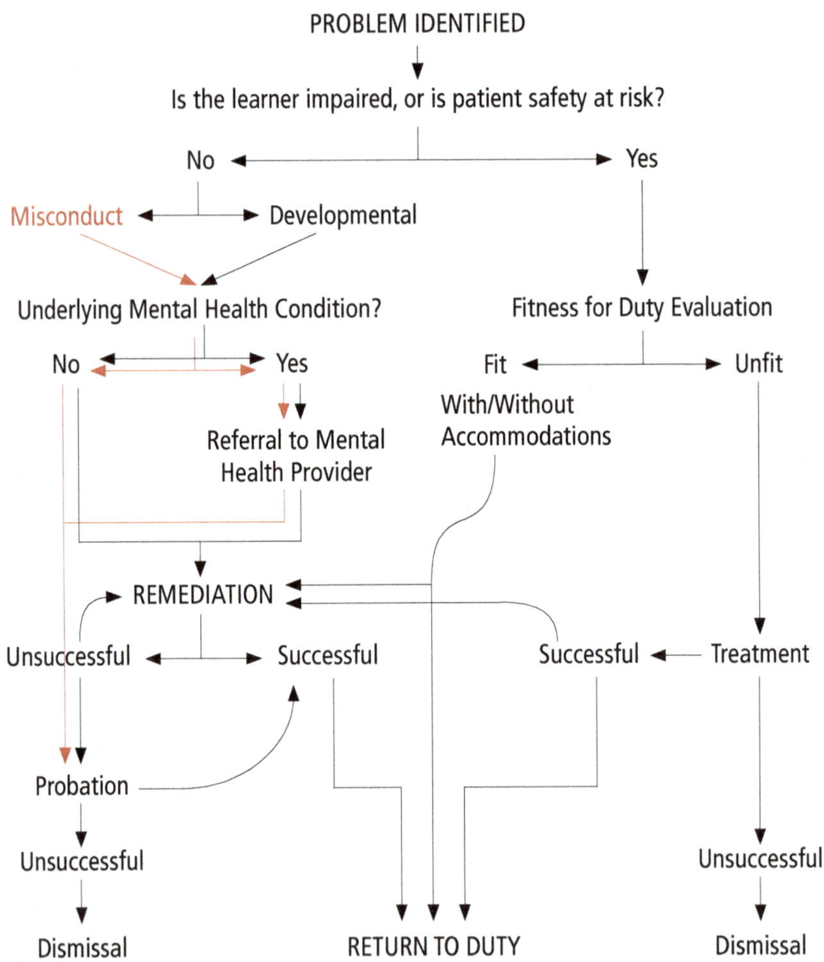

Figure 2.5. Programmatic Approach to the Struggling Learner[5] (Reprinted with permission from ACGME.)

Finally, as discussed in the case of Dr. Mouawad, learners with disabilities protected by the ADA may benefit from formal workplace accommodations; this request should come from the treating clinical provider.[17] Once the program is comfortable that the learner is appropriately accommodated, the learner should be held to the same performance standards as their peers. We recommend that programs involve their legal counsel early and often and adhere to institutional policy when making these decisions.

SUMMARY

In this chapter, we have emphasized the importance of viewing learner performance struggle through a wide developmental lens that considers the diverse etiologic factors that may impede trainee progress. We have shared our approach to categorization of learner deficits and our formative assessment process. Our remediation program is fortunate to have resources—including salary support for a remediation specialist and dedicated mental health team—that facilitate establishment of the supportive space for which we have been advocating. Identifying means to support learners in need can be challenging for smaller programs or programs with limited funding. Institutional and program leaders should familiarize themselves with available options for mental health evaluation and treatment, and these should include a mixture of institutional and community resources. It is important to keep in mind insurance limitations, wait times, and provider familiarity and comfort level with treating health care providers in training. Given the relatively high prevalence of ADHD in our cohort (ADHD is often diagnosed during medical training), we strongly encourage programs to establish a confidential, affordable, expeditious mechanism by which learners can be evaluated for ADHD and learning disorders. All institutions and programs should be carefully vetted to ensure the providers are aware of the legal, ethical, and social community requirements of working with medical learners.

References

1. Howley LD, Wilson WG. Direct Observation of Students during Clerkship Rotations: A Multiyear Descriptive Study: *Acad Med.* 2004;79(3):276-280. doi:10.1097/00001888-200403000-00017

2. Kogan JR, Hatala R, Hauer KE, Holmboe E. Guidelines: The do's, don'ts and don't knows of direct observation of clinical skills in medical education. *Perspect Med Educ.* 2017;6(5):286-305. doi:10.1007/s40037-017-0376-7

3. Hauer KE, Park YS, Bullock JL, Tekian A. "My Assessments Are Biased!" Measurement and Sociocultural Approaches to Achieve Fairness in Assessment in Medical Education. *Acad Med.* 2023;98(8S):S16. doi:10.1097/ACM.0000000000005245

4. Engel GL. The need for a new medical model: a challenge for biomedicine. *Science.* 1977;196(4286):129-136. doi:10.1126/science.847460

5. Warburton K. *The Struggle Is Real.* Warburton, KM, Parsons AS, et al. ACGME Remediation Toolkit. Posted August 31, 2024. Learn at ACGME. https://dl.acgme.org/courses/acgme-remediation-toolkit.

6. Yao DC, Wright SM. National Survey of Internal Medicine Residency Program Directors Regarding Problem Residents. *JAMA.* 2000;284(9):1099-1104. doi:10.1001/jama.284.9.1099

7. Warburton KM, Shahane AA. Mental Health Conditions Among Struggling GME Learners: Results From a Single Center Remediation Program. *J Grad Med Educ.* 2020;12(6):773-777. doi:10.4300/JGME-D-20-00007.1

8. Warburton KM, Goren E, Dine CJ. Comprehensive Assessment of Struggling Learners Referred to a Graduate Medical Education Remediation Program. *J Grad Med Educ.* 2017;9(6):763-767. doi:10.4300/JGME-D-17-00175.1

9. Ds T, Mh M, Rj S. Problem neurology residents: a national survey. *Neurology.* 2011;76(24):2119-2123. doi:10.1212/wnl.0b013e31821f4636

10. Dupras DM, Edson RS, Halvorsen AJ, Hopkins RH, McDonald FS. "Problem Residents": Prevalence, Problems and Remediation in the Era of Core Competencies. *Am J Med.* 2012;125(4):421-425. doi:10.1016/j.amjmed.2011.12.008

11. Guerrasio J, Garrity MJ, Aagaard EM. Learner Deficits and Academic Outcomes of Medical Students, Residents, Fellows, and Attending Physicians Referred to a Remediation Program, 2006–2012. *Acad Med.* 2014;89(2):352-358. doi:10.1097/ACM.0000000000000122

12. Warburton KM, Yost JS, Bajo SD, Martindale JR, Parsons AS, Ryan MS. Characteristics of ADHD in Struggling Residents and Fellows. *J Grad Med Educ.* 2024;16(6):730-734. doi:10.4300/JGME-D-24-00449.1

13. Williams BW, Welindt D, Hafferty FW, Stumps A, Flanders P, Williams MV. Adverse Childhood Experiences in Trainees and Physicians With Professionalism Lapses: Implications for Medical Education and Remediation. *Acad Med.* 2021;96(5):736-743. doi:10.1097/ACM.0000000000003532

14. Williams BW. Professionalism Lapses and Adverse Childhood Experiences: Reflections From the Island of Last Resort. *Acad Med.* 2019;94(8):1081. doi:10.1097/ACM.0000000000002793

15. Sukhera J, Poleksic J, Zaheer J, Pack R. Normalising disclosure or reinforcing heroism? An exploratory critical discourse analysis of mental health stigma in medical education. *Med Educ.* 2022;56(8):823-833. doi:10.1111/medu.14790

16. Brower KJ. Professional Stigma of Mental Health Issues: Physicians Are Both the Cause and Solution. *Acad Med.* 2021;96(5):635-640. doi:10.1097/ACM.0000000000003998

17. The ADA: Your Responsibilities as an Employer. US EEOC. Accessed January 22, 2025. https://www.eeoc.gov/publications/ada-your-responsibilities-employer

18. The Sick Physician: Impairment by Psychiatric Disorders, Including Alcoholism and Drug Dependence. *JAMA.* 1973;223(6):684-687. doi:10.1001/jama.1973.03220060058020

19. Guerrasio J. *Remediation of the Struggling Medical Learner.* 1 edition. Association for Hospital Medical Education; 2013.

20. ACGME Home. Accessed January 22, 2025. https://www.acgme.org/

21. UME Competencies AAMC | AACOM | ACGME. Accessed January 22, 2025. https://engage.aamc.org/UME-Competencies-AAMC-ACGME-AACOM

22. Young G, Meyer J, Crane I, et al. A Longitudinal, Structured Clinical Remediation Program for Medical Students. *Acad Med.* 2023;98(11S):S191. doi:10.1097/ACM.0000000000005401

23. Mak-van der Vossen M, van Mook W, van der Burgt S, et al. Descriptors for unprofessional behaviours of medical students: a systematic review and categorisation. *BMC Med Educ.* 2017;17(1):164. doi:10.1186/s12909-017-0997-x

24. Andrews MA, Kelly WF, DeZee KJ. Why Does This Learner Perform Poorly on Tests? Using Self-Regulated Learning Theory to Diagnose the Problem and Implement Solutions. *Acad Med.* 2018;93(4):612. doi:10.1097/ACM.0000000000001422

25. Broks VMA, Dijk SW, Van den Broek WW, Stegers-Jager KM, Woltman AM. Self-regulated learning profiles including test anxiety linked to stress and performance: A latent profile analysis based across multiple cohorts. *Med Educ.* 2024;58(5):544-555. doi:10.1111/medu.15283

26. Hahn H, Kropp P, Kirschstein T, Rücker G, Müller-Hilke B. Test anxiety in medical school is unrelated to academic performance but correlates with an effort/reward imbalance. *PloS One.* 2017;12(2):e0171220. doi:10.1371/journal.pone.0171220

27. Merry JW, Elenchin MK, Surma RN. Should students change their answers on multiple choice questions? *Adv Physiol Educ.* 2021;45(1):182-190. doi:10.1152/advan.00090.2020

28. Parsons AS, Dreicer JJ, Martindale JR, Young G, Warburton KM. A Targeted Clinical Reasoning Remediation Program for Residents and Fellows in Need. *J Grad Med Educ.* 2024;16(4):469. doi:10.4300/JGME-D-23-00822.1

29. Guerrasio J, Aagaard EM. Methods and Outcomes for the Remediation of Clinical Reasoning. *J Gen Intern Med.* 2014;29(12):1607-1614. doi:10.1007/s11606-014-2955-1

30. Sweller J. CHAPTER TWO—Cognitive Load Theory. In: Mestre JP, Ross BH, eds. *Psychology of Learning and Motivation.* Vol 55. Academic Press; 2011:37-76. doi:10.1016/B978-0-12-387691-1.00002-8

31. Van Merriënboer JJG, Sweller J. Cognitive load theory in health professional education: design principles and strategies. *Med Educ.* 2010;44(1):85-93. doi:10.1111/j.1365-2923.2009.03498.x

32. Young JQ, Van Merrienboer J, Durning S, Ten Cate O. Cognitive Load Theory: implications for medical education: AMEE Guide No. 86. *Med Teach.* 2014;36(5):371-384. doi:10.3109/0142159X.2014.889290

33. Guerrasio J.

Remediation of the Struggling Medical Learner. 2nd Edition. Association for Hospital Medical Education; 2018.

34. Johnson CE, Keating JL, Molloy EK. Psychological safety in feedback: What does it look like and how can educators work with learners to foster it? *Med Educ.* 2020;54(6):559-570. doi:10.1111/medu.14154

35. Bakke BM, Sheu L, Hauer KE. Fostering a Feedback Mindset: A Qualitative Exploration of Medical Students' Feedback Experiences With Longitudinal Coaches. *Acad Med.* 2020;95(7):1057. doi:10.1097/ACM.0000000000003012

36. Percival CS, Maggio LA, Wyatt TR, Martin PC. "The program director's word … it's stronger than the word of God": Epistemic injustice revealed through narratives of remediated graduate medical education residents. *Med Educ.* 2024;58(7):848-857. doi:10.1111/medu.15295

37. Hauer KE, Cate O ten, Boscardin CK, et al. Ensuring Resident Competence: A Narrative Review of the Literature on Group Decision Making to Inform the Work of Clinical Competency Committees. *J Grad Med Educ.* 2016;8(2):156-164. doi:10.4300/JGME-D-15-00144.1

38. Kinnear B, Warm EJ, Hauer KE. Twelve tips to maximize the value of a clinical competency committee in postgraduate medical education. *Med Teach.* 2018;40(11):1110-1115. doi:10.1080/0142159X.2018.1474191

39. Ekpenyong A, Padmore JS, Hauer KE. The Purpose, Structure, and Process of Clinical Competency Committees: Guidance for Members and Program Directors. *J Grad Med Educ.* 2021;13(2 Suppl):45-50. doi:10.4300/JGME-D-20-00841.1

40. Goldhamer MEJ, Martinez-Lage M, Black-Schaffer WS, et al. Reimagining the Clinical Competency Committee to Enhance Education and Prepare for Competency-Based Time-Variable Advancement. *J Gen Intern Med.* 2022;37(9):2280-2290. doi:10.1007/s11606-022-07515-3

41. Keeley MG, Gusic ME, Morgan HK, Aagaard EM, Santen SA. Moving Toward Summative Competency Assessment to Individualize the Postclerkship Phase. *Acad Med.* 2019;94(12):1858-1864. doi:10.1097/ACM.0000000000002830

42. Keeley MG, Bray MJ, Bradley EB, Peterson CM, Waggoner-Fountain LA, Gusic ME. Fidelity to Best Practices in EPA Implementation: Outcomes Supporting Use of the Core Components Framework From the University of Virginia Entrustable Professional Activity Program. *Acad Med.* 2022;97(11):1637. doi:10.1097/ACM.0000000000004944

43. Parsons AS, Greenfield J, Bradley E, et al. Summative Entrustment Decisions in UME: Outcomes of a Binding Entrustment Committee Decision. *Acad Med.* 2023;98(11S):S186. doi:10.1097/ACM.0000000000005391

44. Schenarts PJ, Langenfeld S. The Fundamentals of Resident Dismissal. *Am Surg.* 2017;83(2):119-126.

45. Tulgan H, Cohen SN, Kinne KM. How a Teaching Hospital Implemented Its Termination Policies for Disruptive Residents. *Acad Med.* 2001;76(11):1107.

46. Minicucci RF, Lewis BF. Trouble in Academia: Ten Years of Litigation in Medical Education. *Acad Med.* 2003;78(10):S13.

Section 2

Identification, Characterization, Assessment, and Coaching of Clinical Reasoning

In Section 2, we narrow our focus to clinical reasoning, which is central to the practice of medicine and yet complex and difficult to learn. To set the stage, we delve into the principles and practices essential to identifying, characterizing, and coaching medical learners with clinical reasoning deficits.

Chapter 3, "An Introduction to Clinical Reasoning," defines clinical reasoning in traditional terms, tracing its historical development through distinct intellectual eras and providing a scaffold for use in remediation.

In chapter 4, "Recognition and Characterization of Clinical Reasoning Deficits," we broaden our conceptualization of clinical reasoning to include the overlapping domains of executive functioning, metacognition, and self-regulation and consider the importance of *situativity* in both assessment and coaching.

Chapter 5, "Assessment of Clinical Reasoning," compares and contrasts accepted clinical reasoning assessment strategies, acknowledging both the inherent heterogeneity in learner presentation of struggle and barriers to direct observation.

Finally, we present a learner-centered method for coaching clinical reasoning deficits and describe our clinical reasoning remediation program in chapter 6, "Using a Coaching Approach."

CHAPTER 3

An Introduction to Clinical Reasoning

AN ANALOGY

IMAGINE TWO AIRLINE pilots on two different aircraft preparing for takeoff and a long journey ahead. Both proceed down their own runway, accelerating to high speed before lifting off. Approaching 10,000 feet of elevation, something goes wrong aboard each plane. As alarms fill their cockpits, each pilot attempts to rapidly diagnose the problem. Taking in contextual clues, they generate potential hypotheses to explain the problem with the information available to them. Drawing upon their years of training and experience, these aviation experts recognize patterns in the available data and seek out missing pieces. Each copilot calls out additional information, including heading and altitude, and proceeds to reference a standardized checklist. As more information is gathered, each pilot forms an unconscious representation of the problem before one pilot voices a brief summary of the issue. The pilots each narrow their initial list of potential explanations to fewer and fewer options, hoping to employ an effective intervention and avoid catastrophe.

In the face of great uncertainty, Pilot A diagnoses the problem and enacts a successful management plan to stabilize the aircraft. Unfortunately, Pilot B's plane stalls, falls to the ground, and, tragically, crashes. As in other airline accidents, agents from the National Transportation Safety Board (NTSB) investigate the crash. The agents undertake a similar cognitive process to that of the distressed pilots, attempting to diagnose what went wrong for Pilot B. Was there an error in Pilot B's decision-making? And if so, where in their reasoning process was the cognitive deficit? What were the contextual factors that influenced this decision-making? Agents assess Pilot B's behavior in detail, both during the fatal flight and in previous flights, hoping to gain some insight into what may have led to this tragic outcome.

Parallels between the airline industry and medicine are plentiful, from decision-making under pressure to the utilization of checklists and frameworks to prevent errors and assess performance. In fact, many of the assessment tools introduced later in this book were originally developed for use in the airline industry. In these two fictitious scenarios, the pilots undertook a series of processes to solve a problem similar to those embarked on by a clinician aiming to determine the correct diagnosis, assess prognosis, and enact a management plan for their patient. Though rarely straightforward and always heavily influenced by context, these steps can be delineated, taught, assessed, and refined. In medicine, we call this process clinical reasoning.

WHY CLINICAL REASONING?

Clinical reasoning is defined as the integration, organization, and interpretation of information in order to form a working diagnosis and make management decisions for a patient.[1,2] It is arguably the most critical ability that a clinician possesses. In the case of a routine clinical encounter, when the reasoning process works correctly, the patient leaves the clinical environment with an explanation for their signs and symptoms and an evidence-based plan consistent with their goals and values. When the reasoning process fails, which occurs all too commonly, diagnostic and management errors can result in patient harm. Atypical presentations of disease, patient-specific elements, environmental complexities, resource constraints, and other factors that will be described in later chapters may further limit the clinician's success. In an attempt to reduce these errors, many have dedicated their careers to studying and describing the clinical reasoning process. Although no definitive evidence-based approach to teaching clinical reasoning exists, much has been written about how to apply our understanding of cognitive psychology and decision-making to medical practice. In contrast, little has been published on how to effectively assess and coach learners who struggle in this area.

Clinical teachers can draw upon our current understanding of the cognitive processes and contextual factors that underlie effective clinical reasoning to teach and coach struggling medical learners.

WHERE HAVE WE BEEN?

Education and clinical reasoning have been intertwined from the beginning of modern medicine, evolving through three distinct historical eras shaped by intellectual forces external to the field. In the first era, influenced by the development of pathological anatomy and statistics in the mid-19th century, clinicians argued to what degree reasoning was an inductive scientific process versus a more fundamental exercise in formal logic and problem-solving similar to other domains of knowledge.[3,4] After sitting on the sideline for several generations, these ideas were formally instituted into medical education with the global reforms of the 19th and early 20th centuries. Initially focused on general theories of logic and problem-solving (such as abductive reasoning), medicine evolved with higher education to stress themes from Dewey's critical thinking (such as practical content and context-independent reasoning) that could be more generally employed.[5,6] Probably the most notable artifact of this era is the clinicopathological conference (CPC), a mystery case conference at which discussants are given clinical information and must "think aloud" the diagnostic and management processes.[7,8]

The multidisciplinary intellectual upheaval of World War II ushered in the second era of clinical reasoning. New tools developed or refined during the war (e.g., screening algorithms for selectees, receiver operating characteristic curves for enemy aircraft, and randomized controlled trials) made it clear that human reasoning could be explicitly modeled.[9,10] This new field, called cybernetics (from *kybernētēs*, the Greek root for "helmsman"), sought to understand self-correcting systems, including the human mind as well as artificial intelligence (AI). Clinicians played an active part in the movement, especially with the introduction of decision theory in medical education.[11,12] Decision theory is a formalized approach to understanding how choices are made by weighing options, evaluating probabilities, and calculating the potential risks and benefits of different outcomes.[13] At its core, decision theory asserts that individuals act rationally to maximize positive outcomes.[14] This model provides a systematic framework for decision-making in fields like economics and engineering and has relevance for coaches looking to support medical learners struggling with clinical reasoning. The most prototypical example of decision theory is probabilistic or Bayesian reasoning, sometimes called evidence-based diagnosis.[15–17] Pre-test probabilities of disease are taken from the epidemiological literature, and physicians must continuously update the likelihood of various outcomes as new information becomes available.[18,19] Many of the coaching exercises presented in later chapters are based on probability theory and emphasize the importance of considering pretest probability (common diagnoses are common even when presenting atypically), testing and treatment thresholds, likelihood ratios, and post-test probability.

The third era, which emerged in the 1970s and continues to this day, has been significantly influenced by cognitive psychology which now serves as a lens through which to understand clinical decisions.[20–24] Cognitive psychology acknowledges that clinicians frequently rely on heuristics and intuitive reasoning as understood by Dual Process Theory (DPT).[25] This latest evolution reflects an appreciation for the adaptive, non-linear nature of clinical reasoning, underscoring that human decision-making, especially in medicine, is influenced as much by cognitive frameworks as by logic and probability.[26–28] DPT was popularized by Daniel Kahneman and Amos Tversky and has been investigated extensively in the field of medicine and medical education.[29] DPT posits that decision-making occurs in an individual's mind through two primary information processing pathways: 1) pattern recognition (System 1) is intuitive, heuristically driven, and occurs largely unconsciously; while 2) analytic thinking (System 2) is deliberate and takes place under conscious control. Thousands of papers on DPT have been published in the medical literature. Experts function predominantly in pattern recognition mode, whereas novices spend proportionately more time in analytic mode, engaged in logical thinking due to their lack of knowledge and clinical experience.[30,31] Ideally, both experts and novices toggle back and forth between processes as needed; the extent to which this toggling occurs is dependent on case complexity, prior knowledge and experience, external pressures, situational awareness, and the capacity for cognitive flexibility.[32,33] For most, this ability develops over time. The organization, activation, and real-time application of medical knowledge is central to DPT.[34]

SCRIPTS AND SCHEMAS

The most prominent example of DPT is script theory. Over time, clinicians amass a rich cadre of scripts in their long-term memory.[35,36] An illness script is a high-level, pre-compiled, conceptual knowledge structure that can be activated in appropriate contexts and continually modified through repeated study and relevant experience.[35] Practically, illness scripts—anchored in general disease knowledge and activated and refined by specific patient presentations—contain three components: risk factors or enabling conditions, the underlying pathophysiological process, and the patient's presenting signs and symptoms.[37] Illness scripts inform our understanding of diagnostic reasoning in which biomedical knowledge is used to explain a patient's clinical presentation, and patterns of illness are mapped to diagnostic categories.[38] Similar but distinct, a management script comprises the possible courses of action a clinician may take to treat a medical problem.[39–41] Management scripts are to management reasoning what illness scripts are to diagnostic reasoning. A related term, schema, refers to a more general organizing structure of medical knowledge.[42,43] For example, a diagnostic schema organizes information hierarchically, connecting broad categories to more specific information. Schemas can be structured around any clinical data point (e.g., symptom, sign, or lab result) using parallel higher-level groupings (e.g., organ systems or mechanisms) that facilitate the progressive narrowing to specific diagnoses.[42,44] Scripts and schemas can be moved into working memory as "chunks" of organized knowledge, ensuring that the rather finite processing capacity of working memory is not overloaded.[45,46] The accumulation and refinement of scripts and schemas are key elements of effective clinical reasoning, as is the formation of robust retrieval networks that facilitate rapid access to this stored knowledge by working memory when needed.[47] This organization system helps explain why experts, who tend to spend more time in pattern recognition mode, can fluidly integrate analytic thinking when necessitated by the cognitive demands of a complex case.

KNOWLEDGE *AND* PROCESS

The central role of scripts highlights the critical importance of medical knowledge for effective clinical reasoning.[48,49] In fact, the patient safety literature suggests that knowledge gaps remain a primary factor in diagnostic and management errors.[50,51] Norcini and colleagues found a relationship between learner performance on multiple-choice licensing examinations and later patient outcomes.[52] The worst performers were conservatively four standard deviations below the best performers, which would translate to a 22% difference for the mortality of their patients. However, remediation experts maintain that knowledge quantity, though critical, is not sufficient for effective clinical reasoning. Coaching struggling learners generally involves schematic application of the clinical reasoning process, case-specific knowledge organization, and knowledge transfer within context.[53]

The traditional model of medical education focuses almost exclusively on knowledge acquisition, beginning with the teaching of physiology, then pathophysiology, toward a causal understanding of disease.[54] Though a causal understanding of disease can improve reasoning,[55] when medical learners first encounter patients, they are presented with seemingly disparate signs and symptoms and tasked with synthesizing these data to establish a diagnosis. At some point during or after the diagnostic process, they are also expected to engage in the more complex and uncertain process of determining optimal management for their patient. In 1997, Narayan and Corcoran-Perry introduced the concept of "line of reasoning" (defined as an argument or set of arguments leading to a conclusion), combining both knowledge and cognitive processes to provide a more complete representation of how we use knowledge to make a decision in context.[56] Unfortunately, still to this day, many schools and training programs devote inadequate time to helping learners organize knowledge and apply these processes in clinical contexts.[57–59] Learners are thus left to inherit the cognitive processes of expert clinicians, refined over years of patient-care experience, as they participate in care teams in the clinical environment.[60] Part osmosis and part apprenticeship, this approach is ostensibly sufficient in most cases, as the majority of medical learners complete undergraduate and graduate medical training without the need for remediation.[61] However, some learners require more deliberate teaching and practice to achieve competence.

Though the debate in the literature between the primacy of knowledge or process rages on, effective clinical reasoning requires both. In this book, we offer two distinct strategies to support struggling learners. The first comprises a theory-informed process of identifying and coaching clinical reasoning micro skills with consistent linkage to, and application of, case-specific biomedical knowledge within the relevant context (Section 3). The second centers on recognition of behavioral phenotypes of clinical reasoning difficulty in unique contexts (Section 4). Throughout both sections we propose coaching strategies that center on acquisition and/or reorganization of knowledge in a way that facilitates effective clinical reasoning. The interplay between knowledge deficiencies and clinical reasoning struggle is explored in more detail in chapter 9.

INDUCTIVE VERSUS DEDUCTIVE

The steps leading to formation of a working diagnosis are collectively termed diagnostic reasoning, and the process that results in the creation of a management plan is known as management reasoning.[62,63] Data gathering, often considered the first step of diagnostic reasoning, refers collectively to the activities of asking questions about the patient's history and current experience, performing the physical examination, and collecting initial laboratory and imaging results.[64] For novices and struggling learners, early hypothesis generation is particularly important—as long as the correct hypothesis is included in the differential—because hypotheses inform and streamline subsequent data gathering, consistent with hypothetico-deductive reasoning and the well-described scientific method.[65–70] Pertinent data is synthesized and abstracted into an early problem representation, formed, and then revised through interval conversion of specific features of the patient's presentation into semantic qualifiers.[71–73] Formation of an accurate problem representation, an iterative conceptualization of the clinical problem which can occur unconsciously or through verbal or written communication,[73,74] allows the learner to generate a refined list of possible diagnoses. This, in turn, informs additional data gathering toward selection of a working diagnosis. For experts, early reasoning is typically more inductive (i.e., pattern recognition) before it switches to a deductive approach. Data gathering occurs in concert with problem representation, allowing for the generation of hypotheses through pattern recognition, thus improving efficiency and accuracy of the entire reasoning process.[48,73] With a working diagnosis, the clinician can activate management scripts and then select management options specific to the patient's needs.[39,40,75]

As mentioned, experts inductively generate accurate hypotheses—based on the patient's chief concern and early clinical data—using pattern recognition.[76,77] Data gathering then continues to test these early formed hypotheses.[78] Data is gathered efficiently and deliberately using hypothesis-driven inquiry, and these hypotheses are "tested" by comparing gathered data to existing, stored knowledge that is organized in the form of scripts (more on scripts to follow).[35,36,38] Experts possess a broad and deep repository of organized medical knowledge that allows for early pattern recognition.[30,79,80] In contrast, novices remain reliant on analytical thinking to generate an initial list of diagnostic hypotheses. In other words, they must be deductive from the beginning of the reasoning process. The role of early and accurate hypothesis generation cannot be overstated. One study suggested that when clinicians think of the correct diagnosis early in the encounter, they are correct 96% of the time; when they do not, the number drops to 13%.[81] In an outpatient setting, Gruppen found that the differential diagnosis was correct after receiving the nurse's note in 79% of cases.[82]

The coaching exercises we present throughout will employ other types of reasoning as well. For example, analogical reasoning requires reflection on the similarities between two situations.[4] When comparing and contrasting real-world case experience to a new patient, coach and learner can identify signs and symptoms consistent with atypical presentations of disease, explicitly consider unique contextual features of a case, and refine their illness scripts for subsequent use. Abductive reasoning is a form of inference that seeks the simplest, most likely explanation in the face of incomplete data, a common scenario in the clinical environment.[4,83] The uncertainty that results from incomplete data can cause some struggling learners to freeze, thus limiting their ability to make even provisional diagnoses or management plans. By using abductive reasoning, clinicians can arrive at a working diagnosis to guide early investigation and treatment and revise it as more information becomes available.

THE ROLE OF BIAS

A bias is a cognitive disposition to respond and can be positive or negative.[84] When making decisions, clinicians often rely on simplified information-processing strategies called heuristics, which may lead to systematic—and therefore predictable—errors.[50,85,86] For instance, clinicians (and people in general) tend to overestimate the accuracy of their judgements (overconfidence bias) and to perceive events as being more predictable once they have occurred (hindsight bias).[87] Yet, heuristics are not necessarily a bad thing. Heuristics allow for increased speed and reduced effort when making decisions and allow us to reason even with missing data.[88] The notion that pattern recognition (System 1) is highly error-prone has long been accepted, yet studies reveal that errors occur at similar rates in both intuitive and analytical thinking (System 2).[28,49,50,80] Researchers have focused their error reduction efforts on two major strategies: cognitive debiasing and knowledge enhancement. Cognitive debiasing encourages a deliberate shift to analytical thinking in high-stakes or complex scenarios for which error risk is high.

Common cognitive biases include:[89,90]

1. Anchoring bias: Relying too heavily on the first piece of information encountered (the "anchor") when making decisions
2. Confirmation bias: Focusing on information that supports an existing belief while ignoring evidence to the contrary
3. Availability bias: Overestimating the likelihood of events based on how easily examples come to mind
4. Representative bias: Judging the probability of an event based on how similar it is to a prototype or stereotype, often leading to ignoring base rates
5. Framing bias: Being influenced by the way information is presented, such as viewing a choice differently depending on whether it is framed as a gain or a loss
6. Overconfidence bias: Undue confidence in one's diagnostic abilities, leading to under-appreciation of alternative explanations
7. Sunk cost fallacy: Continuing a course of action due to previously invested resources (time, money, effort) rather than future benefits
8. Loss aversion: Preferring to avoid losses rather than acquiring equivalent gains, as losses are perceived as more impactful

Despite their theoretical appeal, research shows that debiasing strategies have not significantly decreased error rates.[91–93] We do not focus specifically on debiasing strategies in this book. Nonetheless, like many teachers of clinical reasoning, we recognize the central role of metacognition, a foundational principle of these strategies, in any clinical reasoning coaching program.[94]

Metacognition, thinking about one's own thinking, is usually operationalized in the form of reflection. However, to be effective, Mamede's work suggests that reflection must promote recruitment of relevant knowledge (remember the primacy of knowledge), asking questions such as, What findings support your diagnosis? What findings refute your diagnosis? What findings would you expect, given your diagnosis, but are absent from the case?[95–97] Given this understanding, the coaching strategies described hereafter employ targeted exercises requiring application of case-specific biomedical knowledge while promoting metacognitive awareness of the reasoning process. Table 3.1 provides a list of relevant clinical reasoning terminology.

Table 3.1. Relevant Clinical Reasoning Terminology

Term	Definition
Clinical reasoning	The collection, organization, and interpretation of information to arrive at a working diagnosis, forecast prognosis, and make management decisions for a patient
Diagnostic reasoning	The process leading to the formation of a working diagnosis, involving data gathering, hypothesis generation, problem representation, hypothesis refinement, and final selection of the most likely diagnosis.[98] Diagnostic reasoning is inherently a classification task; sometimes inductive—via pattern recognition—and sometimes deductive—via analytic thinking.[33,80]
Prognostic reasoning	The process of judging the severity of a patient's illness or injury and forecasting their clinical course based on disease-specific knowledge, patient-specific factors, and other relevant data
Management reasoning	The process of making decisions about treatment, follow-up visits, further testing, allocation of limited resources, and shared decision-making with patients.[63,99] Often requires prioritizing among multiple "correct" options with consideration of patient-specific factors and context

Table 3.1. Relevant Clinical Reasoning Terminology

Term	Definition
Hypothesis generation	The cognitive process of developing a list of potential diagnoses for a patient's clinical presentation. For novices or those facing an unfamiliar problem, this is often deliberately analytic; for experts, it may occur rapidly via pattern recognition.
Data gathering	The process of collecting clinical information (history, physical examination, initial labs, imaging) in a systematic or hypothesis-driven manner
Problem representation	Iterative conceptualization of the clinical problem which can occur unconsciously or through verbal or written communication.[73,74] Includes a patient's risk factors, time course of illness onset, and clinical presentation using semantic qualifiers. A "summary statement" is just one final form of a problem representation.[100]
Hypothesis refinement	The process of narrowing, prioritizing, and/or reorganizing the differential diagnosis based on newly gathered data and/or deeper reflection on the patient's presentation
Illness script	A high-level, pre-compiled, conceptual knowledge structure stored in long-term memory that represents the typical risk factors, pathophysiology, and presenting features of a particular condition.[35,37] Illness scripts can be rapidly activated (often unconsciously) and continually refined through study and clinical experience.[36]
Management script	Similarly, a high-level, precompiled, conceptual knowledge structure of the courses of action that a clinician may undertake to address a patient's health care problem(s).[39,41] Typically include laboratory tests, imaging, procedures, specialty consultants, medication, monitoring, and follow-up
Working diagnosis	The most likely or provisional diagnosis at a given point in time—sufficiently supported by the data to guide immediate clinical decisions, yet subject to revision as new information emerges

(continued)

Table 3.1. Relevant Clinical Reasoning Terminology

Term	Definition
Pattern recognition (System 1)	A fast, intuitive, heuristic-driven mode of thinking that occurs largely unconsciously and often relies on matching the patient's current presentation to previously stored illness scripts[33,80]
Analytic thinking (System 2)	A systematic, deliberate mode of thinking that occurs under conscious control and relies on logic, the scientific method (e.g., hypothetico-deductive reasoning), and stepwise decision-making to reach conclusions[33,80]
Hypothesis-driven data gathering	A targeted approach to further data gathering—through history, exam, or tests—that systematically tests or refutes a set of previously generated diagnostic hypotheses
Management script activation	The first step in management reasoning, involving retrieval (often unconscious) of a high-level framework or "script" for how to address a patient's particular problem (e.g., treatment pathways, monitoring, follow-up strategies)[39]
Management option selection	The second step in management reasoning in which specific actions or interventions are chosen from the activated script—tailored to the context, patient/provider preferences, and available resources[39]
Semantic qualifiers	Paired, contrasting descriptors (e.g., acute vs. chronic, diffuse vs. localized) used systematically in problem representation to compare and contrast potential diagnoses[98,101]
Framework	A structured external representation of knowledge designed to simplify and clarify complex medical concepts.[43] Frameworks provide an organized way to categorize information, helping learners build and refine schemas. Examples include anatomical frameworks for differential diagnoses and stepwise clinical algorithms.

Table 3.1. Relevant Clinical Reasoning Terminology

Term	Definition
Schema	A cognitive structure that organizes and integrates prior knowledge and experiences, influencing how clinicians interpret new information.[43] Schemas develop over time through education, clinical exposure, and personal experiences. Illness scripts and management scripts are technically considered to be separate types of schemas. Practically speaking, though, schemas are higher-level, hierarchical categories with parallel construction (e.g., organ-based or mechanisms) that narrow to subsidiary categories and eventually terminate at individual diagnoses or management options.[42,45]
Metacognition	Thinking about one's own thinking processes. Involves monitoring one's cognitive activities, evaluating reasoning steps, and adjusting strategies accordingly[94,102]
Structured reflection	A deliberate, often formalized approach to reviewing one's clinical reasoning during or after a patient encounter or case discussion.[96] Aims to identify knowledge gaps, explore alternative diagnoses or interventions, question assumptions, and improve future reasoning by explicitly linking case-specific data to broader knowledge and context[95]

THE ROLE OF CONTEXT

When viewed through the lens of DPT, clinical reasoning is a cognitive task that occurs exclusively within the mind of the clinician. However, research increasingly shows that clinical reasoning extends far beyond individual cognition and is profoundly influenced by context.[103–107] Four theories, collectively known as situativity, guide our understanding of this complex relationship: situated cognition, ecological psychology, embodied cognition, and distributed cognition (discussed with regard to AI later in this chapter).[108–110] Daniel and colleagues propose a transtheoretical model that integrates DPT with these theories of context (Figure 1) to characterize clinical reasoning more broadly.[110,111]

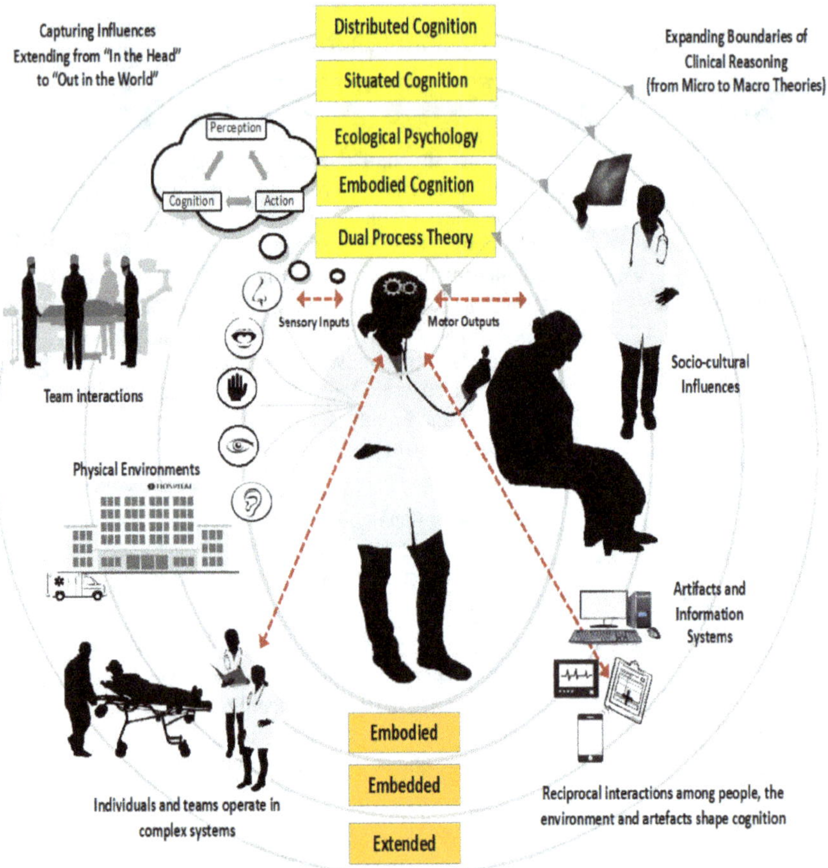

Figure 3.1. A Transtheoretical Model of Clinical Reasoning (Used with permission of the author.)[111]

Situated cognition argues that cognitive processes are inseparably tied to the environment in which they occur.[112,113] In other words, clinical reasoning is not an isolated, abstract task but is deeply embedded in the social and physical context of patient care. This context specificity helps explain why clinicians' reasoning can vary significantly across encounters and settings, even with similar patient presentations or diagnoses.[105] Ecological psychology suggests that clinicians' reasoning is shaped by continuous interactions with their environment, including specific "affordances," or action possibilities, offered by the surrounding milieu.[114,115] For example, the availability of certain diagnostic tools, access to patient information, and even the physical layout of the clinical setting all create affordances that influence clinical decision-making. Clinicians engage in perception-action loops in which perception of environmental cues informs actions; these actions in turn generate new perceptual feedback, creating a dynamic cycle of adaptation and decision-making. In subsequent chapters, we explore how coaches can encourage the struggling learner to relate mindfully to their environment and help them to identify and utilize these affordances and engage in perception-action loops in real-world settings. This includes how learners respond to cues, adapt to situational demands, and leverage available resources to make patient-centered decisions. The related concept of embodied cognition reflects the impact of physical interactions and the sensory environment on clinical judgment. Clinicians gather information by physically examining patients, reading body language, and interpreting environmental factors that shape their understanding of a patient's condition.[26,116] Situated and embodied cognition greatly inform our conceptualization of clinical reasoning during operative procedures, which we explore in chapter 15.

Together, these theories suggest that clinical reasoning is a highly contextualized, interactive process that unfolds within and is shaped by the clinical environment, team dynamics, and available resources. Recognizing these influences underscores the importance of assessing and coaching medical learners not merely as individual decision-makers but also as active participants in complex, collaborative care systems. Effective education and training must, therefore, emphasize not only the cognitive abilities required for individual clinical reasoning but also the abilities to work within care teams, adapt to situational demands, and effectively utilize the resources and tools that support modern patient care. Similarly, successful clinical reasoning coaching requires explicit consideration of context.

MORE ON MANAGEMENT

While the medical education discourse around clinical reasoning has traditionally been dominated by diagnostic reasoning, recognition of the importance of management reasoning is growing. Much of the clinician's role is consumed by decisions related to management reasoning,[117] defined by Cook and colleagues as "the process of making decisions about patient management including choices about treatment, follow-up visits, further testing, and allocation of limited resources."[63,99] Despite this recent unifying definition, the discussion of management reasoning goes back much further in the medical decision-making literature. Lusted published his seminal paper *Decision Making Studies in Patient Management*[118] in 1971, applying the current understanding of decision theory to management decision-making. This work built directly on that of Knowles who, just two years prior, had raised new and concerning questions about the cost vs benefit of diagnostic and therapeutic interventions.[119] In his concluding paragraph, Knowles said:[118,119]

> *One could and should ask how many renal arteriograms in patients with hypertension have resulted directly in the surgical or medical cure of the patients' hypertension. Or one could ask how many lung scans have altered the diagnosis, treatment or prognosis of the patient thought to have a pulmonary embolus. Such studies might conceivably put a discriminatory brake on the use of a technology seemingly run wild. As one looks at the cost of developing modern radiotherapeutic facilities, one must ask what the benefit of radiotherapy is as contrasted with the cost although in this instance even to ask the question, in an affluent, developed country will bring criticism raining down around the shoulders of the questioner.*

Beck revisited this work 20 years later in 1991, emphasizing the need for structured approaches to guide appropriate test selection and manage patient care effectively.[120] As these studies suggest, management is more than simply medical treatment. The successful application of clinical reasoning to the complex social milieu that characterizes modern medicine requires a partnership between clinician, patient, and interprofessional care team that prioritizes shared decision-making and efforts to minimize systemic inequities.[121–123] Arguably more complex than diagnostic reasoning, management reasoning is inherently an exercise of prioritization among many potentially correct options.[63,75] When considering a management plan, the answer is often "it depends." Management planning is influenced by patient preferences, clinician preferences, system factors, and the availability of resources, among other factors. Management reasoning is thought to occur in two cognitive steps: management script activation and management option selection.[39,41] This process is informed by a number of underlying concepts, including uncertainty, value (cost and quality), and risk—all of which influence the threshold to test and treat.[75,124–126] These concepts will be explored in more detail in chapters 8 and 12, in which we discuss coaching exercises to assist learners who are struggling with specific elements of management reasoning.

WHAT ABOUT PROGNOSIS?

Recent literature supports the categorization of prognostic reasoning as a subtype of clinical reasoning, related but distinct from diagnostic and management reasoning (Figure 2).[127–129] Our colleague Dr. Jessica Dreicer defines prognostic reasoning as the process of judging the severity of a patient's illness or injury and forecasting their clinical course. This includes estimating and anticipating the likely outcomes of a patient's condition based on the integration of clinical findings, patient-specific factors, disease-specific knowledge, and clinical context. Prognostic reasoning involves assessing the severity of the current illness, predicting potential future clinical trajectories, and identifying factors that may influence recovery or deterioration. Though comparatively less is known about how learners struggle in this area, clinician estimates of prognosis are generally inaccurate with a tendency towards overoptimism.[130,131] We explore this phenotype of struggle in more detail in chapter 11. For now, it is important to understand that all three subtypes of reasoning are required for effective clinical decision-making, and all are routinely employed in the clinical environment. The relative emphasis of diagnostic, prognostic, and management reasoning in clinical care varies considerably depending on the context, and these subtypes are often deployed in a non-linear fashion as depicted in Figure 2.

WHERE ARE WE GOING? ARTIFICIAL INTELLIGENCE AND CLINICAL REASONING

Clinical reasoning has continuously been buffeted by scientific forces outside of medicine, and many would argue that we are on the cusp of a new era in clinical reasoning. Just as decision theory and cognitive psychology emerged from the cybernetics movement of the 1950s, so did AI. Clinicians were enthusiastic early adopters of these technologies, which largely focused on specific domains of clinical care using computational methods such as Bayesian inference and expert systems. Many of these systems, such as

AAPHELP for acute abdominal pain or MYCIN for antibiotic selection, outperformed humans in limited domains.[132] However, initial attempts to extend AI to more general reasoning processes failed. By the 1980s, INTERNIST-I had been developed as a general-purpose reasoning algorithm, encoding human-like associations between diseases.[133] This new class of AI, termed differential generators, offered helpful suggestions, though the relative inaccuracy and difficulty in inputting data limited clinical implementation.[134] Through the 2010s, tools such as Isabel[135] and Dxplain[136] were primarily utilized in preclinical medical education as an adjunct to more traditional methods of teaching clinical reasoning.

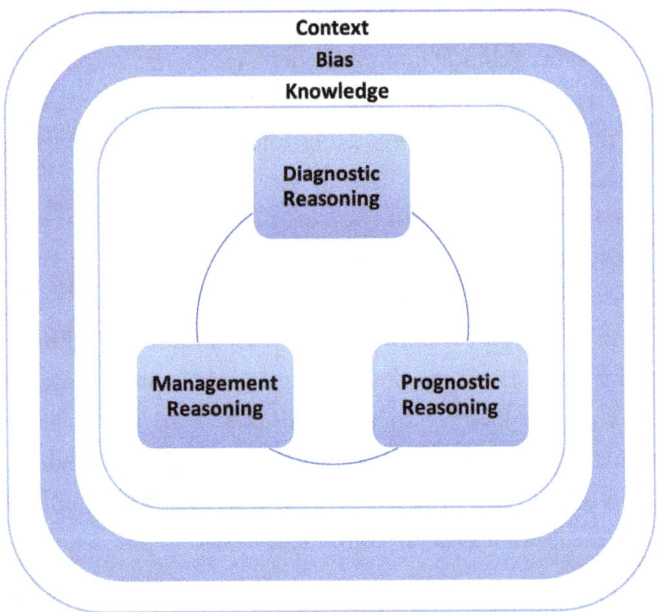

Figure 3.2. Three Related, but Distinct Subtypes of Clinical Reasoning

Machine learning (ML) risk prediction algorithms became more prominent in the 2010s and spurred debates about uninterpretable algorithms in clinical reasoning. Whereas a Bayesian risk prediction model such as a Wells score[137] could be easily understood, ML algorithms were opaque with unclear relationships between data inputs and risk output. Conversations around AI in reasoning drastically shifted in 2022, when the technology company

OpenAI publicly released GPT-3.5, a large language model (LLM).[138] LLMs are ML algorithms trained on vast amounts of human language that can produce realistic-sounding text to natural-language inputs.[139] Studies soon suggested that LLMs could perform reasoning tasks that had previously been exclusively the domain of clinicians (e.g., demonstrating empathy in communication, taking a history, creating problem representations, and making nuanced management decisions including augmenting the decision to operate and improving the quality of informed consent).[140–145] Further, despite not being trained specifically on medical uses, LLMs could outperform any previous differential generator.[146] As of spring 2025, the reasoning abilities of LLMs have continued to improve and now routinely outclass even attending physicians.[147,148] This disruptive technology will likely continue to transform medical education.[149,150]

Stretching back to the stethoscope "seeing with a better eye," medical technology has always informed the nature of clinical reasoning.[151] No technology has been quite so influential, however, as the electronic health record, which serves not only as a means of recording reasoning, but sharing it across different clinicians separated by time and space. New psychological theories such as distributed cognition have been advanced to explain the impact of computing technology on reasoning. Distributed cognition emphasizes that clinical reasoning is often a collaborative task.[152–155] Rather than existing solely in the mind of one clinician, reasoning can be distributed across multiple team members, tools, and even across different physical locations. For instance, a clinician's thought process may depend on contributions from other team members, interactions with electronic health records, data from medical devices, or input from AI-driven support systems. Each team member interacts with distinct pieces of information, has a unique perspective, and may engage with specialized tools, thereby creating what is called a "limited cognitive horizon," an awareness restricted to their particular role. Through the dynamic interplay of these individual roles, distributed cognition suggests that clinical reasoning is co-constructed and emerges across the team over time.

Viewed through a psychological lens, there is little doubt that AI technologies will play a large part in both the clinical care of patients and the education of clinicians and support for struggling medical learners. However, many challenges remain, including important concerns about human-computer interaction, bias encoded into the models, regulatory oversight, and the risk of cognitive deskilling for learners who use these models from the beginning of medical school.

NEXT STEPS...

With this foundational understanding in mind, we can now employ a systematic process for identifying, assessing, and coaching medical learners who struggle with clinical reasoning. Just as the NTSB relies on standardized protocols to determine the root cause of an airline accident— assessing the pilots' thought processes through an analysis of their behavior—we utilize knowledge-linked and context-focused coaching exercises to probe medical learners' decision-making as they work through clinical cases. We then translate our working definition of clinical reasoning to the clinical environment, defining common patterns of difficulty that are often mislabeled and/or misunderstood. These phenotypes represent struggles with the application of knowledge and/or the integration of higher-level abilities within specific contexts. For each phenotype, we describe associated patterns of behavior, potential underlying causes, and targeted coaching strategies. Our method is applicable to learners in a variety of health care specialties across the continuum of medical education.

Acknowledgement: Thank you to Iyob Makonnen (airline pilot) and Paul Malpiedi (experienced flyer) for their help with the opening scenario in this chapter.

References

1. Young M, Thomas A, Lubarsky S, et al. Drawing Boundaries: The Difficulty in Defining Clinical Reasoning. *Acad Med.* 2018;93(7):990. doi:10.1097/ACM.0000000000002142
2. Young M, Thomas A, Gordon D, et al. The terminology of clinical reasoning in health professions education: Implications and considerations. *Med Teach.* 2019;41(11):1277-1284. doi:10.1080/0142159X.2019.1635686
3. A History of Medicine. Volume I: Primitive and Archaic Medicine. *J Am Med Assoc.* 1951;145(14):1107. doi:10.1001/jama.1951.02920320081040
4. Bolton JW. Varieties of clinical reasoning. *J Eval Clin Pract.* 2015;21(3):486-489. doi:10.1111/jep.12309

5. Dewey J. *How We Think.* D C Heath; 1910:vi, 228. doi:10.1037/10903-000
6. Lau JYF. Revisiting the origin of critical thinking. *Educ Philos Theory.* 2024;56(7):724-733. doi:10.1080/00131857.2024.2320199
7. Harris NL, Scully RE. The Clinicopathological Conferences (CPCs).
8. Richard Clarke Cabot and the Clinicopathologic Conference. *N Engl J Med.* 1939;220(21):880-880. doi:10.1056/NEJM193905252202106
9. Lusted LB. Signal Detectability and Medical Decision-Making. *Science.* 1971;171(3977):1217-1219. doi:10.1126/science.171.3977.1217
10. Stigler SM. A Historical View of Statistical Concepts in Psychology and Educational Research. *Am J Educ.* 1992;101(1):60-70. doi:10.1086/444032
11. Hacking I. *The Emergence of Probability: A Philosophical Study of Early Ideas about Probability, Induction and Statistical Inference.* 2nd ed. Cambridge University Press; 2006. doi:10.1017/CBO9780511817557
12. Mazur DJ. A history of evidence in medical decisions: from the diagnostic sign to Bayesian inference. *Med Decis Mak Int J Soc Med Decis Mak.* 2012;32(2):227-231. doi:10.1177/0272989X11434739
13. Lehmann EL. Some Principles of the Theory of Testing Hypotheses. *Ann Math Stat.* 1950;21(1):1-26. doi:10.1214/aoms/1177729884
14. Albert DA. Decision Theory in Medicine: A Review and Critique. *Milbank Mem Fund Q Health Soc.* 1978;56(3):362. doi:10.2307/3349653
15. The Theory That Would Not Die. Yale University Press. Accessed February 3, 2025. https://yalebooks.yale.edu/9780300188226/the-theory-that-would-not-die
16. Fienberg SE. When did Bayesian inference become "Bayesian"? *Bayesian Anal.* 2006;1(1):1-40. doi:10.1214/06-BA101
17. Eddy DM. The Origins of Evidence-Based Medicine: A Personal Perspective. *AMA J Ethics.* 2011;13(1):55-60. doi:10.1001/virtualmentor.2011.13.1.mhst1-1101
18. Stigler SM. The History of Statistics : *The Measurement of Uncertainty before 1900.* Cambridge, Mass. : Belknap Press of Harvard University Press; 1986. Accessed February 3, 2025. http://archive.org/details/historyofstatist0000stig
19. Technology I of M (US) C on HC, Sox H, Stern S, Owens D, Abrams HL. The Use of Diagnostic Tests: A Probabilistic Approach. In: *Assessment of Diagnostic Technology in Health Care: Rationale, Methods, Problems, and Directions: Monograph of the Council on Health Care Technology.* National Academies Press (US); 1989. Accessed February 3, 2025. https://www.ncbi.nlm.nih.gov/books/NBK235178/
20. Kihlstrom JF. The cognitive unconscious. *Science.* 1987;237(4821):1445-1452. doi:10.1126/science.3629249
21. Oatley K, Johnson-Laird PN. Towards a cognitive theory of emotions. *Cogn Emot.* 1987;1(1):29-50. doi:10.1080/02699938708408362
22. Bower GH. Mood and memory. *Am Psychol.* 1981;36(2):129-148. doi:10.1037/0003-066X.36.2.129
23. Dember WN. Motivation and the cognitive revolution. *Am Psychol.* 1974;29(3):161-168. doi:10.1037/h0035907

24. Heyck H. Cognitive Psychology During the Cold War Era, 1955–1975. In: *Oxford Research Encyclopedia of Psychology.* Accessed February 3, 2025.

25. Wason PC, Evans JSTBT. Dual processes in reasoning? *Cognition.* 1974;3(2):141-154. doi:10.1016/0010-0277(74)90017-1

26. Bellini-Leite SC. Dual Process Theory: Embodied and Predictive; Symbolic and Classical. *Front Psychol.* 2022;13:805386. doi:10.3389/fpsyg.2022.805386

27. Evans JStBT. Dual-Processing Accounts of Reasoning, Judgment, and Social Cognition. *Annu Rev Psychol.* 2008;59(1):255-278. doi:10.1146/annurev.psych.59.103006.093629

28. Evans JSBT, Stanovich KE. Dual-Process Theories of Higher Cognition: Advancing the Debate. *Perspect Psychol Sci J Assoc Psychol Sci.* 2013;8(3):223-241. doi:10.1177/1745691612460685

29. Kahneman D. *Thinking, Fast and Slow.* 1st edition. Farrar, Straus and Giroux; 2013.

30. Norman G, Young M, Brooks L. Non-analytical models of clinical reasoning: the role of experience. *Med Educ.* 2007;41(12):1140-1145. doi:10.1111/j.1365-2923.2007.02914.x

31. Hruska P, Hecker KG, Coderre S, et al. Hemispheric activation differences in novice and expert clinicians during clinical decision making. *Adv Health Sci Educ Theory Pract.* 2016;21(5):921-933. doi:10.1007/s10459-015-9648-3

32. Croskerry P. Clinical cognition and diagnostic error: applications of a dual process model of reasoning. *Adv Health Sci Educ Theory Pract.* 2009;14 Suppl 1:27-35. doi:10.1007/s10459-009-9182-2

33. Croskerry P. A Universal Model of Diagnostic Reasoning. *Acad Med.* 2009;84(8):1022-1028. doi:10.1097/ACM.0b013e3181ace703

34. Schmidt HG, Rikers RMJP. How expertise develops in medicine: knowledge encapsulation and illness script formation. *Med Educ.* 2007;41(12):1133-1139. doi:10.1111/j.1365-2923.2007.02915.x

35. Custers EJFM. Thirty years of illness scripts: Theoretical origins and practical applications. *Med Teach.* 2015;37(5):457-462. doi:10.3109/0142159X.2014.956052

36. Charlin B, Boshuizen HPA, Custers EJ, Feltovich PJ. Scripts and clinical reasoning. *Med Educ.* 2007;41(12):1178-1184. doi:10.1111/j.1365-2923.2007.02924.x

37. Gavinski K, Covin YN, Longo PJ. Learning How to Build Illness Scripts. *Acad Med.* 2019;94(2):293. doi:10.1097/ACM.0000000000002493

38. Charlin B, Tardif J, Boshuizen HPA. Scripts and Medical Diagnostic Knowledge: Theory and Applications for Clinical Reasoning Instruction and Research. *Acad Med.* 2000;75(2):182-190.

39. Parsons AS, Wijesekera TP, Rencic JJ. The Management Script: A Practical Tool for Teaching Management Reasoning. *Acad Med.* 2020;95(8):1179-1185. doi:10.1097/ACM.0000000000003465

40. Cook DA, Stephenson CR, Gruppen LD, Durning SJ. Management reasoning scripts: Qualitative exploration using simulated physician-patient encounters. *Perspect Med Educ.* 2022;11(4):196-206. doi:10.1007/s40037-022-00714-y

41. Abdoler EA, O'Brien BC, Schwartz BS. Following the Script: An Exploratory Study of the Therapeutic Reasoning Underlying Physicians' Choice of Antimicrobial Therapy. *Acad Med.* 2020;95(8):1238. doi:10.1097/ACM.0000000000003498

42. Cammarata M, Dhaliwal G. Diagnostic Schemas: Form and Function. *J Gen Intern Med.* 2023;38(2):513-516. doi:10.1007/s11606-022-07935-1

43. Dreicer JJ, Parsons AS, Joudi T, Stern S, Olson APJ, Rencic JJ. Framework and Schema are False Synonyms: Defining Terms to Improve Learning. *Perspect Med Educ.* 12(1):294-303. doi:10.5334/pme.947

44. Martin M, Sedighi Manesh R, Henderson MC, Critchfield JM. Diagnostic Scheming. *J Gen Intern Med.* 2015;30(12):1874-1878. doi:10.1007/s11606-015-3478-0

45. Thalmann M, Souza AS, Oberauer K. How does chunking help working memory? *J Exp Psychol Learn Mem Cogn.* 2019;45(1):37-55. doi:10.1037/xlm0000578

46. Minter DJ, Manesh R, Cornett P, Geha RM. Putting Schemas to the Test: An Exercise in Clinical Reasoning. *J Gen Intern Med.* 2018;33(11):2010-2014. doi:10.1007/s11606-018-4599-z

47. Manesh R, Dhaliwal G. Digital Tools to Enhance Clinical Reasoning. *Med Clin North Am.* 2018;102(3):559-565. doi:10.1016/j.mcna.2017.12.015

48. Mandin H, Jones A, Woloschuk W, Harasym P. Helping students learn to think like experts when solving clinical problems. *Acad Med.* 1997;72(3):173.

49. Norman G, Pelaccia T, Wyer P, Sherbino J. Dual process models of clinical reasoning: The central role of knowledge in diagnostic expertise. *J Eval Clin Pract.* 2024;30(5):788-796. doi:10.1111/jep.13998

50. Norman GR, Monteiro SD, Sherbino J, Ilgen JS, Schmidt HG, Mamede S. The Causes of Errors in Clinical Reasoning: Cognitive Biases, Knowledge Deficits, and Dual Process Thinking. *Acad Med.* 2017;92(1):23-30. doi:10.1097/ACM.0000000000001421

51. Graber ML. The incidence of diagnostic error in medicine. *BMJ Qual Saf.* 2013;22(Suppl 2):ii21-ii27. doi:10.1136/bmjqs-2012-001615

52. Norcini JJ, Boulet JR, Opalek A, Dauphinee WD. The Relationship Between Licensing Examination Performance and the Outcomes of Care by International Medical School Graduates. *Acad Med.* 2014;89(8):1157. doi:10.1097/ACM.0000000000000310

53. LeClair RJ, Cleveland JL, Eden K, Binks AP. An integrated pre-clerkship curriculum to build cognitive medical schema: It's not just about the content. *Front Physiol.* 2023;14:1148916. doi:10.3389/fphys.2023.1148916

54. Rencic J, Trowbridge RL, Fagan M, Szauter K, Durning S. Clinical Reasoning Education at US Medical Schools: Results from a National Survey of Internal Medicine Clerkship Directors. *J Gen Intern Med.* 2017;32(11):1242-1246. doi:10.1007/s11606-017-4159-y

55. Woods NN, Brooks LR, Norman GR. It all make sense: biomedical knowledge, causal connections and memory in the novice diagnostician. *Adv Health Sci Educ Theory Pract.* 2007;12(4):405-415. doi:10.1007/s10459-006-9055-x

56. Narayan SM, Corcoran-Perry S. Line of reasoning as a representation of nurses' clinical decision making. *Res Nurs Health.* 1997;20(4):353-364. doi:10.1002/(sici)1098-240x(199708)20:4<353::aid-nur8>3.0.co;2-f

57. Kononowicz AA, Hege I, Edelbring S, Sobocan M, Huwendiek S, Durning SJ. The need for longitudinal clinical reasoning teaching and assessment: Results of an international survey. *Med Teach.* 2020;42(4):457-462. doi:10.1080/0142159X.2019.1708293

58. Wagner FL, Sudacka M, Kononowicz AA, et al. Current status and ongoing needs for the teaching and assessment of clinical reasoning - an international mixed-methods study from the students` and teachers` perspective. *BMC Med Educ.* 2024;24(1):622. doi:10.1186/s12909-024-05518-8

59. Gold JG, Knight CL, Christner JG, Mooney CE, Manthey DE, Lang VJ. Clinical reasoning education in the clerkship years: A cross-disciplinary national needs assessment. *PloS One.* 2022;17(8):e0273250. doi:10.1371/journal.pone.0273250

60. Harvard Macy Institute - Blog - Teaching Clinical Reasoning: How early is too early? Accessed February 3, 2025. https://harvardmacy.org/blog/teaching-clinical-reasoning

61. Jagannath AD, Dreicer JJ, Penner JC, Dhaliwal G. The cognitive apprenticeship: advancing reasoning education by thinking aloud. *Diagn Berl Ger.* Published online December 1, 2022. doi:10.1515/dx-2022-0043

62. Patel JJ, Bergl PA. Diagnostic vs Management Reasoning. *JAMA.* 2018;320(17):1818. doi:10.1001/jama.2018.13354

63. Cook DA, Sherbino J, Durning SJ. Management Reasoning: Beyond the Diagnosis. *JAMA.* 2018;319(22):2267-2268. doi:10.1001/jama.2018.4385

64. Daniel M, Rencic J, Durning SJ, et al. Clinical Reasoning Assessment Methods: A Scoping Review and Practical Guidance. *Acad Med.* 2019;94(6):902-912. doi:10.1097/ACM.0000000000002618

65. Sisson JC, Donnelly MB, Hess GE, Woolliscroft JO. The characteristics of early diagnostic hypotheses generated by physicians (experts) and students (novices) at one medical school. *Acad Med J Assoc Am Med Coll.* 1991;66(10):607-612. doi:10.1097/00001888-199110000-00015

66. Kostopoulou O, Lionis C, Angelaki A, Ayis S, Durbaba S, Delaney BC. Early diagnostic suggestions improve accuracy of family physicians: a randomized controlled trial in Greece. *Fam Pract.* 2015;32(3):323-328. doi:10.1093/fampra/cmv012

67. Kostopoulou O, Rosen A, Round T, Wright E, Douiri A, Delaney B. Early diagnostic suggestions improve accuracy of GPs: a randomised controlled trial using computer-simulated patients. *Br J Gen Pract J R Coll Gen Pract.* 2015;65(630):e49-54. doi:10.3399/bjgp15X683161

68. Coderre S, Wright B, McLaughlin K. To Think Is Good: Querying an Initial Hypothesis Reduces Diagnostic Error in Medical Students. *Acad Med.* 2010;85(7):1125. doi:10.1097/ACM.0b013e3181e1b229

69. Hasnain M, Bordage G, Connell KJ, Sinacore JM. History-taking Behaviors Associated with Diagnostic Competence of Clerks: An Exploratory Study. *Acad Med.* 2001;76(10):S14.

70. Lawson AE. Hypothetico-deductive Method. In: Gunstone R, ed. *Encyclopedia of Science Education*. Springer Netherlands; 2015:471-472. doi:10.1007/978-94-007-2150-0_260

71. McQuade CN, Simonson MG, Lister J, et al. Characteristics differentiating problem representation synthesis between novices and experts. *J Hosp Med.* 2024;19(6):468-474. doi:10.1002/jhm.13335

72. Auclair F. Problem formulation by medical students: an observation study. *BMC Med Educ.* 2007;7(1):16. doi:10.1186/1472-6920-7-16

73. Nendaz MR, Bordage G. Promoting diagnostic problem representation. *Med Educ.* 2002;36(8):760-766. doi:10.1046/j.1365-2923.2002.01279.x

74. Chang RW, Bordage G, Connell KJ. COGNITION, CONFIDENCE, AND CLINICAL SKILLS: The Importance of Early Problem Representation during Case Presentations. *Acad Med.* 1998;73(10):S109.

75. Cook DA, Stephenson CR, Gruppen LD, Durning SJ. Management Reasoning: Empirical Determination of Key Features and a Conceptual Model. *Acad Med.* 2023;98(1):80. doi:10.1097/ACM.0000000000004810

76. Myung SJ, Kang SH, Phyo SR, Shin JS, Park WB. Effect of enhanced analytic reasoning on diagnostic accuracy: a randomized controlled study. *Med Teach.* 2013;35(3):248-250. doi:10.3109/0142159X.2013.759643

77. Brush JE, Sherbino J, Norman GR. Diagnostic reasoning in cardiovascular medicine. *BMJ.* 2022;376:e064389. doi:10.1136/bmj-2021-064389

78. Evans JSBT. *Hypothetical Thinking: Dual Processes in Reasoning and Judgement.* Psychology Press; 2020. doi:10.4324/9780203947487

79. Brush JE, Sherbino J, Norman GR. How Expert Clinicians Intuitively Recognize a Medical Diagnosis. *Am J Med.* 2017;130(6):629-634. doi:10.1016/j.amjmed.2017.01.045

80. Norman G. Dual processing and diagnostic errors. *Adv Health Sci Educ Theory Pract.* 2009;14 Suppl 1:37-49. doi:10.1007/s10459-009-9179-x

81. Barrows HS, Norman GR, Neufeld VR, Feightner JW. The clinical reasoning of randomly selected physicians in general medical practice. *Clin Investig Med Med Clin Exp.* 1982;5(1):49-55.

82. Gruppen LD, Woolliscroft JO, Wolf FM. The contribution of different components of the clinical encounter in generating and eliminating diagnostic hypotheses. *Res Med Educ Proc Annu Conf Conf Res Med Educ.* 1988;27:242-247.

83. Vertue FM, Haig BD. An abductive perspective on clinical reasoning and case formulation. *J Clin Psychol.* 2008;64(9):1046-1068. doi:10.1002/jclp.20504

84. Croskerry P. Cognitive forcing strategies in clinical decisionmaking. *Ann Emerg Med.* 2003;41(1):110-120. doi:10.1067/mem.2003.22

85. Eva KW, Norman GR. Heuristics and biases--a biased perspective on clinical reasoning. *Med Educ.* 2005;39(9):870-872. doi:10.1111/j.1365-2929.2005.02258.x

86. Tversky A, Kahneman D. Judgment under Uncertainty: Heuristics and Biases. *Science.* 1974;185(4157):1124-1131. doi:10.1126/science.185.4157.1124

87. Berner ES, Graber ML. Overconfidence as a Cause of Diagnostic Error in Medicine. *Am J Med.* 2008;121(5):S2-S23. doi:10.1016/j.amjmed.2008.01.001

88. McLaughlin K, Eva KW, Norman GR. Reexamining our bias against heuristics. *Adv Health Sci Educ Theory Pract.* 2014;19(3):457-464. doi:10.1007/s10459-014-9518-4

89. Croskerry P. Achieving quality in clinical decision making: cognitive strategies and detection of bias. *Acad Emerg Med Off J Soc Acad Emerg Med.* 2002;9(11):1184-1204. doi:10.1111/j.1553-2712.2002.tb01574.x

90. Croskerry P. From Mindless to Mindful Practice — Cognitive Bias and Clinical Decision Making. *N Engl J Med.* 2013;368(26):2445-2448. doi:10.1056/NEJMp1303712

91. Ludolph R, Schulz PJ. Debiasing Health-Related Judgments and Decision Making: A Systematic Review. *Med Decis Mak Int J Soc Med Decis Mak.* 2018;38(1):3-13. doi:10.1177/0272989X17716672

92. Lambe KA, O'Reilly G, Kelly BD, Curristan S. Dual-process cognitive interventions to enhance diagnostic reasoning: a systematic review. *BMJ Qual Saf.* 2016;25(10):808-820. doi:10.1136/bmjqs-2015-004417

93. Korteling JEH, Gerritsma JYJ, Toet A. Retention and Transfer of Cognitive Bias Mitigation Interventions: A Systematic Literature Study. *Front Psychol.* 2021;12:629354. doi:10.3389/fpsyg.2021.629354

94. Merkebu J, Veen M, Hosseini S, Varpio L. The case for metacognitive reflection: a theory integrative review with implications for medical education. *Adv Health Sci Educ Theory Pract.* 2024;29(4):1481-1500. doi:10.1007/s10459-023-10310-2

95. Mamede S, Schmidt HG. Deliberate reflection and clinical reasoning: Founding ideas and empirical findings. *Med Educ.* 2023;57(1):76-85. doi:10.1111/medu.14863

96. Mamede S, Schmidt H. Reflection in Diagnostic Reasoning: What Really Matters? *Acad Med.* 2014;89(7):959-960. doi:10.1097/ACM.0000000000000306

97. Mamede S, van Gog T, Moura AS, et al. Reflection as a strategy to foster medical students' acquisition of diagnostic competence. *Med Educ.* 2012;46(5):464-472. doi:10.1111/j.1365-2923.2012.04217.x

98. Bowen JL. Educational Strategies to Promote Clinical Diagnostic Reasoning. *N Engl J Med.* 2006;355(21):2217-2225. doi:10.1056/NEJMra054782

99. Cook DA, Durning SJ, Sherbino J, Gruppen LD. Management Reasoning: Implications for Health Professions Educators and a Research Agenda. *Acad Med.* 2019;94(9):1310. doi:10.1097/ACM.0000000000002768

100. McQuade CN, Bonifacino E. Reasoning on Rounds: Summary Statement or Problem Representation? *J Gen Intern Med.* Published online December 12, 2023. doi:10.1007/s11606-023-08570-0

101. Steward D, Bordage G, Lemieux M. Semantic Structures and Diagnostic Thinking of Experts and Novices. *Acad Med.* 1991;66(9):S70.

102. Marcum JA. An integrated model of clinical reasoning: dual-process theory of cognition and metacognition. *J Eval Clin Pract.* 2012;18(5):954-961. doi:https://doi.org/10.1111/j.1365-2753.2012.01900.x

103. Croskerry P. Context Is Everything or How Could I Have Been That Stupid? *Healthc Q Tor Ont.* 2009;12 Spec No Patient:e171-6. doi:10.12927/hcq.2009.20945

104. Durning SJ, Artino AR, Boulet JR, Dorrance K, van der Vleuten C, Schuwirth L. The impact of selected contextual factors on experts' clinical reasoning performance (does context impact clinical reasoning performance in experts?). *Adv Health Sci Educ Theory Pract.* 2012;17(1):65-79. doi:10.1007/s10459-011-9294-3

105. Konopasky A, Artino AR, Battista A, et al. Understanding context specificity: the effect of contextual factors on clinical reasoning. *Diagnosis.* 2020;7(3):257-264. doi:10.1515/dx-2020-0016

106. Durning S, Artino AR, Pangaro L, van der Vleuten CPM, Schuwirth L. Context and clinical reasoning: understanding the perspective of the expert's voice. *Med Educ.* 2011;45(9):927-938. doi:10.1111/j.1365-2923.2011.04053.x

107. McBee E, Ratcliffe T, Schuwirth L, et al. Context and clinical reasoning : Understanding the medical student perspective. *Perspect Med Educ.* 2018;7(4):256-263. doi:10.1007/s40037-018-0417-x

108. Durning SJ, Artino AR. Situativity theory: a perspective on how participants and the environment can interact: AMEE Guide no. 52. *Med Teach.* 2011;33(3):188-199. doi:10.3109/0142159X.2011.550965

109. Merkebu J, Battistone M, McMains K, et al. Situativity: a family of social cognitive theories for understanding clinical reasoning and diagnostic error. *Diagn Berl Ger.* 2020;7(3):169-176. doi:10.1515/dx-2019-0100

110. Parsons AS, Wijesekera TP, Olson APJ, Torre D, Durning SJ, Daniel M. Beyond thinking fast and slow: Implications of a transtheoretical model of clinical reasoning and error on teaching, assessment, and research. *Med Teach.* Published online June 5, 2024:1-12. doi:10.1080/0142159X.2024.2359963

111. Daniel M, Wilson E, Seifert C, et al. Expanding boundaries: a transtheoretical model of clinical reasoning and diagnostic error. *Diagn Berl Ger.* 2020;7(3):333-335. doi:10.1515/dx-2019-0102

112. Daniel M, Durning SJ, Wilson E, Abdoler E, Torre D. Situated cognition: clinical reasoning and error are context dependent. *Diagnosis.* 2020;7(3):341-342. doi:10.1515/dx-2020-0011

113. Rencic J, Schuwirth LWT, Gruppen LD, Durning SJ. A situated cognition model for clinical reasoning performance assessment: a narrative review. *Diagn Berl Ger.* 2020;7(3):227-240. doi:10.1515/dx-2019-0106

114. Daniel M, Torre D, Durning SJ, Wilson E, Rencic JJ. Ecological psychology: diagnosing and treating patients in complex environments. *Diagn Berl Ger.* 2020;7(3):339-340. doi:10.1515/dx-2020-0008

115. Perceiving, Acting and Knowing: Toward an Ecological Psychology. Routledge & CRC Press. Accessed November 24, 2023. https://www.routledge.com/Perceiving-Acting-and-Knowing-Toward-an-Ecological-Psychology/Shaw-Bransford/p/book/9781138205055

116. Daniel M, Wilson E, Torre D, Durning SJ, Lang V. Embodied cognition: knowing in the head is not enough. *Diagn Berl Ger.* 2020;7(3):337-338. doi:10.1515/dx-2020-0004

117. Choi JJ, Contractor JH, Patel VL, Shapiro MF. How team clinical reasoning occurs on ward rounds: Implications for learning. *Clin Teach.* 2023;20(4):e13599. doi:10.1111/tct.13599

118. Lusted LB. Decision-Making Studies in Patient Management. *N Engl J Med.* 1971;284(8):416-424. doi:10.1056/NEJM197102252840805

119. Knowles JH. Radiology — A Case Study in Technology and Manpower. *N Engl J Med.* 1969;280(24):1323-1329. doi:10.1056/NEJM196906122802404

120. Beck JR. Decision-making studies in patient management: twenty years later. *Med Decis Mak Int J Soc Med Decis Mak.* 1991;11(2):112-115. doi:10.1177/0272989X9101100207

121. Olson APJ, Durning SJ, Fernandez Branson C, Sick B, Lane KP, Rencic JJ. Teamwork in clinical reasoning - cooperative or parallel play? *Diagn Berl Ger.* 2020;7(3):307-312. doi:10.1515/dx-2020-0020

122. Boyle JG, Walters MR, Jamieson S, Durning SJ. Sharing the Bandwidth in Cognitively Overloaded Teams and Systems: Mechanistic Insights from a Walk on the Wild Side of Clinical Reasoning. *Teach Learn Med.* 2022;34(2):215-222. doi:10.1080/10401334.2021.1924723

123. Olson A, Rencic J, Cosby K, et al. Competencies for improving diagnosis: an interprofessional framework for education and training in health care. *Diagn Berl Ger.* 2019;6(4):335-341. doi:10.1515/dx-2018-0107

124. Wijesekera TP, Parsons AS, Abdoler EA, Trowbridge RL, Durning SJ, Rencic JJ. Management Reasoning: A Toolbox for Educators. *Acad Med.* 2022;97(11):1724. doi:10.1097/ACM.0000000000004796

125. Abdoler EA, Parsons AS, Wijesekera TP. The future of teaching management reasoning: important questions and potential solutions. *Diagn Berl Ger.* Published online November 23, 2022. doi:10.1515/dx-2022-0048

126. Pauker SG, Kassirer JP. The threshold approach to clinical decision making. *N Engl J Med.* 1980;302(20):1109-1117. doi:10.1056/NEJM198005153022003

127. Chiffi D, Zanotti R. Fear of knowledge: Clinical hypotheses in diagnostic and prognostic reasoning. *J Eval Clin Pract.* 2017;23(5):928-934. doi:10.1111/jep.12664

128. Mullen N, Ashby S, Haskins R, Osmotherly P. The prognostic reasoning by physiotherapists of musculoskeletal disorders: A phenomenological exploratory study. *Musculoskelet Sci Pract.* 2025;75:103241. doi:10.1016/j.msksp.2024.103241

129. Daly P. A concise guide to clinical reasoning. *J Eval Clin Pract.* 2018;24(5):966-972. doi:10.1111/jep.12940

130. Christakis NA, Lamont EB. Extent and determinants of error in doctors' prognoses in terminally ill patients: prospective cohort study. *BMJ.* 2000;320(7233):469-472. doi:10.1136/bmj.320.7233.469

131. Malhotra K, Fenton JJ, Duberstein PR, et al. Prognostic accuracy of patients, caregivers, and oncologists in advanced cancer. *Cancer.* 2019;125(15):2684-2692. doi:10.1002/cncr.32127

132. Lea AS, Jones DS. Mind the Gap — Machine Learning, Dataset Shift, and History in the Age of Clinical Algorithms. *N Engl J Med.* 2024;390(4):293-295. doi:10.1056/NEJMp2311015

133. Wolfram DA. An appraisal of INTERNIST-I. *Artif Intell Med.* 1995;7(2):93-116. doi:10.1016/0933-3657(94)00028-Q

134. Bond WF, Schwartz LM, Weaver KR, Levick D, Giuliano M, Graber ML. Differential Diagnosis Generators: an Evaluation of Currently Available Computer Programs. *J Gen Intern Med.* 2012;27(2):213-219. doi:10.1007/s11606-011-1804-8

135. Differential Diagnosis Tool | Isabel Healthcare. Accessed February 3, 2025. https://www.isabelhealthcare.com

136. The Laboratory of Computer Science | DXplain. The Laboratory of Computer Science. Accessed February 3, 2025. http://www.mghlcs.org/projects/dxplain

137. Wells' Criteria for Pulmonary Embolism. MDCalc. Accessed February 3, 2025. https://www.mdcalc.com/calc/115/wells-criteria-pulmonary-embolism

138. OpenAI. Accessed February 6, 2025. https://openai.com/

139. Singhal K, Azizi S, Tu T, et al. Large language models encode clinical knowledge. *Nature.* 2023;620(7972):172-180. doi:10.1038/s41586-023-06291-2

140. Cabral S, Restrepo D, Kanjee Z, et al. Clinical Reasoning of a Generative Artificial Intelligence Model Compared With Physicians. *JAMA Intern Med.* 2024;184(5):581-583. doi:10.1001/jamainternmed.2024.0295

141. Kanjee Z, Crowe B, Rodman A. Accuracy of a Generative Artificial Intelligence Model in a Complex Diagnostic Challenge. *JAMA.* 2023;330(1):78-80. doi:10.1001/jama.2023.8288

142. Rodman A, Buckley TA, Manrai AK, Morgan DJ. Artificial Intelligence vs Clinician Performance in Estimating Probabilities of Diagnoses Before and After Testing. *JAMA Netw Open.* 2023;6(12):e2347075. doi:10.1001/jamanetworkopen.2023.47075

143. Ayers JW, Poliak A, Dredze M, et al. Comparing Physician and Artificial Intelligence Chatbot Responses to Patient Questions Posted to a Public Social Media Forum. *JAMA Intern Med.* 2023;183(6):589-596. doi:10.1001/jamainternmed.2023.1838

144. Strong E, DiGiammarino A, Weng Y, et al. Chatbot vs Medical Student Performance on Free-Response Clinical Reasoning Examinations. *JAMA Intern Med.* 2023;183(9):1028-1030. doi:10.1001/jamainternmed.2023.2909

145. Loftus TJ, Tighe PJ, Filiberto AC, et al. Artificial Intelligence and Surgical Decision-making. *JAMA Surg.* 2020;155(2):148-158. doi:10.1001/jamasurg.2019.4917

146. Busch F, Hoffmann L, Rueger C, et al. Current applications and challenges in large language models for patient care: a systematic review. *Commun Med.* 2025;5:26. doi:10.1038/s43856-024-00717-2

147. Goh E, Gallo R, Hom J, et al. Large Language Model Influence on Diagnostic Reasoning: A Randomized Clinical Trial. *JAMA Netw Open.* 2024;7(10):e2440969. doi:10.1001/jamanetworkopen.2024.40969

148. Goh E, Gallo RJ, Strong E, et al. GPT-4 assistance for improvement of physician performance on patient care tasks: a randomized controlled trial. *Nat Med.* Published online February 5, 2025:1-6. doi:10.1038/s41591-024-03456-y

149. Rodman A, Mark NM, Artino ARJ, Lessing JN. Using Generative Artificial Intelligence in Medical Education. *Acad Med.* 2025;100(2):250. doi:10.1097/ACM.0000000000005937

150. Cooper A, Rodman A. AI and Medical Education - A 21st-Century Pandora's Box. *N Engl J Med.* 2023;389(5):385-387. doi:10.1056/NEJMp2304993

151. Tomos I, Karakatsani A, Manali ED, Papiris SA. Celebrating Two Centuries since the Invention of the Stethoscope. René Théophile Hyacinthe Laënnec (1781-1826). *Ann Am Thorac Soc.* 2016;13(10):1667-1670. doi:10.1513/AnnalsATS.201605-411PS

152. Boyle JG, Walters MR, Jamieson S, Durning SJ. Distributed cognition: Theoretical insights and practical applications to health professions education: AMEE Guide No. 159. *Med Teach.* Published online April 12, 2023:1-11. doi:10.1080/0142159X.2023.2190479

153. Boyle JG, Walters MR, Jamieson S, Durning SJ. Reframing context specificity in team diagnosis using the theory of distributed cognition. *Diagn Berl Ger.* 2023;10(3):235-241. doi:10.1515/dx-2022-0100

154. Wilson E, Daniel M, Rao A, et al. A scoping review of distributed cognition in acute care clinical decision-making. *Diagn Berl Ger.* 2023;10(2):68-88. doi:10.1515/dx-2022-0095

155. Wilson E, Seifert C, Durning SJ, Torre D, Daniel M. Distributed cognition: interactions between individuals and artifacts. *Diagnosis.* 2020;7(3):343-344. doi:10.1515/dx-2020-0012

CHAPTER 4

Recognition and Characterization of Clinical Reasoning Deficits

INSUFFICIENT MEDICAL KNOWLEDGE is often cited as the most common reason that medical learners require remediation. This perception is inaccurate and merely reflects the tendency of many educators to default to knowledge as a culprit whenever they see struggle. The competency of medical knowledge is a natural rallying point because it feels familiar, quantifiable, and remediable. The ubiquitous summative statement "needs to read more" is often a hint that *something* is wrong, but knowledge is not usually it. "Needs to read more" also seems to serve as a default when evaluators need something to say in a written evaluation. We find that learners with a primary clinical reasoning deficit typically have an average global fund of knowledge, with a minority falling above or below average. The real problem, more commonly, is an issue with clinical reasoning, or the application of knowledge in the clinical environment.

Conversely, educators often assume that knowledgeable learners exhibit good clinical judgment which is not always true. While some learners acquire effective reasoning abilities passively with experience, others require explicit instruction. Unfortunately, the formal teaching and assessment of clinical reasoning in medical schools and postgraduate programs is highly variable, meaning that those who fail to develop this ability through knowledge accumulation, organization, and clinical exposure alone may fall through the cracks.[1–3] Identifying struggles in clinical reasoning is particularly challenging due to its nonlinear and iterative nature and its reliance on the dynamic interaction between the clinician and their practice environment.[4,5] Unlike medical knowledge, which can be assessed with standardized tools, clinical reasoning is heavily dependent on context, requiring assessors to make nuanced inferences about a learner's thought processes.[6,7] Thus, without skilled clinician educators equipped to recognize and address reasoning deficits, these struggles may go undetected or be misattributed to other performance issues, thus delaying timely intervention.[8]

In practice, there is overlap between performance deficits in medical knowledge, clinical reasoning, organization and efficiency, and communication, and many learners exhibit more than one fundamental area of deficiency. If a learner struggles to connect and/or communicate with patients, their ability to gather and interpret data may be affected. If knowledge deficits are significant, clinical reasoning will be impacted. Medical knowledge is best assessed through direct observation, review of prior learning history and standardized test performance, assessment of study habits and test-taking behaviors, and consideration of the potential impact of mental health conditions—including performance anxiety.[9–12] When first assessing a learner's clinical reasoning, it is important to observe them working through cases in a content area in which they feel reasonably confident in their medical knowledge. The approach to the learner with co-existing knowledge and reasoning deficits is discussed in chapter 9.

HOW COMMON ARE CLINICAL REASONING DEFICITS?

Outcome or process? Clinical reasoning deficits among practicing clinicians are a major contributor to negative patient outcomes.[13,14] From an outcome standpoint, diagnostic, management, and prognostic errors are the truest measure of faulty clinical reasoning. Diagnostic errors are estimated to affect 10% to 15% of medical cases.[13,15] Management errors can cause patient harm and may result in low-value care.[16–18] In the United States, one in three dollars spent on health care is thought to be wasted in the form of an unnecessary intervention.[19] Clinical reasoning can also be characterized and assessed as a process.[20–23] Common errors stem from points of miscalculation along the pathway, including hypothesis generation (where clinicians overlook critical diagnoses early on) and hypothesis refinement (where they fail to integrate new data to appropriately adjust their differential diagnosis).[24,25] Cognitive biases such as anchoring and premature closure exacerbate these tendencies, leading to over-reliance on an initial diagnosis and insufficient exploration of alternatives.[26–28]

Reports from centralized remediation programs that recognize clinical reasoning as a distinct area of competency support the notion that, when one looks for it, clinical reasoning is a common area of struggle among medical learners across the continuum. Clinical reasoning was the primary deficit in nearly 45% of medical students, 30% of residents, and 35% of post-residency learners referred to the University of Colorado's program over a period of 6 years.[29] Thirty-three percent of residents and fellows referred to our GME program over a 5-year period presented with a primary clinical reasoning deficit,[30] and clinical reasoning was the most commonly identified reason for referral to our longitudinal, structured clinical remediation program for medical students.[31]

HOW DO CLINICAL REASONING DEFICITS MANIFEST IN THE CLINICAL ENVIRONMENT?

Figure 4.1 presents a list of descriptors that characteristically indicate a lesion or lesions in the clinical reasoning process. Often, the clinical supervisor recognizes that a learner is struggling but cannot quite pinpoint the problem. Without an effective framework for analyzing clinical reasoning as a complex cognitive process, many evaluators assume that the learner lacks the requisite knowledge. Simply telling learners to "read more" is typically an ineffective strategy for approaching any of these issues.

CAN'T TELL A STORY	ORDERS TOO MANY TESTS	CAN'T TELL 'SICK V NOT SICK'	INDECISIVE	PRESENTATIONS MISS IMPORTANT DETAILS
DISORGANIZED	CAN'T CALL A CONSULT	OVERWHELMED	ALWAYS BEHIND	ANCHORS
POOR HANDOFFS OF CARE	CAN'T TROUBLESHOOT	MISSES THE BIG PICTURE	CAN'T SEE THE FOREST FOR THE TREES	CAN'T TRIAGE TASKS

Figure 4.1. Commonly Used Phrases to Describe the Medical Learner Struggling with Clinical Reasoning[32]

In two seminal papers published in 2013 and 2017, Audetat and colleagues identified commonly encountered clinical reasoning difficulties and categorized them according to steps in the clinical reasoning process as it was described at the time.[33,34] They emphasized the importance of "diagnosing" a learner's clinical reasoning deficiency, drawing a parallel to the clinical reasoning process used in patient care. This analogy highlighted the need for educators to systematically observe and analyze behaviors that suggest deficits in specific steps of the reasoning process. These principles are foundational to the approach described in this book, which aims to refine the identification of clinical reasoning deficits to allow for targeted coaching.

CASE 1

Dr. Reed is a hard-working intern who is intellectually curious, universally known as a team player, and communicates effectively with patients and their families. She is referred to our remediation program for help with organization and time management after an especially challenging rotation in the intensive care unit (ICU). In retrospect, there have always been concerns about her efficiency, but things significantly worsened with the higher patient census and complexity of the ICU. She was often unprepared for rounds and appeared flustered. Presentations were disorganized and lacked important pieces of information. She struggled to generate plans independently. Notes were entered late, and her supervising residents often had to help her complete her daily work. Particularly after observing her struggle in the role of "resitern" when her senior had the day off, evaluators expressed concern about her ability to progress.

Dr. Reed graduated at the top of her class from an Ivy League university and performed in the middle of her class in medical school. Her board scores were average. She denies any history of learning or attention disorder. She admits to being tired, as she comes in earlier and leaves later than her peers but otherwise reports no mental or physical health concerns. She is quite an organized person in regular life, with good systems for meeting deadlines and taking care of nonwork responsibilities. Her knowledge base is average, and she has a good study plan that involves both acquiring content knowledge and answering test questions. Clinical reasoning was not formally taught at her medical school, and she has never developed effective frameworks for data gathering and presenting patients. She does well enough with straightforward patients but admits feeling unsure about the plans for her patients when their issues are more complex.

THE DISORGANIZED LEARNER

As discussed in chapter 2, the "disorganized learner" may have a primary problem with organization, efficiency, and time management that can be global (affecting many aspects of life) or specific to the clinical learning environment. These learners often benefit from working with a near-peer coach to develop effective organizational systems for common tasks required of a medical trainee.[35] Disorganization and inefficiency may alternatively signify an underlying medical or mental well-being concern such as attention deficit hyperactivity disorder (ADHD), anxiety, depression, or substance use disorder.[36,37]

The disorganized learner often struggles with clinical reasoning. For example, the inability to engage in effective hypothesis-driven data gathering often leads to the appearance that the learner is inefficient. In the inpatient setting, "pre-rounds" are an essential test of this ability, requiring the collection, triage, and synthesis of considerable amounts of data in a compressed time frame. If the learner spends too much time with each patient or spends too much time collecting objective data in the morning, they will not be prepared for rounds. If the process of data gathering is disorganized, the learner may be unable to connect multiple pieces of information. These learners invariably struggle with patient presentations which can lead evaluators to conclude that they are more globally disorganized or have a primary medical knowledge or communication deficit.

There is considerable overlap between these categories, as outlined in Table 4.1, and learners often struggle in more than one area. It is important to differentiate a clinical reasoning problem from those related to mental well-being or organizational systems, as each requires discrete intervention. Many learners (e.g., the learner who struggles with pre-rounds) benefit from coaching that focuses on the concurrent development of effective organizational systems and reasoning frameworks.

Table 4.1. Differential Diagnosis of the Disorganized Learner (adapted)[38]

Type of Deficit or Concert	Historical or Behavioral Clues
I. Organizational systems	• Lacks effective habits, approaches, or systems for completing daily work
A. Global	• Struggles in multiple aspects of life – Difficulty meeting deadlines, bills unpaid, cluttered home or desk • Arrives late to meetings or rounds
B. Specific	• Lack of familiarity with specific information systems (e.g., electronic health record) • Prior educational/training program did not prepare learner for current program (e.g., size, complexity of patients, different expectations) • Unable to describe systems for evaluating new patients, preparation for rounds • Has not seen all patients prior to clinical rounds, unprepared for rounds in general • Spends an atypically long time evaluating new patients • Perpetually behind on all work • Patient presentations and/or notes disorganized

Table 4.1. Differential Diagnosis of the Disorganized Learner (adapted)[38]

Type of Deficit or Concert	Historical or Behavioral Clues
II. Clinical reasoning	• Has not seen all patients prior to clinical rounds, unprepared for rounds in general • Spends an atypically long time evaluating new patients • Struggles to triage tasks in all clinical settings, may lack appreciation of urgency of tasks • Perpetually behind on all work • Scattered history-taking or physical exam • Patient presentations and/or notes disorganized
III. Physical or mental well-being A. Medical impairment (e.g., metabolic disease, neurologic disease, side effect of prescribed medication) B. Fatigue C. Substance use D. Depression E. Anxiety F. Cognitive and/or learning disorder (e.g., ADHD)	• Other signs of impairment (e.g., unsteady gait; slurred speech; lethargic; agitated; withdrawn; fidgety; inappropriate or uninhibited behavior; memory loss or confusion; disheveled appearance; loud, rapid or nonsensical speech) • Known history of mental health condition(s) • Other issues with performance or learning

Table 4.2 provides specific guidance on direct observation to distinguish deficits in organization and efficiency from problems with clinical reasoning.

Table 4.2. Differentiating Clinical Reasoning from Organizational Deficits Through Direct Observation: What to Observe

Organization & Efficiency	Clinical Reasoning
• Global (nonclinical) evidence of disorganization (missed deadlines, late) • Systems for daily work – Admissions, consults, or new clinic patients – Pre-rounding – Note writing – Completion of a task list – Preparation for an operative procedure • Use of electronic health record	• Pre-rounding process • Patient presentations • Written notes • Handoffs of care • Discharge summaries • Ability to triage and prioritize tasks • Response in urgent situations • Preparation for an operative procedure • Troubleshooting during an operative procedure • Shared decision-making/counseling patients

Dr. Reed is paired with a clinical-reasoning coach and undergoes targeted assessment and coaching, described in chapters 7 and 8.

INTELLIGENCE, EXECUTIVE FUNCTIONING, METACOGNITION, AND CLINICAL REASONING

From the most reductionist approach, intelligence is measured through objective testing and represented as an intelligence quotient (IQ) score. Overall IQ comprises four main cognitive domains, the combination of which reflects a person's inherent intellectual aptitude. Domains include verbal comprehension, perceptual reasoning, working memory, and processing speed;

the latter two are also considered components of executive functioning.[39] There is no single, agreed-upon definition of executive functions (EF) in the scientific community.[40,41] In general, EF are thought to rely on various cognitive regulatory processes that provide the foundation to promote other higher-order executive constructs such as the ability to organize and adjust behavior over time, reach future goals, and solve complex problems. The related processes of metacognition and self-regulation are also central to the ability to manage complex tasks, make critical decisions, and generate innovative ideas. While intelligence is largely heritable and stable over the course of a lifetime,[42,43] EF evolve over time, with much of their development occurring between the ages of 20-29 when many medical learners are entering clinical training.

Figure 4.2 describes the relationship between these concepts as a hierarchy (similar to Maslow's hierarchy of needs) in which effective clinical reasoning in the clinical environment requires certain fundamental intellectual, cognitive, and social-emotional capacities. While there is a correlation between IQ and performance, high IQ does not guarantee that a learner will excel at clinical reasoning. Clinical case conceptualization and care planning rely on adequate working memory and focused attention.[44,45] Processing speed and cognitive flexibility contribute to a learner's proficiency at integrating information in the moment and adapting quickly in the face of changing clinical situations.[46,47] Foundational social-emotional factors include emotional awareness, motivation, and inhibitory control. Inhibitory control, the ability to suppress automatic thoughts, emotions, and actions by pausing in the moment, is important when moving from System 1 to System 2 thinking in the face of a complex clinical case. Effective clinical reasoning does not require that one excels in all these domains. In fact, many medical learners have relative deficiencies in one or more of these areas and perform at a high level due to compensatory strengths in other areas.

Executive functioning relies on the network connections between frontal and subcortical brain structures. Any dysfunction within these frontosubcortical projections can lead to challenges with multi-tasking, organizing and expressing thoughts, impulsive responding, regulating emotions, prioritizing tasks, and managing time. EF disorder is not recognized by the DSM-5 as a specific mental-health condition, but EF issues are part

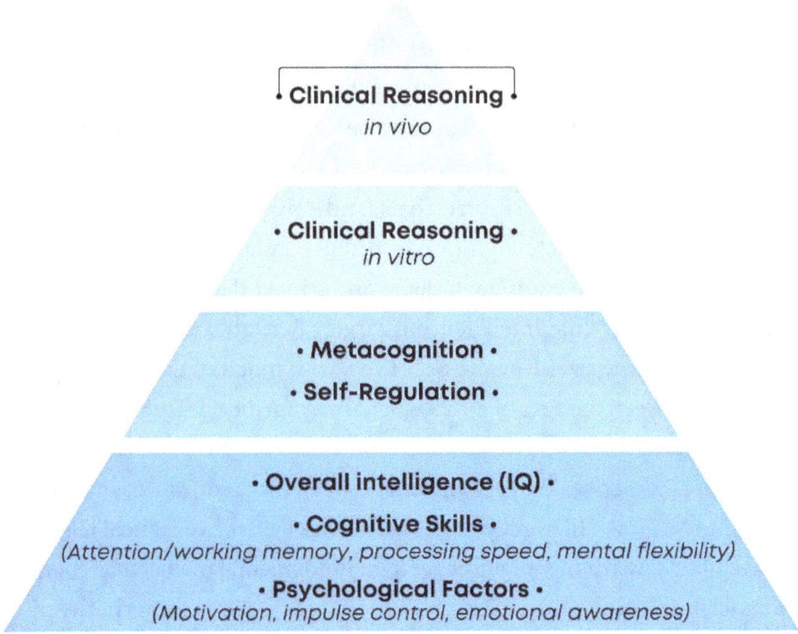

Figure 4.2. Clinical Reasoning and Related Domains as a Hierarchy

of many neurological and mental health disorders (e.g., depression, anxiety, autism spectrum disorder, ADHD, traumatic brain injury, stress, fatigue, and substance use disorder).[48]

The middle layer of the pyramid comprises the higher-order, interrelated constructs of metacognition and self-regulation that are required for effective clinical reasoning.[49–51] In chapter 4 of *Remediation in Medical Education: A Mid-Course Correction*, Howard and Pusic relate expertise to the ability to engage in self-regulatory behaviors.[38] Metacognition refers to knowledge and control over one's own thinking processes.[52] Medical learners should be aware of what they know and what they do not know. Self-regulation includes the processes of establishing goals and, through self-reflection and self-evaluation, selecting goal-directed behaviors and monitoring one's progress toward the achievement of these goals.[53] In the following chapters, self-regulated learning concepts are incorporated into the coaching of clinical reasoning.

Building upon a foundation of emotional awareness in which the learner can recognize and name their own emotions, these higher-order features of emotional intelligence include the ability to monitor one's own and others' feelings, to discriminate between them, and to use this information to guide one's thinking and actions.[54] Evidence supports that emotional intelligence, which is separate from IQ but complementary to academic intelligence, impacts clinical decision-making.[55] While IQ is not considered modifiable, many of these other areas can be taught and honed through interpersonal mindfulness training, interactive learning exercises, and one-on-one work with a coach.

The highest order process of clinical reasoning involves the collection and synthesis of data to manage patients and draws upon the learner's ability to solve novel and complex problems by categorizing, identifying relationships, and drawing inferences. A broader definition of clinical reasoning incorporates the interaction between the learner, the patient, and the clinical environment. In chapter 3 we introduced the importance of integrating *situativity*,[56,57] a collection of psychological theories that describe reasoning as situated in the experience, with the previously discussed internal cognitive processes.[58] Clinical reasoning is impacted by complex interactions between the mind, body, physical environment, sociocultural contexts, and the health care delivery system.[59] In the clinical environment, medical learners are required to care for multiple patients with numerous distractors and competing demands—and in variable environments. They are confronted with the continuous influx of data and the need to make decisions quickly in the face of much uncertainty. These circumstances require the learner to marshal all their lower-order neuropsychological resources (i.e., intellectual, cognitive, and social-emotional) and may expose vulnerabilities in these systems.

It is not uncommon for faulty clinical reasoning to go unnoticed or uncharacterized until postgraduate training. In many cases, these deficits reflect relative deficiencies in EF that become apparent when the work-related demands begin to surpass the learner's previous ability to compensate using other elements of their intelligence. Struggles that come to light later in training often reflect areas of relative weakness (i.e., slow processing speed) that limit ability to demonstrate effective clinical reasoning in a busy clinical environment (*in vivo*). Assuming the learner has not experienced any medical or psychiatric conditions that would better account for a cognitive change, any emergent EF problems may reflect the manifestation of a baseline weakness in the context of higher-performance demands. When confronted with the high level of complexity and role responsibilities required during residency or fellowship training, high IQ and other cognitive strengths alone may be insufficient to keep up with the pace needed to excel.

These findings highlight the importance of investigating underlying issues when confronted with a learner who struggles with clinical reasoning. A comprehensive remediation program should ideally include salary support for, or at least access to, a neuropsychologist to perform individualized evaluations and, when indicated, formal neuropsychological testing for learners suspected of having a cognitive and/or learning disorder. When possible, this testing should be offered confidentially and free of charge. In our experience, ADHD and other cognitive and learning disorders are common in struggling learners and are often previously unrecognized for reasons discussed in chapter 2.[36,37] This more comprehensive characterization of clinical reasoning *in vivo* also underscores the importance of assessing and coaching clinical reasoning in an authentic workplace environment.

References

1. Rencic J, Trowbridge RL, Fagan M, Szauter K, Durning S. Clinical Reasoning Education at US Medical Schools: Results from a National Survey of Internal Medicine Clerkship Directors. *J Gen Intern Med.* 2017;32(11):1242-1246. doi:10.1007/s11606-017-4159-y

2. Connor DM, Durning SJ, Rencic JJ. Clinical Reasoning as a Core Competency. *Acad Med.* 2020;95(8):1166-1171. doi:10.1097/ACM.0000000000003027

3. Hawks MK, Maciuba JM, Merkebu J, et al. Clinical Reasoning Curricula in Preclinical Undergraduate Medical Education: A Scoping Review. *Acad Med.* 2023;98(8):958. doi:10.1097/ACM.0000000000005197

4. Rencic J, Schuwirth LWT, Gruppen LD, Durning SJ. A situated cognition model for clinical reasoning performance assessment: a narrative review. *Diagn Berl Ger.* 2020;7(3):227-240. doi:10.1515/dx-2019-0106

5. Daniel M, Durning SJ, Wilson E, Abdoler E, Torre D. Situated cognition: clinical reasoning and error are context dependent. *Diagnosis.* 2020;7(3):341-342. doi:10.1515/dx-2020-0011

6. Durning SJ, Artino AR, Pangaro LN, Van Der Vleuten C, Schuwirth L. Perspective: Redefining Context in the Clinical Encounter: Implications for Research and Training in Medical Education: *Acad Med.* 2010;85(5):894-901. doi:10.1097/ACM.0b013e3181d7427c

7. Konopasky A, Artino AR, Battista A, et al. Understanding context specificity: the effect of contextual factors on clinical reasoning. *Diagnosis.* 2020;7(3):257-264. doi:10.1515/dx-2020-0016

8. Audétat MC, Dory V, Nendaz M, et al. What is so difficult about managing clinical reasoning difficulties? *Med Educ.* 2012;46(2):216-227. doi:10.1111/j.1365-2923.2011.04151.x

9. Andrews MA, Kelly WF, DeZee KJ. Why Does This Learner Perform Poorly on Tests? Using Self-Regulated Learning Theory to Diagnose the Problem and Implement Solutions. *Acad Med.* 2018;93(4):612. doi:10.1097/ACM.0000000000001422

10. Alfred M, Del Gaizo J, Kanji F, et al. A better way: training for direct observations in healthcare. *BMJ Qual Saf.* 2022;31(10):744-753. doi:10.1136/bmjqs-2021-014171

11. Haight SJ, Chibnall JT, Schindler DL, Slavin SJ. Associations of Medical Student Personality and Health/Wellness Characteristics With Their Medical School Performance Across the Curriculum. *Acad Med.* 2012;87(4):476. doi:10.1097/ACM.0b013e318248e9d0

12. Jeyaraju M, Linford H, Bosco Mendes T, Caufield-Noll C, Tackett S. Factors Leading to Successful Performance on U.S. National Licensure Exams for Medical Students: A Scoping Review. *Acad Med.* 2023;98(1):136. doi:10.1097/ACM.0000000000004877

13. Graber ML, Franklin N, Gordon R. Diagnostic Error in Internal Medicine. *Arch Intern Med.* 2005;165(13):1493. doi:10.1001/archinte.165.13.1493

14. Graber ML, Kissam S, Payne VL, et al. Cognitive interventions to reduce diagnostic error: a narrative review. *BMJ Qual Saf.* 2012;21(7):535-557. doi:10.1136/bmjqs-2011-000149

15. Graber ML. The incidence of diagnostic error in medicine. *BMJ Qual Saf.* 2013;22(Suppl 2):ii21-ii27. doi:10.1136/bmjqs-2012-001615

16. Schauer GF, Robinson DJ, Patel VL. Right diagnosis, wrong care: patient management reasoning errors in emergency care computer-based case simulations. *AMIA Annu Symp Proc AMIA Symp.* 2011;2011:1224-1232.

17. Erath A, Mitchell M, Salwi S, Liu Y, Sherry A. The Sooner the Better: High-Value Care Education in Medical School. *Acad Med.* 2019;94(11):1643-1645. doi:10.1097/ACM.0000000000002881

18. Shah N, Arora V, Moriates C. *Understanding Value Based Healthcare.* McGraw-Hill Education; 2015.

19. Shrank WH, Rogstad TL, Parekh N. Waste in the US Health Care System: Estimated Costs and Potential for Savings. *JAMA.* 2019;322(15):1501-1509. doi:10.1001/jama.2019.13978

20. Young M, Thomas A, Lubarsky S, et al. Drawing Boundaries: The Difficulty in Defining Clinical Reasoning. *Acad Med.* 2018;93(7):990. doi:10.1097/ACM.0000000000002142

21. Young M, Thomas A, Gordon D, et al. The terminology of clinical reasoning in health professions education: Implications and considerations. *Med Teach.* 2019;41(11):1277-1284. doi:10.1080/0142159X.2019.1635686

22. Barrows HS, Feltovich PJ. The clinical reasoning process. *Med Educ.* 1987;21(2):86-91. doi:10.1111/j.1365-2923.1987.tb00671.x

23. Charlin B, Lubarsky S, Millette B, et al. Clinical reasoning processes: unravelling complexity through graphical representation. *Med Educ.* 2012;46(5):454-463. doi:10.1111/j.1365-2923.2012.04242.x

24. Committee on Diagnostic Error in Health Care, Board on Health Care Services, Institute of Medicine, The National Academies of Sciences, Engineering, and Medicine. *Improving Diagnosis in Health Care.* (Balogh EP, Miller BT, Ball JR, eds.). National Academies Press (US); 2015. Accessed October 1, 2020. http://www.ncbi.nlm.nih.gov/books/NBK338596/

25. Auerbach AD, Lee TM, Hubbard CC, et al. Diagnostic Errors in Hospitalized Adults Who Died or Were Transferred to Intensive Care. *JAMA Intern Med.* 2024;184(2):164-173. doi:10.1001/jamainternmed.2023.7347

26. Norman GR, Monteiro SD, Sherbino J, Ilgen JS, Schmidt HG, Mamede S. The Causes of Errors in Clinical Reasoning: Cognitive Biases, Knowledge Deficits, and Dual Process Thinking. *Acad Med.* 2017;92(1):23-30. doi:10.1097/ACM.0000000000001421

27. Croskerry P, Singhal G, Mamede S. Cognitive debiasing 1: origins of bias and theory of debiasing. *BMJ Qual Saf.* 2013;22(Suppl 2):ii58-ii64. doi:10.1136/bmjqs-2012-001712

28. Croskerry P, Singhal G, Mamede S. Cognitive debiasing 2: impediments to and strategies for change. *BMJ Qual Saf.* 2013;22(Suppl 2):ii65-ii72. doi:10.1136/bmjqs-2012-001713

29. Guerrasio J, Garrity MJ, Aagaard EM. Learner Deficits and Academic Outcomes of Medical Students, Residents, Fellows, and Attending Physicians Referred to a Remediation Program, 2006–2012. *Acad Med.* 2014;89(2):352-358. doi:10.1097/ACM.0000000000000122

30. Parsons AS, Dreicer JJ, Martindale JR, Young G, Warburton KM. A Targeted Clinical Reasoning Remediation Program for Residents and Fellows in Need. *J Grad Med Educ.* 2024;16(4):469. doi:10.4300/JGME-D-23-00822.1

31. Young G, Meyer J, Crane I, et al. A Longitudinal, Structured Clinical Remediation Program for Medical Students. *Acad Med.* 2023;98(11S):S191. doi:10.1097/ACM.0000000000005401

32. Parsons AS. *Remediation of Clinical Reasoning.* Warburton, KM, Parsons AS, et al. ACGME Remediation Toolkit. Posted August 31, 2024. Learn at ACGME. https://dl.acgme.org/courses/acgme-remediation-toolkit.

33. Audétat MC, Laurin S, Sanche G, et al. Clinical reasoning difficulties: A taxonomy for clinical teachers. *Med Teach.* 2013;35(3):e984-e989. doi:10.3109/0142159X.2012.733041

34. Audétat MC, Laurin S, Dory V, Charlin B, Nendaz MR. Diagnosis and management of clinical reasoning difficulties: Part II. Clinical reasoning difficulties: Management and remediation strategies. *Med Teach.* 2017;39(8):797-801. doi:10.1080/0142159X.2017.1331034

35. DeKosky AS, Sedrak MS, Goren E, Dine CJ, Warburton KM. Simple Frameworks for Daily Work: Innovative Strategies to Coach Residents Struggling With Time Management, Organization, and Efficiency. *J Grad Med Educ.* 2018;10(3):325-330 . doi:10.4300/JGME-D-17-00756.1

36. Warburton KM, Shahane AA. Mental Health Conditions Among Struggling GME Learners: Results From a Single Center Remediation Program. *J Grad Med Educ.* 2020;12(6):773-777. doi:10.4300/JGME-D-20-00007.1

37. Warburton KM, Yost JS, Bajo SD, Martindale JR, Parsons AS, Ryan MS. Characteristics of ADHD in Struggling Residents and Fellows. *J Grad Med Educ.* 2024;16(6):730-734. doi:10.4300/JGME-D-24-00449.1

38. Kalet A, Chou CL, eds. *Remediation in Medical Education: A Mid-Course Correction.* Springer International Publishing; 2023. doi:10.1007/978-3-031-32404-8

39. Foverskov E, Mortensen EL, Holm A, Pedersen JLM, Osler M, Lund R. Socioeconomic Position Across the Life Course and Cognitive Ability Later in Life: The Importance of Considering Early Cognitive Ability. *J Aging Health.* 2019;31(6):947-966. doi:10.1177/0898264317742810

40. Zink N, Lenartowicz A, Markett S. A new era for executive function research: On the transition from centralized to distributed executive functioning. *Neurosci Biobehav Rev.* 2021;124:235-244. doi:10.1016/j.neubiorev.2021.02.011

41. Karr JE, Areshenkoff CN, Rast P, Hofer SM, Iverson GL, Garcia-Barrera MA. The unity and diversity of executive functions: A systematic review and re-analysis of latent variable studies. *Psychol Bull.* 2018;144(11):1147-1185. doi:10.1037 /bul0000160

42. Plomin R, Deary IJ. Genetics and intelligence differences: five special findings. *Mol Psychiatry.* 2015;20(1):98-108. doi:10.1038/mp.2014.105

43. Deary IJ, Pattie A, Starr JM. The stability of intelligence from age 11 to age 90 years: the Lothian birth cohort of 1921. *Psychol Sci.* 2013;24(12):2361-2368. doi:10.1177/0956797613486487

44. Zanto TP, Gazzaley A. Neural suppression of irrelevant information underlies optimal working memory performance. *J Neurosci Off J Soc Neurosci.* 2009;29(10):3059-3066. doi:10.1523/JNEUROSCI.4621-08.2009

45. Hruska P, Krigolson O, Coderre S, et al. Working memory, reasoning, and expertise in medicine-insights into their relationship using functional neuroimaging. *Adv Health Sci Educ Theory Pract.* 2016;21(5):935-952 . doi:10.1007/s10459-015-9649-2

46. Tong K, Chan YN, Cheng X, et al. Study protocol: How does cognitive flexibility relate to other executive functions and learning in healthy young adults? *PloS One.* 2023;18(7):e0286208. doi:10.1371/journal.pone.0286208

47. Moretti L, Semenza C, Vallesi A. General Slowing and Education Mediate Task Switching Performance Across the Life-Span. *Front Psychol.* 2018;9:630 . doi:10.3389/fpsyg.2018.00630

48. Diamond A. Executive Functions. *Annu Rev Psychol.* 2013;64(Volume 64, 2013):135-168. doi:10.1146/annurev-psych-113011-143750

49. Marcum JA. An integrated model of clinical reasoning: dual-process theory of cognition and metacognition. *J Eval Clin Pract.* 2012;18(5):954-961. doi:https://doi.org/10.1111/j.1365-2753.2012.01900.x

50. Artino AR, Cleary TJ, Dong T, Hemmer PA, Durning SJ. Exploring clinical reasoning in novices: a self-regulated learning microanalytic assessment approach. *Med Educ.* 2014;48(3):280-291. doi:10.1111/medu.12303

51. Berkhout JJ, Helmich E, Teunissen PW, Berg JW van den, Vleuten CPM van der, Jaarsma ADC. Exploring the factors influencing clinical students' self-regulated learning. *Med Educ.* 2015;49(6):589-600. doi:10.1111/medu.12671

52. Medina MS, Castleberry AN, Persky AM. Strategies for Improving Learner Metacognition in Health Professional Education. *Am J Pharm Educ.* 2017;81(4):78 . doi:10.5688/ajpe81478

53. Zimmerman BJ. Attaining self-regulation: A social cognitive perspective. In: *Handbook of Self-Regulation.* Academic Press; 2000:13-39. doi:10.1016 /B978-012109890-2/50031-7

54. Agnoli S, Mancini G, Andrei F, Trombini E. The Relationship Between Trait Emotional Intelligence, Cognition, and Emotional Awareness: An Interpretative Model. *Front Psychol.* 2019;10:1711. doi:10.3389/fpsyg.2019.01711

55. Kozlowski D, Hutchinson M, Hurley J, Rowley J, Sutherland J. The role of emotion in clinical decision making: an integrative literature review. *BMC Med Educ.* 2017;17(1):255. doi:10.1186/s12909-017-1089-7

56. Durning SJ, Artino AR. Situativity theory: a perspective on how participants and the environment can interact: AMEE Guide no. 52. *Med Teach.* 2011;33(3):188-199. doi:10.3109/0142159X.2011.550965

57. Merkebu J, Battistone M, McMains K, et al. Situativity: a family of social cognitive theories for understanding clinical reasoning and diagnostic error. *Diagn Berl Ger.* 2020;7(3):169-176. doi:10.1515/dx-2019-0100

58. Parsons AS, Wijesekera TP, Olson APJ, Torre D, Durning SJ, Daniel M. Beyond thinking fast and slow: Implications of a transtheoretical model of clinical reasoning and error on teaching, assessment, and research. *Med Teach.* Published online June 5, 2024:1-12. doi:10.1080/0142159X.2024.2359963

59. Linzer M, Sullivan EE, Olson APJ, Khazen M, Mirica M, Schiff GD. Improving diagnosis: adding context to cognition. *Diagn Berl Ger.* 2023;10(1):4-8 . doi:10.1515/dx-2022-0058

CHAPTER 5

Assessment of Clinical Reasoning

ASSESSING CLINICAL REASONING IS CHALLENGING

Assessing clinical reasoning is inherently challenging due to its complexity and the contextual factors that shape how reasoning occurs in practice.[1–6] Early methods of reasoning assessment such as think-aloud protocols sought to make learners' cognitive processes visible by asking them to verbalize their thought process while solving clinical problems.[7,8] These approaches largely focused on how clinicians prioritized data and justified decisions. For instance, educators could identify when a learner failed to include critical diagnoses in their differential or relied on faulty assumptions. However, think-aloud methods often capture only a fraction of the reasoning process, omitting the unconscious, automatic processes employed by experts as understood by dual process theory.

Cydulka and colleagues highlighted these limitations in their study of clinical reasoning assessment. By directly observing learners in authentic clinical environments, they uncovered deficits that traditional case discussions or think-aloud exercises missed.[9] For example, learners might order unnecessary diagnostic tests not because of a lack of knowledge, but due to an inability to appropriately prioritize or synthesize clinical information under time pressure. Similarly, learners who struggle to adapt their reasoning in response to subtle changes in a patient's condition may reveal their difficulties only in dynamic, real-time settings. Remember that, as introduced in chapter 3, context specificity (as understood by situated cognition) explains why reasoning deficits often manifest inconsistently; a learner might perform well in routine cases but falter when confronted with diagnostic uncertainty or ambiguous clinical presentations.[10–12]

Although national organizations and landmark publications such as the National Academy of Medicine's *Improving Diagnosis in Healthcare* have advocated for more explicit teaching and assessment of clinical reasoning, these efforts have largely focused on reducing diagnostic error.[13] Unfortunately, the rate of diagnostic, management, and prognostic errors is difficult to determine in the routine assessment of learners and is of questionable utility in guiding coaching efforts. Even experienced educators may lack specific training in the teaching and assessment of clinical reasoning. As discussed in earlier chapters, clinical reasoning deficits are often mis-"diagnosed," a reality that highlights the inherent complexities of assessing clinical reasoning *in vivo*. Furthermore, clinical teachers are hindered by a lack of validated tools to assess the reasoning process in real time. Although a number of approaches have been proposed, each has inherent limitations and none have been widely adopted for use in the clinical setting. For a more in-depth discussion of this topic, we direct the reader to Wijesekera, Durning, Boyle, and Holmboe's chapters 7 and 8 in *Practical Guide to the Assessment of Clinical Competence.*[14] A summary of the evidence supporting existing clinical reasoning methods can be found in an excellent scoping review by Daniel and colleagues[4] which divides clinical reasoning assessment methods into three domains: (1) non-workplace-based assessments, (2) simulated environments, and (3) workplace-based assessments.

Non-workplace-based assessments: Examples include multiple-choice questions, extended matching questions, key feature examinations, and script concordance testing (SCT). These tools evaluate reasoning in hypothetical scenarios, focusing on how learners organize and apply knowledge to specific clinical problems.

Originally developed in 2000,[15] SCT has been investigated by multiple medical and surgical subspecialties as a clinical reasoning assessment and teaching method.[16–24] SCT allows for insight into the reasoning process, including both intuitive and analytical thinking.[25] Here, the learner is presented with a short clinical vignette accompanied by a series of potential diagnoses and/or treatment interventions, then given a new piece of information and asked how this piece of information affects their decision-making. Unlike multiple-choice examinations, there is no single right answer to a given question. Instead, responses are compared to those provided by a group of content experts, and scoring relies on concordance with this reference group. SCT recognizes that effective clinical reasoning requires medical knowledge to be organized in scripts, a principle that is emphasized in multiple subsequent chapters of this book. When faced with the "what if" question, multiple scripts are activated and learners must make a selection quickly and without the full dataset. SCT thus captures the learner's decision-making amid uncertainty, attempting to mimic the realities of the clinical setting. Although the time-intensiveness of creating and grading these scenarios limits the widespread use of SCT as an assessment tool,[26] the theory underlying its use has greatly informed our approach to coaching struggling learners.

Similarly, mock oral examinations are helpful for assessing clinical reasoning by encouraging learners to verbalize their thought process as they work through hypothetical clinical cases. Using structured frameworks (e.g., let's contrast items on the differential diagnosis based on epidemiology) and scaffolding (e.g., what are the three most concerning causes of this symptom?), this approach also informs the teaching of clinical reasoning. In subsequent chapters, multiple applications of the mock oral exam are suggested for coaching the struggling medical learner.

Simulated environments: OSCEs (Objective Structured Clinical Examinations) and technology-enhanced simulations allow learners to demonstrate decision-making in settings that mimic the complexities of the clinical environment—without risk to a patient and with the flexibility to control variables depending on learner level and skill being assessed.[27–29] OSCEs allow for a greater focus on assessment and management of one medical problem at a time but are limited by the inherent constraints of a simulated environment. Advances in simulation-based education (SBE) in recent years have resulted in more widespread use of simulation as a method of teaching, assessing, and coaching clinical reasoning for medical learners. Newer technology means that much of this learning can take place asynchronously. In most situations, learners are given real-time feedback about their performance; however, a recent systematic review highlights the limitations of virtual patients in providing meaningful feedback on clinical reasoning.[30] Table 5.1 summarizes the modalities of simulation that are applicable to clinical reasoning education.[31,32]

Table 5.1. Types of Simulation Used to Teach and Assess Clinical Reasoning in Health Care Education

Standardized patients	actors are trained to portray patients with a specific diagnosis (e.g., OSCE)
Traditional, high-fidelity simulation	manikins and patient simulators replicate clinical scenarios that assess learners' diagnostic and management reasoning
Virtual reality (VR)	learners interact with a virtual world with varying degrees of immersion (e.g., computer-generated patient)
Augmented reality (AR)	learners interact with computer-generated content superimposed on real-world environments or objects, often using glasses or projectors (frequently used for procedural teaching)
Alternate reality	learners interact with a computer-generated parallel world over which they have influence by virtue of their decision making; often gamified (e.g., EHR-based simulation)

The use of standardized patients, manikins, and virtual patients holds appeal for the assessment and teaching of triage (chapter 13), response to clinical urgency (chapter 14), and operative reasoning (chapter 15). For instance, an OSCE station could be designed to challenge learners to recognize and manage a deteriorating patient, testing the learners' ability to synthesize data and act decisively under pressure.[33] In virtual reality, a learner might enter a simulated emergency department and encounter five incoming patients, each of whom needs to be rapidly assessed and prioritized. Artificial intelligence (AI) holds promise as a component of simulated-based assessment of clinical reasoning, leveraging machine learning algorithms to personalize and adapt the learner's experience. Given the limited performance correlation with other standard methods, these resource-intensive tools are best used for formative, rather than summative, assessment.

Workplace-based assessments: Direct observations and global assessments capture reasoning as it unfolds in authentic clinical settings. These methods provide rich, context-specific data but are often time-intensive and subject to variability across assessors. Assessments are also specific to the particulars of the patient and the setting in which the patient is seen. Effective workplace-based assessments require trained observers who can distinguish reasoning deficits from other performance issues such as poor communication or lack of medical knowledge.[34]

In the clinical environment, workplace-based assessment relies on direct observation of actual clinical encounters. Ultimately, this is necessary to assess learners at the top of Miller's pyramid to see not just what a learner can do, but what they actually do. Miller's Pyramid hierarchically categorizes competencies from foundational knowledge ("knows") to integration of knowledge ("knows how") to demonstration in simulated environments ("shows how") to performance in real-world settings ("does").[35] This framework provides a clear structure for mapping assessments to the learner's developmental stage, thus ensuring a logical progression from knowledge acquisition to practical application. By aligning assessment strategies with this framework, educators can better evaluate learners' readiness for increasingly complex clinical responsibilities.

Most medical educators recognize the importance of direct observation for assessing clinical reasoning, but several barriers make it challenging to implement routinely and effectively:

- Lack of clarity regarding what to observe
- Time constraints
- Lack of training in direct observation techniques
- Struggles around integration into the workflow

The incomplete connection between theory and observable behaviors in real-world clinical settings highlights a critical gap in the clinical reasoning literature. In Sections 3 and 4, we bridge this gap and these barriers by offering two complementary and yet distinct approaches to the recognition, assessment, and coaching of clinical reasoning struggles. Throughout our exploration of the many varied ways in which clinical reasoning struggles present in the clinical environment, we provide practical strategies for direct observation, highlighting both cognitive and behavioral components of clinical reasoning.

Workplace-based assessments are on the verge of a major transformation, as the integration of ambient scribes and AI-guided chart review will eliminate prior limitations and revolutionize how we assess clinical performance.[6] No longer constrained by incomplete observations or fragmented feedback, we will have comprehensive visibility into every case a learner encounters, promoting the generation of rich, continuous data streams. This shift should allow us to move beyond episodic assessments toward a dynamic, real-time understanding of clinical reasoning. This also means that we can study situated and distributed cognition, as introduced in chapter 3, *in vivo* with a depth and granularity previously unimaginable.[36,37] These developments are particularly important within the context of competency-based education (CBE) in which workplace-based assessments serve as a cornerstone for judging authentic performance over time. As CBE emphasizes longitudinal, criterion-based progression toward independence, high-quality workplace-based data will be essential for making defensible advancement decisions and ensuring learners are prepared for unsupervised practice. The future of reasoning assessment must therefore be tightly aligned with CBE principles, enabling more accurate, context-rich judgments of competence.

References

1. Torre D, Durning SJ, Rencic J, Lang V, Holmboe E, Daniel M. Widening the lens on teaching and assessing clinical reasoning: from "in the head" to "out in the world." *Diagn Berl Ger.* 2020;7(3):181-190. doi:10.1515/dx-2019-0098

2. Durning S, Artino AR, Pangaro L, van der Vleuten CPM, Schuwirth L. Context and clinical reasoning: understanding the perspective of the expert's voice. *Med Educ.* 2011;45(9):927-938. doi:10.1111/j.1365-2923.2011.04053.x

3. McBee E, Ratcliffe T, Picho K, et al. Consequences of contextual factors on clinical reasoning in resident physicians. *Adv Health Sci Educ Theory Pract.* 2015;20(5):1225-1236. doi:10.1007/s10459-015-9597-x

4. Daniel M, Rencic J, Durning SJ, et al. Clinical Reasoning Assessment Methods: A Scoping Review and Practical Guidance. *Acad Med.* 2019;94(6):902-912. doi:10.1097/ACM.0000000000002618

5. Guth TA, Wolfe RM, Martinez O, et al. Assessment of Clinical Reasoning in Undergraduate Medical Education: A Pragmatic Approach to Programmatic Assessment. *Acad Med.* 2024;99(8):912. doi:10.1097/ACM.0000000000005665

6. Parsons AS, Wijesekera TP, Olson APJ, Torre D, Durning SJ, Daniel M. Beyond thinking fast and slow: Implications of a transtheoretical model of clinical reasoning and error on teaching, assessment, and research. *Med Teach.* Published online June 5, 2024:1-12. doi:10.1080/0142159X.2024.2359963

7. Kassirer JP. Teaching clinical medicine by iterative hypothesis testing. Let's preach what we practice. *N Engl J Med.* 1983;309(15):921-923. doi:10.1056/NEJM198310133091511

8. Developing Clinical Problem-Solving Skills: A Guide to More Effective Diagnosis and Treatment. *Ann Intern Med.* 1992;116(7):607-607. doi:10.7326/0003-4819-116-7-607_2

9. Cydulka RK, Emerman CL, Jouriles NJ. Evaluation of Resident Performance and Intensive Bedside Teaching during Direct Observation. *Acad Emerg Med.* 1996;3(4):345-351. doi:10.1111/j.1553-2712.1996.tb03448.x

10. Konopasky A, Artino AR, Battista A, et al. Understanding context specificity: the effect of contextual factors on clinical reasoning. *Diagnosis.* 2020;7(3):257-264. doi:10.1515/dx-2020-0016

11. Daniel M, Durning SJ, Wilson E, Abdoler E, Torre D. Situated cognition: clinical reasoning and error are context dependent. *Diagnosis.* 2020;7(3):341-342. doi:10.1515/dx-2020-0011

12. Croskerry P. Context Is Everything or How Could I Have Been That Stupid? *Healthc Q Tor Ont.* 2009;12 Spec No Patient:e171-6. doi:10.12927/hcq.2009.20945

13. Committee on Diagnostic Error in Health Care, Board on Health Care Services, Institute of Medicine, The National Academies of Sciences, Engineering, and Medicine. *Improving Diagnosis in Health Care.* (Balogh EP, Miller BT, Ball JR, eds.). National Academies Press (US); 2015. Accessed October 1, 2020. http://www.ncbi.nlm.nih.gov/books/NBK338596/

14. *Practical Guide to the Assessment of Clinical Competence.*; 2023. Accessed January 31, 2025. https://shop.elsevier.com/books/practical-guide-to-the-assessment-of-clinical-competence/holmboe/978-0-443-11226-3

15. Charlin B, Roy L, Brailovsky C, Goulet F, van der Vleuten C. The Script Concordance test: a tool to assess the reflective clinician. *Teach Learn Med.* 2000;12(4):189-195. doi:10.1207/S15328015TLM1204_5

16. Meterissian SH. A novel method of assessing clinical reasoning in surgical residents. *Surg Innov.* 2006;13(2):115-119. doi:10.1177/1553350606291042

17. Kania RE, Verillaud B, Tran H, et al. Online script concordance test for clinical reasoning assessment in otorhinolaryngology: the association between performance and clinical experience. *Arch Otolaryngol Head Neck Surg.* 2011;137(8):751-755. doi:10.1001/archoto.2011.106

18. Sibert L, Darmoni SJ, Dahamna B, Hellot MF, Weber J, Charlin B. On line clinical reasoning assessment with Script Concordance test in urology: results of a French pilot study. *BMC Med Educ.* 2006;6:45. doi:10.1186/1472-6920-6-45

19. Park AJ, Barber MD, Bent AE, et al. Assessment of intraoperative judgment during gynecologic surgery using the Script Concordance Test. *Am J Obstet Gynecol.* 2010;203(3):240.e1-6. doi:10.1016/j.ajog.2010.04.010

20. Ducos G, Lejus C, Sztark F, et al. The Script Concordance Test in anesthesiology: Validation of a new tool for assessing clinical reasoning. *Anaesth Crit Care Pain Med.* 2015;34(1):11-15. doi:10.1016/j.accpm.2014.11.001

21. Omega A, Wijaya Ramlan AA, Soenarto RF, Heriwardito A, Sugiarto A. Assessing clinical reasoning in airway related cases among anesthesiology fellow residents using Script Concordance Test (SCT). *Med Educ Online.* 2022;27(1):2135421. doi:10.1080/10872981.2022.2135421

22. Humbert AJ, Besinger B, Miech EJ. Assessing clinical reasoning skills in scenarios of uncertainty: convergent validity for a Script Concordance Test in an emergency medicine clerkship and residency. *Acad Emerg Med Off J Soc Acad Emerg Med.* 2011;18(6):627-634. doi:10.1111/j.1553-2712.2011.01084.x

23. Lambert C, Gagnon R, Nguyen D, Charlin B. The script concordance test in radiation oncology: validation study of a new tool to assess clinical reasoning. *Radiat Oncol.* 2009;4(1):7. doi:10.1186/1748-717X-4-7

24. Ottolini MC, Chua I, Campbell J, Ottolini M, Goldman E. Pediatric Hospitalists' Performance and Perceptions of Script Concordance Testing for Self-Assessment. *Acad Pediatr.* 2021;21(2):252-258. doi:10.1016/j.acap.2020.10.003

25. Gawad N, Wood TJ, Cowley L, Raiche I. How do cognitive processes influence script concordance test responses? *Med Educ.* 2021;55(3):354-364. doi:10.1111/medu.14416

26. Dory V, Gagnon R, Vanpee D, Charlin B. How to construct and implement script concordance tests: insights from a systematic review. *Med Educ.* 2012;46(6):552-563. doi:10.1111/j.1365-2923.2011.04211.x

27. Durning SJ, Artino A, Boulet J, et al. The feasibility, reliability, and validity of a post-encounter form for evaluating clinical reasoning. *Med Teach.* 2012;34(1):30-37. doi:10.3109/0142159X.2011.590557

28. Park WB, Kang SH, Lee YS, Myung SJ. Does Objective Structured Clinical Examinations Score Reflect the Clinical Reasoning Ability of Medical Students? *Am J Med Sci.* 2015;350(1):64-67. doi:10.1097/MAJ.0000000000000420

29. Lafleur A, Côté L, Leppink J. Influences of OSCE design on students' diagnostic reasoning. *Med Educ.* 2015;49(2):203-214. doi:10.1111/medu.12635

30. Jay R, Sandars J, Patel R, et al. The Use of Virtual Patients to Provide Feedback on Clinical Reasoning: A Systematic Review. *Acad Med.* 2025;100(2):229. doi:10.1097/ACM.0000000000005908

31. Kassutto SM, Baston C, Clancy C. Virtual, Augmented, and Alternate Reality in Medical Education: Socially Distanced but Fully Immersed. *Sch.* 2021;2(4):651-664. doi:10.34197/ats-scholar.2021-0002RE

32. Elendu C, Amaechi DC, Okatta AU, et al. The impact of simulation-based training in medical education: A review. *Medicine (Baltimore).* 2024;103(27):e38813. doi:10.1097/MD.0000000000038813

33. White CB, Ross PT, Gruppen LD. Remediating Students' Failed OSCE Performances at One School: The Effects of Self-Assessment, Reflection, and Feedback. *Acad Med.* 2009;84(5):651. doi:10.1097/ACM.0b013e31819fb9de

34. Govaerts MJB, Schuwirth LWT, Van der Vleuten CPM, Muijtjens AMM. Workplace-based assessment: effects of rater expertise. *Adv Health Sci Educ Theory Pract.* 2011;16(2):151-165. doi:10.1007/s10459-010-9250-7

35. Miller GE. The assessment of clinical skills/competence/performance. *Acad Med.* 1990;65(9):S63.

36. Rencic J, Schuwirth LWT, Gruppen LD, Durning SJ. A situated cognition model for clinical reasoning performance assessment: a narrative review. *Diagn Berl Ger.* 2020;7(3):227-240. doi:10.1515/dx-2019-0106

37. Boyle JG, Walters MR, Jamieson S, Durning SJ. Distributed cognition: Theoretical insights and practical applications to health professions education: AMEE Guide No. 159. *Med Teach.* Published online April 12, 2023:1-11. doi:10.1080/0142159X.2023.2190479

CHAPTER 6

Using a Coaching Approach

CASE

Dr. Jones is a general surgery intern. In medical school, he was noted to be very bright, though he did not speak up much. His presentations often trailed off, with supervising residents interrupting or taking over the discussion of his assessment and plan. Evaluators warned that he would need to increase his confidence level if he wanted to become a surgeon. During the first months of residency, Dr. Jones covered many patients in the surgical ICU. He was diligent in reading his patients' charts and accessed multiple resources to understand each surgical procedure and the underlying pathophysiology. On rounds, however, he remained quiet while others talked over him and proposed diagnostic and management plans for his patients. During feedback sessions, supervisors encouraged him to speak up more often and take greater ownership of his patients. It subsequently became clear that Dr. Jones struggles to generate a differential diagnosis for common postoperative complications and create care plans independently. He is referred for clinical reasoning coaching by his program's clinical competency committee.

DEFINING THE ROLE OF COACH

Distinct from more traditional educational methods such as mentoring, advising, and teaching, coaching has emerged as a transformative approach in medical education.[1,2] Borrowed from other fields, coaching is rooted in the principle of guided discovery in which the focus is on fostering learners' self-awareness and insight through active inquiry rather than direct instruction.[3]

The roles of mentor, advisor, and teacher are well established. However, these terms are commonly used interchangeably and imprecisely. Mentors are experts who share their knowledge and experiences to guide learners in specific domains, often within a hierarchical relationship.[4] Advisors provide oversight and direction, often around a specific goal (e.g., helping learners navigate academic requirements and career pathways).[5] Teachers, on the other hand, focus on imparting knowledge and assessing learners' performance in structured settings. While there is overlap, these roles are broadly characterized by the following verbs, respectively: shows, tells, and explains.[6]

In contrast, coaching is non-hierarchical and emphasizes the learner's agency.[3] Coaches are skilled facilitators who help learners reflect on their strengths, identify growth areas, and develop actionable plans to achieve self-defined or co-created (learner and coach) goals. This process is inherently collaborative and relies on creating a supportive environment in which learners can evaluate their performance without fear of judgment. While mentors and advisors may offer solutions or specific guidance, coaches empower learners to explore their own motivations and reasoning processes and generate solutions tailored to their individual needs. This shift from directive guidance to facilitation of insight makes coaching uniquely suited to address the nuanced challenges of remediating clinical reasoning deficits.

The role of coach in a remediation setting is unique in that the goals of coaching are often externally determined (e.g., by the learner's program, in the case of a remediation plan).[7] However, in all other respects, the approach for which we advocate in this book aligns with traditional coaching in that it is a developmental process that aims to foster insight and a growth mindset as the coach works with the learner to identify strategies to manage their existing challenges. In our program, coaches do not play a role in formal or summative assessment of the struggling learner and do not inform the outcomes of remediation. This creates a supportive space in which the learner can develop.

As discussed in chapters 3 and 4, clinical reasoning involves the synthesis of complex information, integration of knowledge, and application of knowledge to patient care. Struggling learners frequently exhibit difficulties with metacognitive abilities such as self-monitoring and reflection that limit their ability to reason in dynamic and uncertain clinical environments. Coaching directly addresses these deficits by promoting three key areas: insight and metacognition, self-regulated learning, and deliberate practice.

DEVELOPMENT OF LEARNER INSIGHT AND METACOGNITION

Insight, when considered in medical education, refers to a learner's ability to accurately perceive their own strengths and weaknesses as well as the implications of their decisions in clinical and educational contexts.[8] Insight into one's own cognitive processes is a foundational step in addressing clinical reasoning deficits. Coaching facilitates the development of insight by encouraging learners to engage in structured reflection on their thought processes and subsequent actions.[9,10] In subsequent chapters specific frameworks are provided for structured reflection on clinical reasoning. As discussed in chapter 1, insight is a valuable prognostic marker for remediation success. Coaches can often predict the trajectory of remediation efforts based on the learner's level of insight. A learner who demonstrates early signs of self-awareness and reflective capacity is more likely to respond positively to coaching.[3,11]

Effective coaching emphasizes open-ended, reflective questions that begin with "how" or "what."[12] These types of questions guide learners to think critically about their thought processes and consider alternatives. For example, instead of prescribing solutions, a coach might ask questions like this: What strategies have you considered to address this challenge? How did you decide on this differential diagnosis? These questions encourage the learner to articulate their reasoning, recognize gaps or biases, and develop strategies to address them. Over time, this reflective practice enhances the learner's ability to self-assess and adapt and builds the metacognition to support independent and effective clinical reasoning. By emphasizing "how" and "what" questions, the coach encourages a dialogue that is collaborative and growth-oriented, thus empowering the learner to take ownership and internalize the habit of analyzing their thought processes and actions independently.[13]

Insight is closely linked to motivation, which similarly informs learner performance and receptivity to coaching.[14] Many struggling learners begin the coaching process with a fixed mindset, or performance orientation, characterized by the beliefs that mistakes are a sign of failure and competence is intrinsic and/or relatively static.[9,15] These learners may be distrustful of authority figures and tend to be easily discouraged, exclusively seeking out reinforcing feedback. In contrast, learners who adopt a mastery orientation are intrinsically driven to learn and believe that competence grows gradually through effort and practice. These observations can be viewed through the lens of self-determination theory which asserts that human beings possess three innate psychological needs: competence, autonomy, and relatedness.[16] When these needs are met, humans experience a natural inclination toward self-motivation and curiosity. Conversely, in unsupportive conditions, these characteristics are subject to disruption.

Thus, coaching the struggling learner who lacks insight or appears indifferent should prioritize interpersonal connection and learner agency. Effective coaching begins from a perspective of curiosity about the learner's underlying beliefs and fears. Together, coach and learner seek to uncover and remove barriers to learner insight and motivation. Over time, they work as a team to reframe learner perceptions around success and failure, with the coach supporting the learner in their efforts to actively seek out challenges and begin to direct their own learning process.

PROMOTION OF SELF-REGULATED LEARNING (SRL)

SRL has been defined as "self-generated thoughts, feelings, and actions that are planned and cyclically adapted to attain a learner's personal goals."[17] Gruppen and colleagues' multidimensional framework of SRL, which encompasses planning, performance, assessment, and adjustment (Figure 6.1), lends itself naturally to our coaching paradigm.[18] High-performing clinicians intuitively employ SRL strategies, but struggling learners often lack these skills. This results in inconsistent performance and difficulty adapting to new challenges. Coaching can explicitly target these deficiencies by guiding learners through the cyclical phases of SRL. Techniques such as SRL microanalysis are effective in identifying specific areas in which learners falter.[19] Microanalytic protocols use structured interviews composed of context-specific questions to address SRL subprocesses.[20,21] This approach is customizable to a specific task such as the targeted clinical reasoning assessment described in chapter 7 and includes goal setting and metacognitive monitoring.

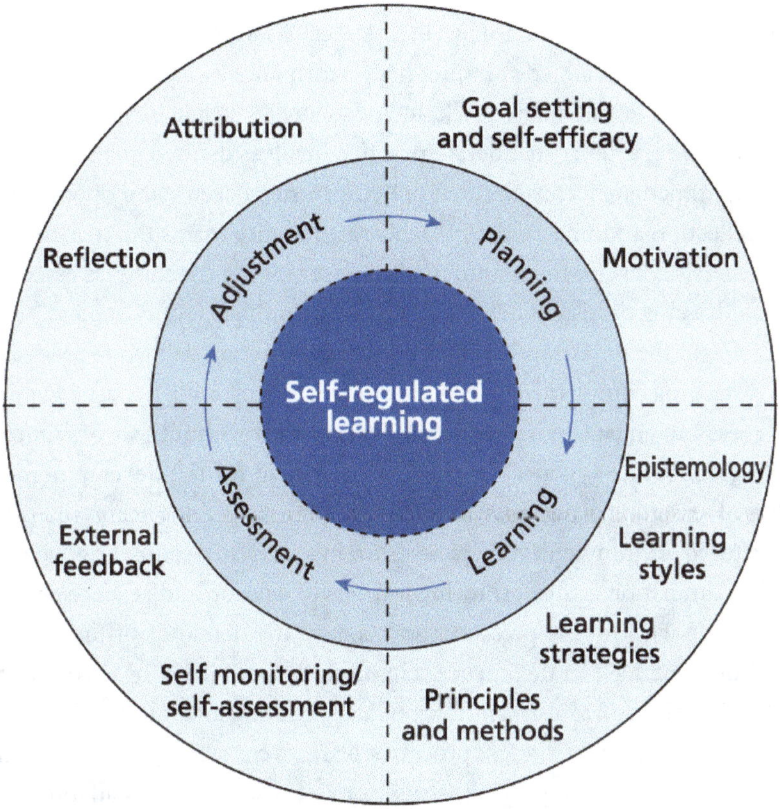

Figure 6.1. The Four Sequential Phases of SRL and Associated Subcomponents [18]

In the planning phase, learners set specific, measurable, and attainable goals, such as mastering a diagnostic algorithm. During the learning and assessment phases, they implement and monitor strategies, adjusting their approach as needed in real time. Finally, in the adjustment phase, learners reflect and refine their tactics for future tasks. The iterative nature of SRL aligns seamlessly with the goals of coaching as it allows learners to build confidence and competence through structured, goal-oriented practice. Coaches play a pivotal role in reinforcing these cycles, providing feedback and fostering a growth mindset.

APPLYING THE PRINCIPLES OF DELIBERATE PRACTICE to Coaching

Deliberate practice, as defined by Dr. K. Anders Ericsson, refers to a structured training approach aimed at improving performance by focusing on specific skills through repetition, feedback, and refinement.[22,23] Unlike routine practice or passive experience, deliberate practice involves defined goals, targeted effort, immediate feedback (even better if from a coach), and opportunity for reflection and fine-tuning.[24] Deliberate practice forms the cornerstone of expertise development and, in clinical reasoning coaching, is essential for addressing persistent deficits and building proficiency.[25] Chapters 7 and 8 highlight the importance of frameworks to structure deliberate practice.

Coaching complements deliberate practice by creating a space in which learners can engage in iterative skill development without fear of failure.[26] While deliberate practice "in context" is critical for the development of clinical reasoning proficiency, we recommend that coaching begins in a calm, structured environment. We typically start in a simulated setting (e.g., coach's office, simulation center), allowing learners to develop and practice clinical reasoning without the pressures and competing demands of the clinical environment. Deliberate practice reinforces metacognition by encouraging reflection and self-assessment. Through exploration and, ultimately, understanding of their own thought processes, learners can self-regulate and refine their decision-making.[27] Deliberate practice also promotes adaptability by providing the opportunity for learners to apply knowledge and skills encountered in one situation to other, related, situations. When the process is successful, learners develop the cognitive flexibility required to reliably put their skills to use in real-world contexts.[28] Chapters 7 to 15 present myriad applications of deliberate practice to clinical reasoning coaching in a variety of environments.

BUILDING THE RELATIONSHIP BETWEEN COACH AND LEARNER

Early meetings between coach and learner should occur one-on-one and focus on building the relationship. The first interaction sets the tone for trust, collaboration, and psychological safety—all of which are critical for learners to engage openly and productively.[29,30] Open body language, active listening, genuine curiosity, and a nonjudgmental tone signal respect for the learner's individuality and a shared commitment to their growth. The coach is encouraged to begin by delineating roles, emphasizing their own role as a partner in the learner's development rather than an evaluator, and setting expectations. Thereafter, the interaction becomes more of a discussion. We advocate for an inquiry-based approach in which the learner is encouraged to share their perspective and their goals. When they trust the relationship, learners are more likely to engage authentically, share vulnerabilities, and approach challenges with a growth mindset.[31]

GIVING FEEDBACK TO STRUGGLING LEARNERS

Medical education has witnessed a shift in the conceptualization of feedback from a one-way conversation—centered on comparing learner performance to a standard—to a collaborative, learner-centered process.[32,33] There are many accepted frameworks for structuring feedback in the moment.[34,35] Experts agree that setting the stage is critical.[36,37] According to our mentor, Dr. Jennifer Kogan, the learner must view the feedback as both credible and trustworthy, further highlighting the importance of relationship-building between coach and learner. Consistent with the fundamental principles of deliberate practice, feedback must be timely, occurring close in timing to the observed performance, and should take place in a private and quiet setting to promote reflection.

We like the ADAPT (Ask, Discuss, Ask, Plan Together) framework (Figure 6.2)[38] developed at the University of Washington; specific examples of its application are provided in Section 4. The coach begins by asking the learner to assess their own performance and identify areas for improvement. This gauges insight and promotes learner buy-in, respectively. Questions such as these are all reasonable places to begin: What are you working on? What isn't going as well as you had hoped? What would you do differently next time? The coach continues to ask probing questions, resisting the urge to interject their own observations and letting the learner do most of the talking. In the discuss phase, the coach reflects what they have heard and offers their observations, beginning with learner strengths and followed by suggested areas for improvement. Feedback should be specific and behavior-based.[39] It is important to avoid making judgments about a learner's character or intention. For example, rather than saying, "You are not paying attention to detail, and your presentations are sloppy. You should be more responsible when presenting cases," a more effective approach is: "I noticed, in your presentation just now, that you described the patient's symptoms but didn't mention the vital signs or the timeline of symptom progression. Including these details would help the team quickly grasp the severity of the case." The coach then clarifies learner understanding and asks for their thoughts on the feedback. "What are your thoughts on this? Is there anything that doesn't make sense?" Together, coach and learner then co-create an action plan with specific and actionable goals.

Learner Initiates	↓	**Coach Initiates**
• Reflect on learning goals • Communicate your goals	**PREPARE** FOR THE OBSERVATION	• Reflect on program & learner goals • Orient learner to expectations
• Try to be natural	**PERFORM** THE OBSERVATION	• Try to be neutral
• Reflect on the observation • ASK for feedback	**ASK** ⟷	• Reflect on learner's readiness • ASK for his/her thoughts about the observation
• Have a conversation about the observation	**DISCUSS** ⟷	• Coach observed, modifiable, specific behaviors related to the task(s)
•ASK for clarification	**ASK** ⟷	•ASK learner to clarify points, as necessary
• Plan next steps with your coach	**PLAN TOGETHER** ⟷	• Plan next steps with your learner

Developed at the University of Washington, UW Medicine, by Susan S. Johnston, EdD; Judith Pauwels, MD; Kristen Patton, MD; Tyra Fainstad, MD; Adelaide McClintock, MD.

Figure 6.2. The ADAPT Framework for Giving Feedback[38] *(Reprinted with permission from the authors.)*

More recently, Mills and colleagues have adapted the SPIKES model (commonly used in the clinical setting for breaking bad news to patients) for use in delivering feedback to the struggling learner (illustrated in Figure 6.3).[40]

Framework Component	Description in the Patient Care BBN Conversation Protocol	Recommendation for Use in BBN Conversations with Learners
Set-up	Gather all necessary information (e.g., test results) to inform the discussion. Identify a space and time for the conversation that will maximize patient comfort and privacy.	Prepare by considering as much as possible what information the learner may need to understand the situation, and what might help them feel most comfortable as they receive the news. Recognize these will vary across learners.
Perception	Elicit the patient's understanding of their condition and what it may mean for their future health.	Ask the learner for their perception of the assessment and their overall performance.
Invitation	Allow patients to share preferences around receiving the news, including the level of detail they'd like to know and who else to involve.	Though learners may have fewer options than patients (i.e., learners cannot defer all decision-making to the educator the way a patient could to a provider or surrogate), maximizing learners' ability to share their preferences for the conversation can advance learner autonomy.
Knowledge	Share the information in clear terms without jargon or euphemisms. Some experts recommend preceding the actual news with a 'warning shot' so patients feel more prepared.	Emphasize clarity of language. Currently cannot recommend for or against avoidance of euphemisms.
Emotion	Expect, make space for, and validate/respond to patients' emotions with empathy	Though learners may have fewer options than patients (i.e., learners cannot defer all decision-making to the educator the way a patient could to a provider or surrogate), maximizing learners' ability to share their preferences for the conversation can advance learner autonomy.
Summarize/ Strategize	Summarize the discussion, ideally in a way patients can reference later. Discuss next steps and work together to develop a plan. Indicate ongoing involvement and support for the patient.	Learners are often well-equipped to engage in shared decision-making on next steps.

Figure 6.3. SPIKES Protocol[40]

PROMOTING LEARNER RECEPTIVITY TO COACHING

In earlier chapters we have considered a variety of emotional and cognitive barriers to insight and engagement in coaching that can also be applied to accepting and actualizing feedback. Drawing from Stone and Heen's framework in *Thanks for the Feedback*,[41] three common triggers—truth, relationship, and identity—frequently obstruct learner receptivity to feedback.

Truth triggers arise when learners perceive feedback as inaccurate, irrelevant, or unfair. For instance, a learner might reject a coach's comment about their communication skills if they believe it doesn't align with their self-assessment or past experiences. Truth triggers can be mitigated when coaches focus on behavior-based observations and avoid making judgments when delivering feedback. If the learner does dispute the observation, the coach should approach the challenge with curiosity rather than confrontation. Questions such as these (remember "what" and "how" questions) create an open space for learners to reflect on the feedback's potential validity and identify actionable insights: What about this feedback feels inaccurate to you? How do you think this perception might have arisen?

Relationship triggers are tied to the credibility or trustworthiness of the feedback. A learner may resist feedback if they mistrust the coach's intentions, feel judged, or perceive a lack of understanding of their perspective. Similarly, the learner may discount the feedback if they do not respect the coach. Relationship triggers highlight the importance of building rapport between the feedback giver and the receiver. The coach should seek to understand and validate the learner's perspective even if they do not agree with it. Phrasing feedback as a collaborative observation rather than a directive can also help mitigate relationship triggers.

Finally, identity triggers show that feedback can challenge a learner's self-concept and evoke strong emotional reactions such as embarrassment, anger, or self-doubt. For example, a learner who takes pride in their organizational skills may react defensively to feedback suggesting they are disorganized, perceiving the assertion as a threat to their core identity. As discussed, coaches can address identity triggers by focusing on behaviors rather than generalizations and by leading with curiosity rather than judgment. Asking questions such as the following shifts the focus from personal inadequacy to professional development: What part of this feedback might be most helpful for your growth? How can you use this feedback to become even more effective? Additionally, coaches can normalize the discomfort of receiving constructive criticism, thus reassuring learners that growth often stems from feedback that is challenging.

DEVELOPING A CLINICAL REASONING REMEDIATION PROGRAM

Building on these principles, Table 6.1 outlines the components of a successful remediation program for struggling medical learners. In chapter 2 we underscore the importance of considering learner deficits in the biopsychosocial context in which they occur and describe our assessment process for struggling learners. Coaching plans should be individualized and, to the extent possible, co-created between learner and coach. We recognize that goals of coaching are often externally derived for struggling learners, as in the case of some formal remediation plans or programs. Even then, learners can still be involved in selection of coaches and observers as well as identification of opportunities for deliberate practice. Coaching itself consists of repeated cycles of deliberate practice of the deficient skill(s), in a variety of settings, under direct observation. As discussed, we typically begin in a simulated setting (e.g., the coach's office, a simulation center) where variables can be controlled and mistakes can be made without risk of harm to a patient. Eventually deliberate

Table 6.1. Elements of a Successful Remediation Program for Struggling Medical Learners

- Biopsychosocial assessment
- Individualized coaching plan
- Opportunities for direct observation + real-time feedback + time for reflection with a coach are emphasized
- Deliberate practice occurs across a variety of settings, with a variety of observers, under guidance from a coach
  - Simulated environment (e.g., coach's office, simulation center)
  - Clinical environment
- Clear boundary between coaching and programmatic assessment

practice moves to the clinical environment with the coach providing oversight for direct observation or, when possible, observing the learner themself. To guarantee the safe space for which we have advocated throughout this book, a firm boundary should be placed between the formative process of coaching and the summative process of programmatic assessment.

Figure 6.4 describes our clinical reasoning remediation program at the University of Virginia. This program supports graduate medical learners (e.g., residents [physicians and nonphysicians] and fellows).[42] We have also adapted this program structure for undergraduate medical learners.[43]

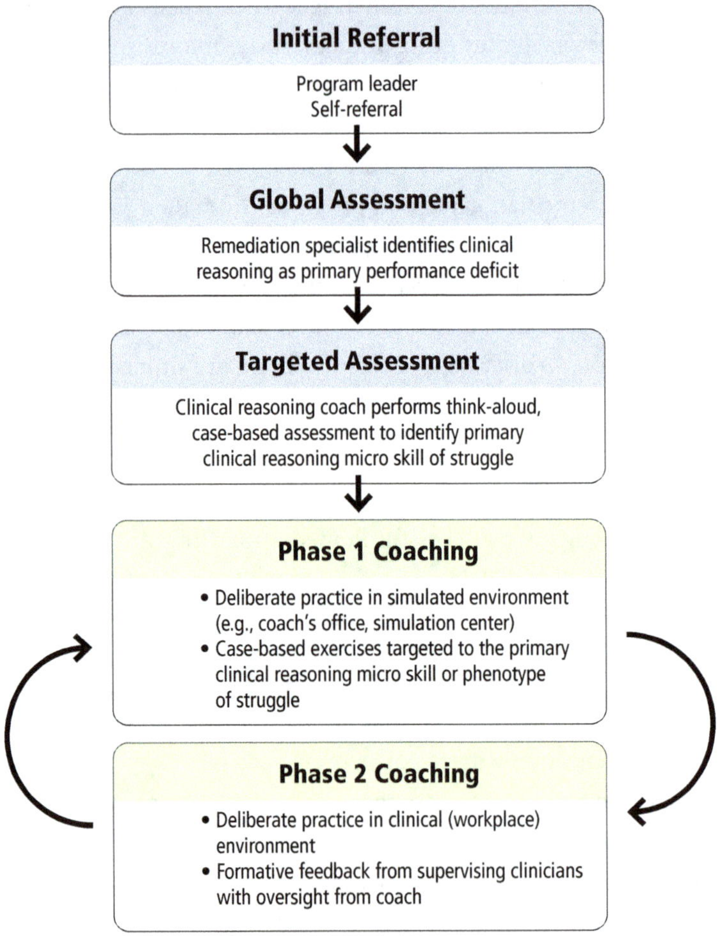

Figure 6.4. Example Clinical Reasoning Remediation Program (Adapted with permission from the *Journal of Graduate Medical Education.*)[42]

In our program, referred learners initially undergo a comprehensive, formative biopsychosocial assessment by a physician remediation expert (as described in chapter 2). Learners identified with a clinical reasoning deficiency are then referred to a physician clinical reasoning remediation coach who performs an additional targeted assessment to define the primary micro-skill deficit (detailed in chapters 7 and 8) and/or the relevant behavioral phenotype of struggle (described in chapters 9 to 15). Coaching is individualized and occurs in two additional phases. Phase 1 incorporates a case-based approach with deliberate practice targeted to the specific clinical reasoning deficit(s) in a simulated (nonworkplace) environment. Here, the coach can individualize and standardize variables in a low-stakes, low(er)-stress setting in which the learner should feel comfortable making mistakes and asking for help and in which the coach and learner can gain a deeper understanding of the learner's reasoning process. Alternatively, coaching can be targeted to the behavioral phenotype of struggle. Once a learner has repeatedly demonstrated competence in a one-on-one setting with the coach, we transition coaching to the clinical (workplace) environment. In Phase 2, which may extend over a period of months to years in some cases, direct observation is undertaken by the coach, when possible, or by clinical supervisors with oversight by the coach. Deliberate practice in the clinical environment is a critical aspect of clinical reasoning development, given the situated nature of cognition and the importance of context in clinical decision-making.[44,45] Learners must be assessed in the complex and dynamic environment in which they work; throughout the book we discuss strategies for performing direct observations in the workplace while being mindful of stigma and logistical constraints. Our hope is that this approach will facilitate earlier detection of, and intervention for, struggling learners and enhance teaching for all medical learners.

CASE, CONTINUED:

Dr. Jones undergoes global assessment which identifies clinical reasoning as the primary performance concern. Additional, targeted assessment and Phase 1 coaching focus on constructing differential diagnoses and formulating management plans. Dr. Jones has shown improvement in these skills and seems to be building consistency in the simulated environment. The coach now feels that it is time to transition Dr. Jones' coaching to the authentic clinical environment.

Transitioning struggling learners from the controlled environment of simulation to the clinical setting is a critical step in the coaching process that requires careful planning and structured implementation. The workplace introduces unique challenges that reflect the complexities of real-world practice. From the learner's perspective, the clinical environment is characterized by competing demands, unpredictability, and variable levels of supervision. These factors may hinder their ability to consistently enact newly acquired skills, which can be both disheartening and highly instructive. Additionally, as we will discuss, numerous barriers to direct observation often complicate this transition. Supervisors inevitably vary in their assessment approaches and skill level. Stigma around remediation may impact the learner's confidence and/or willingness to engage in continued coaching. From the perspective of the clinical supervisor, finding time for coaching amidst clinical responsibilities can be difficult. Acknowledging these challenges and integrating targeted strategies to overcome them are essential for a successful transition.

CLINICAL REASONING COACHING IN THE WORKPLACE ENVIRONMENT

A well-executed transition plan is characterized by clearly defined communication, ongoing direct observation and feedback, independent review of progress, and availability of resources (Table 6.2).

Table 6.2. Requirements for Successful Transition of Coaching from Simulated to Workplace Environment

1. **Well-defined communication between constituents**
2. **Ongoing direct observation and feedback**
3. **Independent review of progress**
4. **Continued availability of coaching resources**

WELL-DEFINED COMMUNICATION

Clear communication between constituents is critical for successful remediation. When possible, the learner should participate in, or at least be aware of, all discussions about their progress, thus ensuring transparency and alignment among all parties involved. Figure 6.5 illustrates the relationships between key team members—learner, coach, institutional or program leadership, and supervising clinicians—emphasizing the importance of coordination.

Though the specifics will depend on learner level and programmatic policy, we advocate for some form of handoff prior to the transfer of coaching activities to the clinical environment. The handoff might highlight coaching areas of focus, opportunities for continued development, and a structured plan for integrating coaching into clinical practice. In our program, the coach and clinical supervisors continue to communicate (with learner permission)

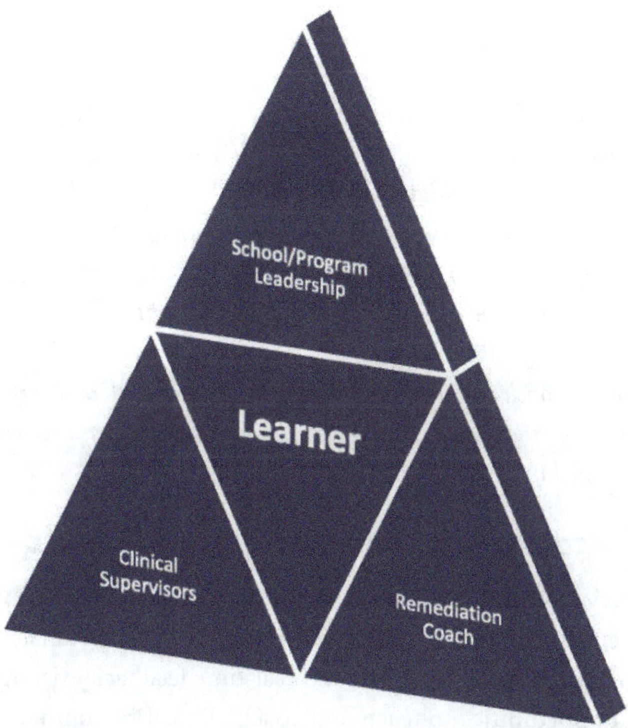

Figure 6.5. Relationship Between Constituents in Coaching Efforts

with the coach providing guidance around direct observation, feedback, and coaching exercises and with the clinical supervisors updating the coach about the learner's progress. Over time, the coach works to empower the learner to lead this communication. Ideally, the learner gains comfort in "feeding forward" their own goals and objectives as they approach a new rotation, leading the encounter with a new clinical supervisor with a statement such as, "I am working on developing clear and concise problem representations with my patients and would like your feedback on how I am doing. Can we touch base after rounds tomorrow so that I can get your thoughts on my presentations?"

As we have discussed, the school or program leadership should not be privy to details regarding learner performance in coaching exercises and should rely on standardized programmatic evaluations to make decisions about summative performance. Thus, we restrict communication between coaches and leadership to reflections on the learner's engagement in the process.

CASE, CONTINUED:

Dr. Jones trusts his coach and has embraced the importance of a team effort in his coaching plan. He still struggles with assertiveness on rounds and admits that he is intimidated by many of his supervisors. He has agreed to let the coach speak with one of the younger attending physicians in his department with whom he feels comfortable. This attending has agreed to coach Dr. Jones in the clinical environment as he continues to work on his clinical reasoning skills. With Dr. Jones' permission and, when possible, in his presence, the coach and faculty member continue to touch base on a regular basis to ensure that Dr. Jones is making progress and efforts are synergistic between coaching and workplace environment.

ONGOING DIRECT OBSERVATION AND FEEDBACK

Direct observation and real-time feedback are critical as learners work to improve their reasoning in the clinical environment.[46–49] Unfortunately, many barriers to both direct observation and real-time feedback exist, resulting in missed opportunities to teach and coach clinical reasoning. Clinical environments are fast-paced, and supervisors often juggle multiple roles.

The responsibility of clinical reasoning assessment is often inadvertently delegated to peers or near-peers without attending oversight. Instead of watching how learners make decisions, faculty often assess the outcome of these decisions (e.g., diagnosis, management plan). Finally, many faculty feel unprepared or uncomfortable evaluating and critiquing a learner's clinical reasoning in real time, especially if they lack formal training or are unaware of tools and frameworks for structuring these activities.[50] To overcome these challenges, we encourage widespread faculty development focused on the delivery of feedback, taking advantage of the frameworks discussed earlier in this chapter. We also advocate for time being carved out on a regular basis (e.g., daily, weekly) for the delivery of clear, specific, and actionable feedback for all learners. Throughout the remaining chapters of this book, we offer guidance on structured direct observation and feedback.

The unfortunate reality is that even with faculty development, finding time and space to coach in the clinical environment is challenging. An additional early hurdle involves the ability to communicate the learner's needs to the next supervisor. Given the stigma associated with remediation, there can be reluctance for this information to be fed forward.[51] There is also very real concern that this knowledge will bias future assessments. To address these issues, the coach may continue to meet with the learner outside of clinical duties. Given the asynchronous nature of clinical encounters and coaching, some creativity is required. Examples that illustrate this often-complex navigation between environments follow:

- Ask the learner to document 5 to 10 patient chief concerns and the differential diagnosis they formed for each concern. This list can be sent to the coach in advance and reviewed at an upcoming meeting.
- Ask the learner to de-identify a new patient evaluation which can be presented to the coach later if presentation organization and communication skills need development. Such presentations can occur in a meeting or in recorded format. Alternatively, a written note could be sent to the coach for feedback.
- Join the learner to directly observe patient encounters in the flow of their usual work. This approach gives higher fidelity translation to direct patient care; however, feasibility may be limited by concerns about stigma and learner privacy.

INDEPENDENT REVIEW OF PROGRESS

A clear separation between coaching and evaluation is essential to maintain the integrity of the remediation process. While the coach facilitates growth, institutional or program leadership and supervising clinicians should independently evaluate the learner's progress in the clinical environment. In our program, coaches do not participate in summative assessment of the struggling learner. In graduate medical education, standardized evaluations by peers and attending clinicians are the primary method of ongoing assessment. In theory, these tools provide organic, real-time insights into performance during patient care. In practice, as we have discussed, consistency and reliability may be negatively impacted by lack of faculty expertise in assessment and/or inadequate direct observation—which underscores the need for faculty development in these areas. It is critical that leaders employ a broad array of assessment modalities. Examples include OSCEs, oral exams, or written tests that target specific deficits and offer structured evaluation opportunities.[52] Because they may not fully capture performance in authentic clinical settings, these methods of assessment should supplement, rather than replace, workplace-based evaluations.[53,54] Assessment of clinical reasoning is discussed in more detail in chapter 5.

CASE, CONTINUED:

With permission, Dr. Jones' coach has provided guidance to the supervising attending around structuring direct observation and feedback of relevant diagnostic and management reasoning skills. Over the next few months, Dr. Jones receives formative feedback from his supervising attending, who notes improvement in diagnostic reasoning but identifies persistent gaps in management plan detail. Weekly coaching sessions reinforce these observations, helping Dr. Jones set actionable goals and informing the coaching process. Following another period of continued coaching, a summative programmatic evaluation indicates progress consistent with his training level, reflecting the efficacy of the targeted coaching intervention.

CONTINUED AVAILABILITY OF COACHING RESOURCES

Ongoing access to coaching resources is critical to support learners as they are coached in the clinical environment. Coaching may occur asynchronously to accommodate the demands of clinical schedules. In some cases, a dedicated coaching rotation, pairing the learner with a coach in a structured clinical setting, may be warranted (Table 6.3). While sometimes logistically challenging, this approach allows for high-fidelity coaching and evaluation and fosters skill integration in real-world contexts.

Table 6.3. Ten Recommendations for a Structured Clinical Reasoning Coaching Rotation

	Recommendation	Example
1	Define specific objectives and goals	Focus on improving hypothesis generation or diagnostic refinement as defined by competency thresholds Improve ability to triage tasks in the busy clinical environment
2	Partner coach and clinical supervisor (i.e., attending)	Ensure the remediation coach collaborates closely with the clinical supervisor to align feedback and support
3	Emphasize direct observation	Observe the learner during patient rounds and use structured tools like mini-CEX
4	Tailor the clinical environment	Place a pediatric resident in a pediatric clinical setting with appropriate case complexity Reduce patient census
5	Provide frequent feedback and reflection opportunities	Hold daily debriefing sessions to review clinical encounters and decision-making
6	Separate coaching rotation evaluation from summative assessment (when possible)	Have a different faculty member assess the learner's progress post-rotation
7	Use blended assessment strategies	Combine direct observation, case discussions, and OSCEs for a comprehensive evaluation
8	Foster psychological safety	Normalize struggles and emphasize growth as part of the professional journey
9	Continuously improve the rotation	Collect feedback from coaches and learners to refine rotation logistics and content
10	Carry the individualized coaching plan through to the clinical environment	Encourage the learner to practice coaching exercises on upcoming rotations

STRATEGIES FOR SUCCESSFUL COACHING TRANSITION TO THE AUTHENTIC CLINICAL ENVIRONMENT

To overcome the barriers discussed in this chapter, we offer the following strategies for ensuring a successful transition from the simulated environment to the workplace environment:

- Cultivating a Growth-Oriented Culture: Normalize remediation as part of professional development to reduce stigma. Leaders should champion a culture that values feedback and continuous growth by sharing success stories and promoting transparency.
- Strategic Supervisor Assignments: Pair learners with supervisors known for high-quality evaluations and a commitment to education. These supervisors are more likely to create an environment of trust and mutual respect in which learners feel supported in addressing their challenges.
- Blended Assessment Strategies: Combine clinical evaluations with standardized assessments to capture a holistic view of learner progress. Clinical evaluations allow supervisors to observe real-world application of skills, while standardized assessments such as simulation-based scenarios or OSCEs provide a controlled environment to assess clinical reasoning.
- Enhanced Resource Allocation: Addressing time constraints and improving access to coaching tools requires innovative solutions. We recommend translating lessons learned from clinical reasoning coaching to clinical supervisors through faculty development efforts.

THE PITCHFORK EFFECT

Effectively the converse of the halo effect discussed in chapter 1, the pitchfork effect refers to a cognitive bias in which a single negative trait or mistake disproportionately influences overall judgment. Struggling learners are exquisitely sensitive to the idea that, once labeled as "struggling," all aspects of their performance will be viewed more critically and result in lower marks. If a learner perceives that they are perpetually "under the microscope," they may demonstrate less willingness to ask for help, think aloud, or engage in coaching efforts out of fear that doing so will reinforce the image that they are struggling. In some cases, the pitchfork effect can create a self-fulfilling prophecy in which learners are more prone to errors related to second-guessing or overly conservative decision-making. Mitigation strategies include framing remediation as skill-building, not punishment, and normalizing the process of coaching using all the principles outlined in this chapter. Acknowledging the very real existence of the pitchfork effect can be quite validating for struggling learners.

CASE, CONTINUED:

Dr. Jones' evaluations from supervising clinicians and peers continue to demonstrate that he is meeting competency standards. The program director, informed by input from standardized programmatic evaluations, determines that Dr. Jones has successfully met the goals of his remediation plan.

ASSESSMENT OF REMEDIATION SUCCESS

Assessing the overall success of remediation is often more challenging than it initially appears. While in a pure coaching relationship, goals of coaching are ideally co-created by the coach and learner, goals for the learner on formal remediation are typically externally derived. As previously discussed, the leader or committee tasked with assessing the overall success of remediation should maintain separation from the coaching process to avoid conflicts of interest. Decisions about advancement, competency, and/or further deployment of remediation resources should be made solely based on standardized programmatic evaluations.

Possible outcomes of remediation include:

- Improvement of deficits, achievement of competency threshold or progression at expected level of performance, thus signaling an end to the remedial period
- Insufficient improvement and progression requiring continuation of remediation efforts or dismissal from the program

As discussed in chapter 1, the policies and practices around formal remediation vary between programs and institutions, and a detailed discussion of remediation outcomes is beyond the scope of this book. It is critical that educators adhere to their own internal policies, document religiously, and consult legal counsel early and often in the process. While not all learners are remediable, with appropriate deployment of resources most struggling learners can be helped if programs adhere to the principles of coaching outlined in this and subsequent chapters.

References

1. Deiorio NM, Carney PA, Kahl LE, Bonura EM, Juve AM. Coaching: a new model for academic and career achievement. *Med Educ Online.* 2016;21. doi:10.3402/meo.v21.33480
2. Deiorio NM, Foster KW, Santen SA. Coaching a Learner in Medical Education. *Acad Med.* 2021;96(12):1758. doi:10.1097/ACM.0000000000004168
3. Association AM. *Coaching in Medical Education : A Faculty Handbook.* American Medical Assn.; 2017.
4. Ramani S, Kusurkar RA, Lyon-Maris J, et al. Mentorship in health professions education—an AMEE guide for mentors and mentees: AMEE Guide No. 167. *Med Teach.* 2024;46(8):999-1011. doi:10.1080/0142159X.2023.2273217
5. Wolff M, Deiorio NM, Miller Juve A, et al. Beyond advising and mentoring: Competencies for coaching in medical education. *Med Teach.* 2021;43(10):1210-1213. doi:10.1080/0142159X.2021.1947479
6. Marcdante K, Simpson D. Choosing When to Advise, Coach, or Mentor. *J Grad Med Educ.* 2018;10(2):227-228. doi:10.4300/JGME-D-18-00111.1
7. Love LM, Simonsen KA, Bowler C, Dallaghan GLB. Archetypes of Coaching Across the Medical Education Continuum. *Acad Med.* 2021;96(12):1757. doi:10.1097/ACM.0000000000004169
8. Ng IKS, Lin NHY, Goh WGW, Teo DB, Tan LF, Ban KHK. "Insight" in medical training: what, why, and how? *Postgrad Med J.* 2024;100(1181):196-202. doi:10.1093/postmj/qgad115
9. Bakke BM, Sheu L, Hauer KE. Fostering a Feedback Mindset: A Qualitative Exploration of Medical Students' Feedback Experiences With Longitudinal Coaches. *Acad Med.* 2020;95(7):1057. doi:10.1097/ACM.0000000000003012
10. Armson H, Lockyer JM, Zetkulic M, Könings KD, Sargeant J. Identifying coaching skills to improve feedback use in postgraduate medical education. *Med Educ.* 2019;53(5):477-493. doi:10.1111/medu.13818
11. Moos C, Spranz-Fogasy T. "Now once again this idea of yours (…) how does it sound when I say that?"—Changing the perspective: how coach's questioning practices elicit self-reflecting processes in clients. *Front Psychol.* 2024;15:1241489. doi:10.3389/fpsyg.2024.1241489
12. Batista E. How Great Coaches Ask, Listen, and Empathize. *Harv Bus Rev.* Published online February 18, 2015. Accessed February 9, 2025. https://hbr.org/2015/02/how-great-coaches-ask-listen-and-empathize
13. Deiorio NM, Wolff M, Miller Juve A, Moore M, Santen SA, Hammoud MM. The Development of a Set of Coaching Competencies for Medical Education Using a Modified Delphi Approach. *Acad Med.* 2021;96(11S):S181. doi:10.1097/ACM.0000000000004333
14. Sargeant J, Armson H, Chesluk B, et al. The Processes and Dimensions of Informed Self-Assessment: A Conceptual Model. *Acad Med.* 2010;85(7):1212. doi:10.1097/ACM.0b013e3181d85a4e

15. Dweck CS. *Mindset: The New Psychology of Success.* Random House; 2006:x, 276.

16. Ryan RM, Deci EL. Self-determination theory and the facilitation of intrinsic motivation, social development, and well-being. *Am Psychol.* 2000;55(1):68-78. doi:10.1037//0003-066x.55.1.68

17. Zimmerman BJ. Attaining self-regulation: A social cognitive perspective. In: *Handbook of Self-Regulation.* Academic Press; 2000:13-39. doi:10.1016/B978-012109890-2/50031-7

18. White CB, Gruppen LD, Fantone JC. Self-regulated learning in medical education. In: *Understanding Medical Education.* John Wiley & Sons, Ltd; 2013:201-211. doi:10.1002/9781118472361.ch15

19. Artino AR, Cleary TJ, Dong T, Hemmer PA, Durning SJ. Exploring clinical reasoning in novices: a self-regulated learning microanalytic assessment approach. *Med Educ.* 2014;48(3):280-291. doi:10.1111/medu.12303

20. Durning SJ, Cleary TJ, Sandars J, Hemmer P, Kokotailo P, Artino AR. Perspective: Viewing "Strugglers" Through a Different Lens: How a Self-Regulated Learning Perspective Can Help Medical Educators With Assessment and Remediation. *Acad Med.* 2011;86(4):488. doi:10.1097/ACM.0b013e31820dc384

21. Cleary TJ, Durning SJ, Artino ARJ. Microanalytic Assessment of Self-Regulated Learning During Clinical Reasoning Tasks: Recent Developments and Next Steps. *Acad Med.* 2016;91(11):1516-1521. doi:10.1097/ACM.0000000000001228

22. Ericsson KA. Deliberate Practice and the Acquisition and Maintenance of Expert Performance in Medicine and Related Domains. *Acad Med.* 2004;79(10):S70.

23. Ericsson KA, Prietula MJ, Cokely ET. The Making of an Expert. *Harv Bus Rev.* Published online July 1, 2007. Accessed March 7, 2023. https://hbr.org/2007/07/the-making-of-an-expert

24. Sauer CG, Newman LR, Leichtner AM. Training in Endoscopy: Coaching, Deliberate Practice, and Reflection. *J Pediatr Gastroenterol Nutr.* 2019;68(3):298-300. doi:10.1097/MPG.0000000000002231

25. Kassirer JP. Teaching Clinical Reasoning: Case-Based and Coached. *Acad Med.* 2010;85(7):1118. doi:10.1097/ACM.0b013e3181d5dd0d

26. Gifford KA, Fall LH. Doctor Coach: A Deliberate Practice Approach to Teaching and Learning Clinical Skills. *Acad Med.* 2014;89(2):272. doi:10.1097/ACM.0000000000000097

27. Merkebu J, Veen M, Hosseini S, Varpio L. The case for metacognitive reflection: a theory integrative review with implications for medical education. *Adv Health Sci Educ Theory Pract.* 2024;29(4):1481-1500. doi:10.1007/s10459-023-10310-2

28. Cho KK, Marjadi B, Langendyk V, Hu W. Medical student changes in self-regulated learning during the transition to the clinical environment. *BMC Med Educ.* 2017;17(1):59. doi:10.1186/s12909-017-0902-7

29. Johnson CE, Keating JL, Molloy EK. Psychological safety in feedback: What does it look like and how can educators work with learners to foster it? *Med Educ.* 2020;54(6):559-570. doi:10.1111/medu.14154

30. Theoretical Foundations of Learning Environments. Routledge & CRC Press. Accessed November 24, 2023. https://www.routledge.com/Theoretical-Foundations-of-Learning-Environments/Land-Jonassen/p/book/9780415894227

31. Memari M, Gavinski K, Norman MK. Beware False Growth Mindset: Building Growth Mindset in Medical Education Is Essential but Complicated. *Acad Med.* 2024;99(3):261. doi:10.1097/ACM.0000000000005448

32. Ramani S, Könings KD, Ginsburg S, van der Vleuten CPM. Meaningful feedback through a sociocultural lens. *Med Teach.* 2019;41(12):1342-1352. doi:10.1080/0142159X.2019.1656804

33. Ramani S, Könings KD, Ginsburg S, van der Vleuten CP. Feedback Redefined: Principles and Practice. *J Gen Intern Med.* 2019;34(5):744-749. doi:10.1007/s11606-019-04874-2

34. Kogan J. The Adapt Model for Feedback. ACGME Remediation Toolkit. Learn at ACGME. August 31, 2024. Accessed February 4, 2025. https://dl.acgme.org/courses/acgme-remediation-toolkit

35. Sargeant J, Lockyer J, Mann K, et al. Facilitated Reflective Performance Feedback: Developing an Evidence- and Theory-Based Model That Builds Relationship, Explores Reactions and Content, and Coaches for Performance Change (R2C2). *Acad Med.* 2015;90(12):1698. doi:10.1097/ACM.0000000000000809

36. Natesan S, Jordan J, Sheng A, et al. Feedback in Medical Education: An Evidence-based Guide to Best Practices from the Council of Residency Directors in Emergency Medicine. *West J Emerg Med.* 2023;24(3):479-494. doi:10.5811/westjem.56544

37. Lockyer J, Lee-Krueger R, Armson H, et al. Application of the R2C2 Model to In-the-Moment Feedback and Coaching. *Acad Med.* 2023;98(9):1062. doi:10.1097/ACM.0000000000005237

38. Prepare to ADAPT | UW Graduate Medical Education. Accessed February 9, 2025. https://sites.uw.edu/uwgme/adapt/

39. Larson EL, Patel SJ, Evans D, Saiman L. Feedback as a Strategy to Change Behavior: The Devil Is in the Details. *J Eval Clin Pract.* 2013;19(2):230-234. doi:10.1111/j.1365-2753.2011.01801.x

40. Mills LM, Cate OT, Boscardin C, O'Sullivan PS. Breaking Bad News to Learners: How Well Does the SPIKES Clinical Model Translate? *Perspect Med Educ.* 2024;13(1):684-692. doi:10.5334/pme.1521

41. Thanks for the Feedback by Douglas Stone, Sheila Heen: 9780143127130 | PenguinRandomHouse.com: Books. PenguinRandomhouse.com. Accessed February 9, 2025. https://www.penguinrandomhouse.com/books/313485/thanks-for-the-feedback-by-douglas-stone-and-sheila-heen/

42. Parsons AS, Dreicer JJ, Martindale JR, Young G, Warburton KM. A Targeted Clinical Reasoning Remediation Program for Residents and Fellows in Need. *J Grad Med Educ.* 2024;16(4):469. doi:10.4300/JGME-D-23-00822.1

43. Young G, Meyer J, Crane I, et al. A Longitudinal, Structured Clinical Remediation Program for Medical Students. *Acad Med.* 2023;98(11S):S191. doi:10.1097/ACM.0000000000005401

44. Daniel M, Durning SJ, Wilson E, Abdoler E, Torre D. Situated cognition: clinical reasoning and error are context dependent. *Diagnosis.* 2020;7(3):341-342. doi:10.1515/dx-2020-0011

45. Konopasky A, Artino AR, Battista A, et al. Understanding context specificity: the effect of contextual factors on clinical reasoning. *Diagnosis.* 2020;7(3):257-264. doi:10.1515/dx-2020-0016

46. Burgess A, van Diggele C, Roberts C, Mellis C. Feedback in the clinical setting. *BMC Med Educ.* 2020;20(2):460. doi:10.1186/s12909-020-02280-5

47. Veloski J, Boex JR, Grasberger MJ, Evans A, Wolfson DB. Systematic review of the literature on assessment, feedback and physicians' clinical performance: BEME Guide No. 7. *Med Teach.* 2006;28(2):117-128. doi:10.1080/01421590600622665

48. Lefroy J, Watling C, Teunissen PW, Brand P. Guidelines: the do's, don'ts and don't knows of feedback for clinical education. *Perspect Med Educ.* 2015;4(6):284-299. doi:10.1007/s40037-015-0231-7

49. Kogan JR, Hatala R, Hauer KE, Holmboe E. Guidelines: The do's, don'ts and don't knows of direct observation of clinical skills in medical education. *Perspect Med Educ.* 2017;6(5):286-305. doi:10.1007/s40037-017-0376-7

50. Audétat MC, Dory V, Nendaz M, et al. What is so difficult about managing clinical reasoning difficulties? *Med Educ.* 2012;46(2):216-227. doi:10.1111/j.1365-2923.2011.04151.x

51. Castanelli DJ, Molloy E, Bearman M. The stigma of underperformance in assessment and remediation. *Adv Health Sci Educ Theory Pract.* Published online October 16, 2024. doi:10.1007/s10459-024-10382-8

52. Daniel M, Rencic J, Durning SJ, et al. Clinical Reasoning Assessment Methods: A Scoping Review and Practical Guidance. *Acad Med.* 2019;94(6):902-912. doi:10.1097/ACM.0000000000002618

53. Guth TA, Wolfe RM, Martinez O, et al. Assessment of Clinical Reasoning in Undergraduate Medical Education: A Pragmatic Approach to Programmatic Assessment. *Acad Med.* 2024;99(8):912. doi:10.1097/ACM.0000000000005665

54. Misra S, Iobst WF, Hauer KE, Holmboe ES. The Importance of Competency-Based Programmatic Assessment in Graduate Medical Education. *J Grad Med Educ.* 2021;13(2 Suppl):113-119. doi:10.4300/JGME-D-20-00856.1

Section 3

Cognitive Micro Skill Assessment and Targeted Coaching

In Section 3, we characterize clinical reasoning as a set of cognitive processes that we term micro skills. We outline our method of assessing and coaching the struggling learner using these micro skills along with context-focused prompts.

This case-based approach requires some expertise in the theoretical foundations of clinical reasoning but is easily teachable. As is true with all the coaching strategies presented in this book, coaching micro skills aligns with the principles of deliberate practice, occurring first in a one-on-one, non-workplace setting and, ultimately, in the authentic clinical environment.

CHAPTER 7

Micro Skill Assessment of Clinical Reasoning

DESPITE THEORETICAL ADVANCES in assessment methods, clinical reasoning deficits often remain subtle and difficult to detect. Learners may exhibit behaviors such as hesitancy to commit to a diagnosis, ambivalence in decision-making, or overconfidence despite overlooking key details. These issues require skilled assessors who can identify patterns of error and probe deeper to uncover the underlying cognitive processes. For example, a learner's reliance on irrelevant details during a patient presentation might signal struggles with problem representation, while a failure to adjust hypotheses after receiving new data could indicate difficulties with hypothesis refinement. In addition, most clinical reasoning assessment occurs subjectively as part of the direct clinical care experience—if it is explicitly evaluated at all. Failure to identify clinical reasoning deficits represents a lost opportunity for just-in-time, meaningful feedback to learners. Feedback is universally regarded by medical educators as a vital part of the learning process and is also a common area of perceived shortcoming. As discussed in chapter 4, feedback is most successful when it promotes self-regulated learning (SRL). Learners who employ metacognition and specific goal setting identify more accurate diagnoses in exercises designed to assess clinical reasoning.[1–3] It would follow that feedback that helps learners develop SRL could also lead to improved clinical reasoning. For educators to provide this sort of specific, meaningful feedback they must first be able to accurately, and in real-time, recognize clinical reasoning struggles in the clinical learning environment.

SELF-REGULATED LEARNING MICROANALYSIS

SRL microanalysis is a relatively new method of workplace-based clinical reasoning assessment that emphasizes learner centeredness. Here, learners are presented with a structured interview protocol designed to gather real-time, task-level information on their thoughts as they approach, perform, and reflect on an activity.[1,4] Questions are aligned with temporal phases of a task (e.g., before, during, after). Validity evidence supports the use of SRL microanalysis in the context of clinical reasoning remediation (Figure 7.1);[5–7] SRL microanalysis has greatly informed our work.

Phases of Cyclical Feedback Loop	Self-regulation Processes	SRL Micoranalytic Assessment Questions
Forethought (before)	Goal setting	"Do you have a goal(s) in mind as you prepare to do this activity?"[2,3]
	Strategic planning	"What do you think you need to do to perform well on this activity?"[2,3]
	Self-efficacy	"How confident are you that you can determine the most likely diagnosis for this patient on your first attempt?"[4]
Performance (during)	Metacognitive monitoring	"As you have been going through this process, what has been the primary thing that you have been thinking about or focusing on?"[2,3]
Self-reflection (after)	Self-evaluation	"In your opinion, what percentage of questions that you asked while conducting the patient history would an expert clinician say were essential questions for this case?"[9]

Figure 7.1. Phase-specific SRL Microanalytic Assessment Questions for Clinical Reasoning Tasks[7]

As described later in this chapter, our targeted clinical reasoning assessment process encourages learners to think aloud about the specifics of their reasoning related to a case. We ask questions related to goal setting, strategic planning, metacognitive monitoring, and self-evaluation. The aim is to capture in-the-moment insights into a learner's thinking and actions during clinical encounters. We know that learners with focused, strategic planning during such tasks tend to achieve better academic and clinical outcomes.[5,7,8] For example, medical students using strategies like prioritizing symptoms or comparing diagnoses outperformed peers who lacked such approaches.[1] Incorporating SRL microanalysis into our assessment process has allowed for effective assessment by the clinical reasoning coach while simultaneously promoting development of learner insight and self-assessment skills. A limitation inherent in this approach is the prominent role of context,[9,10] which we discuss in more detail below.

CLINICAL REASONING ASSESSMENT TO GUIDE COACHING

As introduced in chapters 3 and 4, clinical reasoning is a complex, multifaceted process that involves integrating knowledge, analyzing patient data, and making decisions that are responsive to evolving information. This intricate exercise encompasses numerous cognitive tasks such as recognizing patterns, prioritizing differential diagnoses, and managing uncertainty—all while adapting to clinical context. Despite its inherent complexity, clinical reasoning can be broken down into a set of discrete processes, each referred to as a micro skill. This is a simplification that, while not fully capturing the fluid and dynamic nature of real-world reasoning, provides a practical framework for coaching learners. In other words, given the challenges of assessing clinical reasoning holistically, breaking the process into discrete micro skills provides a structured and actionable approach for both assessment and coaching. These micro skills allow learners and educators to focus on specific aspects of reasoning that can be taught, assessed, deliberately practiced, and coached.

We have developed a unique remediation program that provides individualized assessment and coaching of clinical reasoning in phases.[11,12] Phase 1 refers to the global assessment introduced in chapter 2 which culminates in identification of the clinical performance deficit (e.g., clinical reasoning). For learners struggling with clinical reasoning, Phase 2 incorporates targeted, formative assessment to identify the deficient micro skill(s) and/or relevant behavioral phenotype of struggle. We share our targeted assessment tool below.

The micro skills approach is rooted in research on the reasoning strategies used by expert clinicians which highlights how experts efficiently organize and retrieve knowledge, recognize salient clinical features, and adapt their reasoning dynamically as cases unfold.[13] We have adapted the approach based on our experience working with struggling learners who often display fragmented reasoning or difficulty integrating new information. By breaking clinical reasoning into discrete micro skills, coaches can identify specific areas where learners falter, thus enabling targeted interventions that build the foundational components of sound clinical reasoning. This chapter and the next explicitly acknowledge how expert and novice reasoning differ and illustrate the value of focusing on individual micro skills, in context, to bridge these gaps.

WHICH MICRO SKILLS?

Bordage introduced an early taxonomy in his 1999 address, "*Why did I miss the diagnosis? Some cognitive explanations and educational implications.*"[14] He categorized diagnostic errors as data gathering, data integration, and situational factors, and stressed the roles of pattern recognition, analytical thinking, and problem representation in clinical reasoning. In a landmark paper published six years later, Graber and colleagues catalogued errors as system-related, no-fault, or cognitive.[15] The most common type, cognitive errors, was further subdivided into faulty knowledge, faulty data gathering, faulty information processing, and faulty verification. Norman and Eva built on this approach, viewing errors through the commonly described prism of knowledge, skills, and attitudes.[16] Though mentioned in some of these taxonomies, we credit Durning and colleagues with emphasizing the importance of contextual factors, including clinician factors, patient factors, and setting factors, in reasoning and error.[17]

In her seminal 2006 paper,[18] Bowen described clinical reasoning as an iterative cycle involving:

1. **Data gathering**: Collect clinical information guided by the clinician's initial hypotheses, beginning with the chief concern
2. **Problem representation**: Synthesize the data into a concise, accurate summary that captures the essence of the clinical problem

3. **Hypothesis generation**: Develop an initial differential diagnosis based on pattern recognition and analytical reasoning
4. **Additional data gathering**: Collect additional data to distinguish and/or discriminate among hypotheses

Throughout this iterative cycle, the clinician searches for an illness script that matches the patient's presentation while revising their initial differential diagnosis. Lacking robust illness scripts, novices may struggle to link clinical features to underlying pathophysiology or to revise their thinking in response to contradictory evidence.

In their widely read book *Learning Clinical Reasoning*, Kassirer, Wong, and Kopelman defined the process of clinical reasoning as follows: diagnostic hypothesis generation, refinement of diagnostic hypotheses, use and interpretation of diagnostic tests, assembling a working diagnosis, therapeutic decision-making, and examining and applying evidence as the processes of clinical reasoning.[19]

Audetat and colleagues studied clinical teachers in their authentic environment, constructing a model based on their understanding of clinical and educational reasoning processes.[20] The result was a taxonomy for learners that includes three components: (1) hypothesis generation and direction of data gathering, (2) refinement of hypotheses and hypothesis testing, and (3) final diagnosis or characterization of problem and development of a management plan. This classification system allowed the research group to uncover five categories of clinical reasoning difficulties among their learners (Figure 7.2).[21,22]

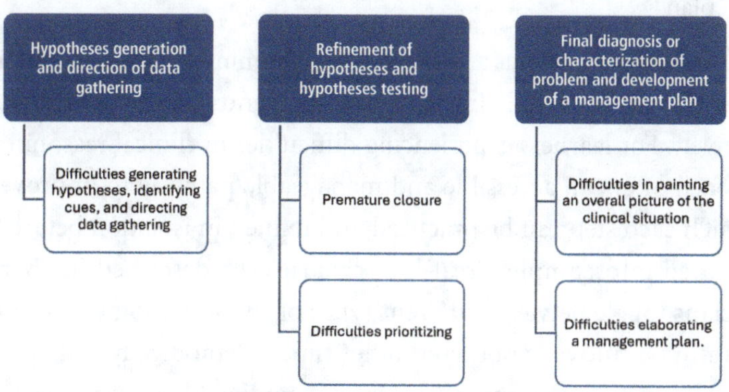

Figure 7.2. Three Discrete Clinical Reasoning Processes and Associated Areas of Learner Difficulty[21,22]

Weinstein and colleagues incorporated these five categories into a framework for case-based faculty development.[23] Faculty "diagnosed" learners as struggling most in one of the five domains, focusing on the root cause of difficulty before employing targeted remediation strategies. More specifically, breaking clinical reasoning into its core components (e.g., hypothesis generation, data gathering, problem representation, hypothesis refinement, and management) allowed educators to address distinct areas of learner difficulty.

Building on this previous work, we utilize the latest evidence-based understanding of the clinical reasoning process to inform an assessment framework that employs the following micro skills:

1. **Early Hypothesis Generation:** Formulating an initial differential diagnosis based on the initial chief concern and demographic information
2. **Hypothesis-Driven Data Gathering:** Collecting information that directly informs or challenges initial hypotheses
3. **Problem Representation:** Iteratively synthesizing data into a concise summary that captures the clinical essence of the case
4. **Hypothesis Refinement:** Narrowing and prioritizing the differential diagnosis in response to new findings
5. **Management Script Activation:** Drawing on illness-specific knowledge of relevant management strategies and their application to the patient's context
6. **Management Option Selection:** Weighing the risks, benefits, and feasibility of testing and treatment options to develop a comprehensive plan

Each micro skill represents a key step in the reasoning process and contributes to the clinician's overall ability to assess, diagnose, and manage patients effectively. For learners experiencing difficulties in clinical reasoning, this approach offers an accessible and manageable pathway to improvement in which each step can be practiced and refined in isolation before being integrated into complex, real-life scenarios. As described in chapter 3, clinicians toggle between different types of thinking, sometimes rapidly generating intuitive hypotheses, other times methodically gathering and reassessing data in response to unexpected findings. However, for coaching purposes, this simplification allows learners to focus on and improve specific cognitive abilities, thus fostering clarity and building confidence. By achieving competence in each micro skill, learners can incrementally develop a more complex, integrated reasoning process.

MICRO SKILL ASSESSMENT USING SRL MICROANALYSIS

Rooted in the principles of SRL microanalysis, our novel assessment process enables access to a learner's thinking as they work through an activity and thus evaluates the metacognitive aspects of clinical reasoning. The struggling learner is presented with a clinical case and asked to articulate their thoughts at each step, revealing their processes for approaching and prioritizing information. Coaches observe how the learner generates hypotheses, gathers and interprets data, constructs iterative problem representations, refines their differential, arrives at a working diagnosis, and suggests a management plan. Consistent with SRL microanalysis, the coach's inquiry focuses on forethought, performance, and self-reflection for each micro skill.[1,7] This approach allows the assessor to identify specific areas on which to focus the coaching intervention. For example, if a learner fails to adjust their differential diagnosis in response to new findings, this could indicate difficulties in hypothesis refinement. Alternatively, struggling to develop a concise problem representation may signal a need for more support in synthesizing and prioritizing information.

This Phase 2 assessment is completed in a controlled setting outside of the busy clinical environment, thus removing the pressure to act quickly and allowing for in-depth exploration of each step.[11] Beginning the work in the simulated environment also allows the coach to standardize cases across sessions and learners, ensuring the consistency and comparability which permit tracking of progress over time. This method aligns with a deliberate practice model for which identification of the specific micro skill deficit becomes the foundation for an individualized coaching plan. Focused practice on the micro skill most in need of improvement leads ultimately to more effective coaching that builds the learner's competence and confidence. We explore the coaching process itself in chapter 8.

Table 7.1 outlines our micro skill assessment process in a step-by-step format along with the aforementioned coaching questions and a developmental scale. The developmental scale is not learner specific and is provided only for relative comparison of performance across cases and between micro skills. We recommend conducting this assessment across multiple cases comprising a broad array of clinical conditions, ideally in areas of learner content familiarity. Cases should employ patient chief concerns specific to the struggling learner's level and/or specialty in a variety of hypothetical clinical contexts. The coach begins with typical presentations of common problems that progressively increase in complexity. As the learner thinks aloud, the coach employs frequent "stops" to determine the reasoning behind their verbalized decisions while promoting reflection and forethought towards the next step. The goal of this assessment process is to determine the primary micro skill or micro skills in which the learner struggles which will ultimately allow for targeted coaching.

SRL MICROANALYSIS AND CONTEXT

An inherent limitation of the SRL microanalysis approach is its sensitivity to context. As described previously, clinical reasoning is fundamentally situated, meaning that a learner's ability to generate hypotheses, synthesize data, and refine diagnostic or management decisions is influenced by multiple contextual factors. These include complexity, clinical setting, time constraints, and the availability of support structures such as faculty guidance or electronic decision aids.[10,24–28] Because SRL microanalysis is initially conducted in a structured, low-stakes environment, it may not fully capture the cognitive demands learners face when reasoning under real-world pressures. A learner who demonstrates effective problem representation in a controlled case discussion, for example, may struggle to maintain the same clarity when managing multiple patients in a busy emergency department. Additionally, clinical reasoning is often assessed through the lens of a given specialty's priorities which can lead to variability in how an expert assesses a learner's reasoning. A family medicine physician, for instance, may prioritize the most common and likely diagnoses, while an emergency medicine physician may focus on identifying life-threatening conditions first. This variability underscores the importance of moving away from an idealized notion of a single "correct" decision in favor of a more nuanced, context-aware approach to assessment. To address these limitations, coaching questions should explicitly incorporate contextual factors aligned with the phases of SRL. During the forethought phase, questions should prompt learners to anticipate challenges related to time pressure, uncertainty, and the need for rapid decision-making. In the performance phase, questions should explore whether learners recognize and adapt to evolving clinical cues. Finally, during the self-reflection phase, learners should be asked to evaluate how context influenced their reasoning and decision-making. Additionally, given the distributed nature of cognition in clinical environments, assessments should consider how learners leverage available resources—including interprofessional team members and informatics tools—to arrive at sound clinical decisions. We discuss these issues more in Section 4.

"DIAGNOSING" THE MICRO SKILL DEFICIT

Our emphasis on narrowing the areas of clinical reasoning struggle to a specific micro skill is informed by our understanding of the remediation literature.[29–33] As discussed in chapter 2, directing coaching effort towards the most significant performance deficit allows for the most effective and efficient allocation of limited remediation resources. Bearman and colleagues described this diagnostic process as "identifying discrepancy between the expected performance and the demonstrated performance and then trying to establish the reason for this underperformance."[34] Subsequent coaching can be ineffective and disorganized if the targeted assessment process is superficial or overlooked.[35] This point cannot be stressed enough: Matching coaching with the specific underlying clinical reasoning deficit is critical.[36]

Clinical evaluation data and behavioral insights from other educators, though likely also limited and incomplete in nature, provide a more holistic view of the learner's struggles. In fact, we know that subjective input, both from one-on-one assessment and formal or informal clinical evaluation data, can sufficiently inform effective remediation.[35] To support this process, Table 7.2 provides behavioral clues as to how a learner might struggle with each micro skill in the clinical environment. This information can serve as a reference when reviewing clinical performance data. In addition, with the rapid advancements in AI-driven clinical documentation and AI-guided chart review, we are likely entering a new era in which clinical performance data will be richer and more continuous.[10,37,38] AI should allow us to systematically capture every case a learner engages with, providing new insights into their reasoning across a broad spectrum of clinical scenarios. By integrating these

AI-enhanced data streams with SRL microanalysis and behavioral insights, we expect coaches will have a more comprehensive and nuanced understanding of a learner's challenges.

In chapter 8, we examine clinical reasoning micro skills in detail, exploring their respective roles in the reasoning process. We provide targeted coaching exercises for each micro skill to support struggling learners.

Table 7.1. Micro Skill Assessment Using SRL Microanalysis to Identify the Primary Clinical Reasoning Deficit

Step 1	Early Hypothesis Generation
	How well does the learner generate early hypotheses based on a provided chief concern and demographic information?
Forethought Coaching Questions Before the learner engages in hypothesis generation, these questions help them consider contextual influences on their reasoning	*What process do you typically use to generate an early differential when first encountering a patient?* *How might the clinical setting (ED vs. inpatient vs. outpatient) impact your expectations for this case?* *What assumptions might you be making based on the way the case is initially presented to you?*
System 1 Thinking **(Instruct: *Tell me what's on the top of your mind.*): Rapid, intuitive hypothesis generation based on pattern recognition** 1. Unable to generate any diagnostic possibilities 2. Generates a **few** early diagnostic possibilities using pattern recognition based on their level of education/training 3. Generates an **expected** early list of diagnostic possibilities using pattern recognition based on their level of training 4. Generates a list of early diagnostic possibilities based on pattern recognition **beyond** what would be expected for their level of education/training	**System 2 Thinking** **(Ask: *How would you build on your differential diagnosis?*): Deliberate, structured reasoning to expand initial hypotheses** 1. Disorganized and lacks a systematic way of approaching generation of diagnostic possibilities 2. Identifies partial systematic framework (e.g., just reviewing common **or** "can't miss" **or** systems-based vs anatomic-based vs known schema) 3. Identifies a more complete generic systematic framework (e.g., common **and** "can't miss" **and** systems-based vs anatomic-based vs known schema)

Table 7.1. Micro Skill Assessment Using SRL Microanalysis to Identify the Primary Clinical Reasoning Deficit *(continued)*

Performance Coaching Questions Guide the learner to consider the real-time influences on their decision-making	*As you are formulating your differential diagnosis, what factors are influencing your selection of diagnoses?* *As you are formulating your differential diagnosis, what external information (e.g., triage note, EMS handoff, nursing report, or electronic health record [EHR]) might be influencing your thinking?* *How does the setting (emergency department, clinic, ICU) shape the way you prioritize certain diagnoses?* *What aspects of the patient's presentation are most salient to you right now? Why?*
Reflection Coaching Questions Encourage self-assessment of the learner's reasoning process	*How confident are you that your initial differential diagnosis captures the most likely possibilities given the setting and available data?* *What role did external factors (e.g., triage note, EMS report, EHR summary) play in shaping your initial differential? Did they help or mislead you?* *How would you approach this chief concern differently in subsequent cases or encounters?* *What actions do you need to take to improve your ability to generate an early differential in different clinical contexts?* *How would you approach this chief concern differently in subsequent cases or encounters?*
Step 2	**Hypothesis-Driven Data Gathering**

How well does the learner gather data in a hypothesis-driven manner? This step assesses the learner's ability to gather pertinent signs and symptoms of disease that will support or refute initial hypotheses

(continued)

Table 7.1. Micro Skill Assessment Using SRL Microanalysis to Identify the Primary Clinical Reasoning Deficit *(Step 2 continued)*

<table>
<tr><td>Forethought Coaching Questions

Before the learner begins data gathering, these questions help them consider contextual influences on their approach</td><td>What data do you plan to collect to confirm or refute your initial hypotheses, and how does the clinical setting (ED, inpatient, outpatient) influence what's available?

Beyond the patient's symptoms, what external sources (e.g., nursing report, EMS handoff, EHR notes, family history) could provide crucial context for your data gathering?

Are there limitations in this clinical setting that could impact how you obtain history or perform a physical exam?

How might the way the patient presents (e.g., altered mental status, language barrier, incomplete history) shape your data collection strategy?</td></tr>
<tr><td>History Gathering

(Ask: What are 5 to 10 history items that you would need to further evaluate your differential? Tell me why you selected a particular symptom.): Provide data in a sequential fashion.

1. History is generic and not targeted to their differential diagnosis, does not adapt data gathering to reflect consideration of previously gathered data
2. History is focused on key features of diseases in their differential diagnosis but does not adapt to updated data
3. History is focused on key features of diseases in their differential diagnosis and adapts to updated information</td><td>Physical Exam

(Ask: What are 3 to 5 physical exam items that you would need to further evaluate your differential? Tell me why you want a particular item.):

1. Physical exam is generic and not targeted to key features of the differential diagnosis and does not adapt to reflect consideration of previously gathered data
2. Physical exam is targeted to key features of their differential diagnosis but does not articulate how certain exam findings change the likelihood of disease presence. Clinician does not examine systems unrelated to current care of the patient.
3. Physical exam is targeted to key features of the differential diagnosis and is able to articulate how exam findings change current likelihood of disease presence. Clinician does not examine systems unrelated to current care of the patient.</td></tr>
</table>

Table 7.1. Micro Skill Assessment Using SRL Microanalysis to Identify the Primary Clinical Reasoning Deficit *(continued)*

Performance Coaching Questions Guide the learner to consider the real-time influences on their decision-making	*As you gather data, how are external sources (e.g., EHR notes, nursing input, EMS report) influencing what you focus on?* *Are there constraints—such as time pressure, patient stability, or resource limitations—that are affecting what data you can collect?* *What assumptions did you initially make about the patient's history or physical exam, and how is new information reinforcing or challenging those assumptions?* *Are there unexpected findings that are shifting your priorities, and how are you adapting?* *As you gather data, how are you deciding which findings are most relevant?*
Reflection Coaching Questions Encourage self-assessment of the learner's reasoning process	*What specific data points helped confirm or challenge your initial hypotheses, and where did they come from (e.g., patient history, EHR, EMS, nursing)?* *In hindsight, were there any external data sources (e.g., collateral history, prior medical records) that you underutilized?* *How did the setting (e.g., busy ED vs. structured clinic) influence what information you could obtain?* *Did any unexpected findings lead you to reconsider your approach? If so, how?* *What knowledge or resources (e.g., clinical guidelines, team discussions, specialty input) would have improved your data collection?*
Step 3	**Problem Representation**

How well does the learner create a clear, useful problem representation in the form of a summary statement?
This step assesses the learner's ability to succinctly abstract and summarize relevant features of the case at various time points in the case progression

(continued)

Table 7.1. Micro Skill Assessment Using SRL Microanalysis to Identify the Primary Clinical Reasoning Deficit *(Step 3 continued)*

Forethought Coaching Questions Before the learner constructs a summary statement, these questions help them consider the purpose and contextual influences	*What do you aim to achieve by creating a summary statement for this case, and who is your intended audience (e.g., consultant, attending, handoff team)?* *How will you ensure that your summary captures the clinical essence of the problem while remaining adaptable to different contexts (e.g., ED vs. inpatient vs. rounds)?* *What factors, such as the acuity of the case, time constraints, or communication setting (verbal vs. written), might influence how you structure your summary?* *How does the patient's background (e.g., complex comorbidities, limited available history, language barrier) impact how you frame the case?*

Ask learner:

Can you summarize this patient in 1 to 2 lines?

Epidemiology (e.g., relevant demographics, past medical history, social history, etc):

1. No relevant epidemiology is included
2. Some relevant or some irrelevant epidemiology is included
3. Most relevant and no irrelevant epidemiology is included

Semantic qualifiers (e.g., acute/chronic/subacute, constant/intermittent, etc):

1. No relevant semantic qualifiers are included
2. Some relevant or some irrelevant semantic qualifiers are included
3. Most relevant and no irrelevant semantic qualifiers are included

Clinical syndrome (e.g., relevant history, physical exam, data):

1. No relevant aspects of the clinical syndrome are included
2. Some relevant or some irrelevant aspects of the clinical syndrome are included
3. Most relevant and no irrelevant aspects of the clinical syndrome are included

Table 7.1. Micro Skill Assessment Using SRL Microanalysis to Identify the Primary Clinical Reasoning Deficit *(continued)*

Performance Coaching Questions Guide the learner to refine their problem representation in real time by considering contextual influences	*As you create your summary, how are you deciding which details to include or omit, and how might that change if you were presenting to a consultant vs. an inpatient team?* *Does your current problem representation align with the data you've gathered, or are there inconsistencies that need clarification?* *How does the acuity of the case affect the level of detail in your summary statement?* *If you had to relay this information urgently (e.g., rapid response, sign-out), how would you adjust your approach?* *How might different team members interpret your summary differently?*
Reflection Coaching Questions Encourage self-assessment of the learner's reasoning and communication process	*How effectively does your problem representation capture the key features of the case, and how might it be perceived by different team members?* *Is there a more concise or efficient way to summarize the information you want to convey, especially in a high-acuity setting?* *Did your summary statement evolve as new data emerged? If not, what prevented you from adjusting it?* *What contextual factors made this task more or less challenging?* *What strategies can you use to refine your problem representation skills for different clinical contexts (e.g., written documentation vs. verbal handoff)?*

(continued)

Table 7.1. Micro Skill Assessment Using SRL Microanalysis to Identify the Primary Clinical Reasoning Deficit *(continued)*

Step 4	Hypothesis Refinement
How well does the learner refine and prioritize the differential diagnosis based on the evolving clinical scenario?	
Forethought Coaching Questions Before the learner engages in hypothesis refinement, these questions help them consider their approach and contextual influences	*What is your strategy for narrowing and prioritizing your differential diagnosis, and how does the clinical setting (e.g., ICU vs. outpatient vs. ED) impact this process?* *What criteria will you use to decide which hypotheses to keep or eliminate, and how do time pressures or resource availability influence these choices?* *How do external factors such as consultant input, prior documentation, or clinical team discussions affect your hypothesis refinement?* *Are there any patient-specific factors (e.g., comorbidities, social determinants, medication history) that should play a role in refining your differential?*

Ask:
Based on the information you have gathered, how would you update your differential at this point?

Appropriate differential refinement:

1. Anchors on single diagnostic possibility or maintains inappropriately broad differential
2. Can identify 2 to 3 diagnoses of high likelihood **but** struggles to justify thought processes
3. Can identify 2 to 3 diagnoses of high likelihood **and** can justify thought processes

Can prioritize a working diagnosis for management decisions (Ask: *Of your list, what is your top concern and why?*):

1. Lacks ability to prioritize narrowed differential
2. Accurately prioritizes differential and may even choose a working diagnosis to guide management decisions

Table 7.1. Micro Skill Assessment Using SRL Microanalysis to Identify the Primary Clinical Reasoning Deficit *(continued)*

Performance Coaching Questions Guide the learner to refine their differential in real time while considering contextual influences	*As you review your differential, what process are you using to adjust the ranking of your diagnoses, and how does this compare to team input or consultant feedback?* *Are you considering how disease prevalence in this specific setting (e.g., hospital vs. community clinic) influences which diagnoses are most likely?* *How do time-sensitive decisions (e.g., need for empiric treatment, awaiting test results) impact your prioritization of hypotheses?*
Reflection Coaching Questions Encourage self-assessment of the learner's reasoning and adaptability	*What changes to your differential diagnosis were most influenced by new findings, and why?* *Did any contextual factors (e.g., patient acuity, test availability, consultant recommendations) alter your thought process?* *Looking back, were there any biases or assumptions that influenced how you refined your hypotheses? If so, how might you mitigate these in the future?* *Were there alternative approaches to refining your differential that you overlooked? If so, why?* *What strategies can you implement to improve your ability to adjust hypotheses dynamically in different clinical settings?*
Step 5	**Management Script Activation**
How well does the learner generate a management plan for a working diagnosis or for a focused set of possible diagnoses?	

(continued)

Table 7.1. Micro Skill Assessment Using SRL Microanalysis to Identify the Primary Clinical Reasoning Deficit *(Step 5 continued)*

Forethought Coaching Questions Before the learner constructs a management plan, these questions help them consider relevant knowledge and experiences	*What illness-specific knowledge will guide your management plan for this patient?* *What prior cases or clinical experiences are informing your understanding of management strategies for this patient?*
Creates a general management script template (labs, imaging, medications, consultants, procedures, monitoring, etc) based on working diagnosis (Ask: *For your current working diagnosis/leading diagnoses what are all your possible options for management?*) 1. Partial or incomplete management script template for working diagnosis 2. Detailed and comprehensive management script for working diagnosis	
Performance Coaching Questions	*As you consider management strategies, how are you prioritizing the options?* *Are you encountering any challenges in applying your knowledge to this patient's case?*
Reflection Coaching Questions Encourage self-assessment of the learner's ability to develop management scripts effectively	*What additional knowledge or preparation would enhance your approach in similar cases, particularly in different clinical settings?* *Did you rely too heavily on pattern recognition, or did you critically assess all management options before making decisions?* *Looking back, were there any management options you underutilized or overlooked? What led to that?*

Table 7.1. Micro Skill Assessment Using SRL Microanalysis to Identify the Primary Clinical Reasoning Deficit *(continued)*

Step **6**	**Management Option Selection**
	How well does the learner generate a patient- and context-specific management plan?
Forethought Coaching Questions Before selecting management options, these questions help the learner consider patient-specific and contextual influences	*How will you tailor the management approach to fit the patient's unique clinical and social context (e.g., comorbidities, functional status, health literacy, support systems)?* *What factors will you consider when weighing risks and benefits of treatment options, and how might these change depending on the setting (e.g., ICU vs. general ward vs. outpatient)?* *How will you decide on the feasibility of different management strategies given resource availability, financial constraints, and system limitations?* *What role do patient goals, preferences, or cultural considerations play in shaping your management decisions?*
Select from created menu of management options based on patient-specific considerations (Ask: *Based on your management script (above), what next steps in* management *would you pursue for this patient and why? Provide patient-specific and* context-*specific features of the case that would impact management.*) 1. Unable to select appropriate options specific to the patient and/or context 2. Selects **some** appropriate and **some** inappropriate options based on **some** relevant patient-specific and/or context-specific features of the case 3. Selects **all** appropriate options with consideration of **all** relevant patient-specific and context-specific features of the case	

(continued)

Table 7.1. Micro Skill Assessment Using SRL Microanalysis to Identify the Primary Clinical Reasoning Deficit *(Step 6 continued)*

Performance Coaching Questions Guide the learner to refine their management decisions by considering real-world constraints and patient-centered factors	*How are your management strategies impacted by cost, risk, system constraints, uncertainty in the diagnosis, patient preferences, or other influencing factors?* *Are there any institutional policies, clinical guidelines, or decision-support tools that you are using to inform your approach? How are you applying them to this case?* *If your preferred management plan is not feasible due to system limitations (e.g., medication shortages, lack of specialty access), how would you modify your approach?* *How would you explain your management choices to the patient or their family to ensure shared decision-making?* *If your management approach is challenged by a consultant, supervisor, or colleague, how would you justify or adapt your plan?*
Reflection Coaching Questions Encourage metacognition and self-assessment of the learner's ability to select appropriate, patient-centered management options	*How well did your chosen management plan address the patient's condition and unique circumstances?* *Did you fully consider system constraints, cost, or feasibility when making management decisions? If not, what could you do differently next time?* *How effectively did you integrate patient goals, values, and preferences into your decision-making process?* *Looking back, did you adjust your management plan as new information emerged, or did any biases limit your flexibility?* *What steps can you take to strengthen your ability to select effective, patient-centered management options in future cases?*

Table 7.2. Behavioral Clues to Assist in Identifying the Primary Micro Skill Deficit[11,22,23]

Early Hypothesis Generation

- Limited differential diagnosis based on chief concern and patient demographics
- Fails to ask defining or discriminating features **early** in the encounter
- Differential diagnoses begin and remain overly narrow
- Overly reliant on previous experience, recent case examples, or diagnostic momentum
- Fails to consider common diagnoses
- Struggles to justify why a question was asked or exam maneuver was performed

Hypothesis-Driven Data Gathering

- History taking and/or physical examination is scattered, disorganized, or overly exhaustive
- Persists in irrelevant lines of inquiry
- Fails to ask clarifying questions
- Fails to **ever** ask defining or discriminating features
- Presentations and documentation contain irrelevant information or lack relevant data (including pertinent negatives)

Problem Representation

- Unable to summarize the case using key information
- Considers each data point in isolation or remains fixated on individual pieces of clinical data
- Cannot convert patient language to abstract medical terminology
- Cannot adapt to new information in real-time
- Summary statements (final problem representations) inconsistent with primary diagnoses
- Struggles with presentations, calling consults, and/or handoffs of care
- Cannot integrate the patient's context into decision-making or clinical communication
- Struggles to triage

(continued)

Table 7.2. Behavioral Clues to Assist in Identifying the Primary Micro Skill Deficit[11,22,23] *(continued)*

Hypothesis Refinement

- Spends excessive time exploring a minor point
- Patient encounter is rigid, or supervisor needs to intervene to shift the focus of the encounter
- Diagnoses, each supported by relevant data, remained siloed
- Differential diagnosis is disorganized, and learner struggles to justify each diagnosis
- Fails to update and reprioritize differential diagnosis as new information is obtained
- Struggles with uncertainty
- Consistent overtesting

Management Script Activation

- Limited or simplistic plan for treatment or additional testing
- Suggested interventions lack specificity to the diagnosis or syndrome
- Each issue's management is addressed in isolation
- Consistent undertesting
- Struggles during urgent/emergent clinical encounters
- Applies guidelines in an inappropriate or rigid manner
- Unable to describe or adjust management plan to changing clinical course/trajectory

Management Option Selection

- Suggested interventions lack specificity to the patient's goals and values
- Suggested interventions lack consideration of system restraints or affordances
- Chooses interventions without consideration of risk, uncertainty, or cost
- Struggles to deal with clinical uncertainty
- Failure to appreciate the complex bio-psycho-social aspects of the case
- Failure to appreciate the longitudinal nature of clinical care or inappropriate follow-up
- Struggles to explain the plan to the patient or family

References

1. Artino AR, Cleary TJ, Dong T, Hemmer PA, Durning SJ. Exploring clinical reasoning in novices: a self-regulated learning microanalytic assessment approach. *Med Educ.* 2014;48(3):280-291. doi:10.1111/medu.12303
2. Mamede S, Figueiredo-Soares T, Elói Santos SM, de Faria RMD, Schmidt HG, van Gog T. Fostering novice students' diagnostic ability: the value of guiding deliberate reflection. *Med Educ.* 2019;53(6):628-637. doi:10.1111/medu.13829
3. Wang F, Liu D, Zhang M. Metacognitive processes, situational factors, and clinical decision-making in nursing education: a quantitative longitudinal study. *BMC Med Educ.* 2024;24(1):1530. doi:10.1186/s12909-024-06467-y
4. Cecilio-Fernandes D, Carvalho DRDS, Sandars J, Santos TM. Self-regulated learning microanalysis feedback for developing clinical skills: A pilot study. *Med Teach.* 2024;46(10):1356-1361. doi:10.1080/0142159X.2024.2308060
5. Durning SJ, Cleary TJ, Sandars J, Hemmer P, Kokotailo P, Artino AR. Perspective: Viewing "Strugglers" Through a Different Lens: How a Self-Regulated Learning Perspective Can Help Medical Educators With Assessment and Remediation. *Acad Med.* 2011;86(4):488. doi:10.1097/ACM.0b013e31820dc384
6. Andrews MA, Kelly WF, DeZee KJ. Why Does This Learner Perform Poorly on Tests? Using Self-Regulated Learning Theory to Diagnose the Problem and Implement Solutions. *Acad Med.* 2018;93(4):612. doi:10.1097/ACM.0000000000001422
7. Cleary TJ, Durning SJ, Artino ARJ. Microanalytic Assessment of Self-Regulated Learning During Clinical Reasoning Tasks: Recent Developments and Next Steps. *Acad Med.* 2016;91(11):1516-1521. doi:10.1097/ACM.0000000000001228
8. Gandomkar R, Mirzazadeh A, Jalili M, Yazdani K, Fata L, Sandars J. Self-regulated learning processes of medical students during an academic learning task. *Med Educ.* 2016;50(10):1065-1074. doi:10.1111/medu.12975
9. Torre D, Durning SJ, Rencic J, Lang V, Holmboe E, Daniel M. Widening the lens on teaching and assessing clinical reasoning: from "in the head" to "out in the world." *Diagn Berl Ger.* 2020;7(3):181-190. doi:10.1515/dx-2019-0098
10. Parsons AS, Wijesekera TP, Olson APJ, Torre D, Durning SJ, Daniel M. Beyond thinking fast and slow: Implications of a transtheoretical model of clinical reasoning and error on teaching, assessment, and research. *Med Teach.* Published online June 5, 2024:1-12. doi:10.1080/0142159X.2024.2359963
11. Parsons AS, Dreicer JJ, Martindale JR, Young G, Warburton KM. A Targeted Clinical Reasoning Remediation Program for Residents and Fellows in Need. *J Grad Med Educ.* 2024;16(4):469. doi:10.4300/JGME-D-23-00822.1
12. Warburton KM, Goren E, Dine CJ. Comprehensive Assessment of Struggling Learners Referred to a Graduate Medical Education Remediation Program. *J Grad Med Educ.* 2017;9(6):763-767. doi:10.4300/JGME-D-17-00175.1
13. Steward D, Bordage G, Lemieux M. Semantic Structures and Diagnostic Thinking of Experts and Novices. *Acad Med.* 1991;66(9):S70.
14. Bordage G. Why did I miss the diagnosis? Some cognitive explanations and educational implications. *Acad Med.* 1999;74(10):S138.

15. Graber ML, Franklin N, Gordon R. Diagnostic Error in Internal Medicine. *Arch Intern Med.* 2005;165(13):1493. doi:10.1001/archinte.165.13.1493

16. Norman GR, Eva KW. Diagnostic error and clinical reasoning. *Med Educ.* 2010;44(1):94-100. doi:10.1111/j.1365-2923.2009.03507.x

17. Durning S, Artino AR, Pangaro L, van der Vleuten CPM, Schuwirth L. Context and clinical reasoning: understanding the perspective of the expert's voice. *Med Educ.* 2011;45(9):927-938. doi:10.1111/j.1365-2923.2011.04053.x

18. Bowen JL. Educational Strategies to Promote Clinical Diagnostic Reasoning. *N Engl J Med.* 2006;355(21):2217-2225. doi:10.1056/NEJMra054782

19. Kassirer, Wong, and Kopelman. *Learning Clinical Reasoning.* Wolters Kluwer Lippincott Williams & Wilkins Health; 2010. Accessed February 13, 2025. http://archive.org/details/learningclinical00kass

20. Audétat MC, Laurin S, Sanche G, et al. Clinical reasoning difficulties: A taxonomy for clinical teachers. *Med Teach.* 2013;35(3):e984-e989. doi:10.3109/0142159X.2012.733041

21. Charlin B, Lubarsky S, Millette B, et al. Clinical reasoning processes: unravelling complexity through graphical representation. *Med Educ.* 2012;46(5):454-463. doi:10.1111/j.1365-2923.2012.04242.x

22. Audétat MC, Laurin S, Dory V, Charlin B, Nendaz MR. Diagnosis and management of clinical reasoning difficulties: Part II. Clinical reasoning difficulties: Management and remediation strategies. *Med Teach.* 2017;39(8):797-801. doi:10.1080/0142159X.2017.1331034

23. Weinstein Adam, Gupta Shanu, Pinto-Powell Roshini, et al. Diagnosing and Remediating Clinical Reasoning Difficulties: A Faculty Development Workshop. *MedEdPORTAL.* 13. doi:10.15766/mep_2374-8265.10650

24. Konopasky A, Artino AR, Battista A, et al. Understanding context specificity: the effect of contextual factors on clinical reasoning. *Diagnosis.* 2020;7(3):257-264. doi:10.1515/dx-2020-0016

25. Daniel M, Durning SJ, Wilson E, Abdoler E, Torre D. Situated cognition: clinical reasoning and error are context dependent. *Diagnosis.* 2020;7(3):341-342. doi:10.1515/dx-2020-0011

26. Croskerry P. Context Is Everything or How Could I Have Been That Stupid? *Healthc Q Tor Ont.* 2009;12 Spec No Patient:e171-6. doi:10.12927/hcq.2009.20945

27. Rencic J, Schuwirth LWT, Gruppen LD, Durning SJ. A situated cognition model for clinical reasoning performance assessment: a narrative review. *Diagn Berl Ger.* 2020;7(3):227-240. doi:10.1515/dx-2019-0106

28. Durning SJ, Artino AR, Pangaro LN, Van Der Vleuten C, Schuwirth L. Perspective: Redefining Context in the Clinical Encounter: Implications for Research and Training in Medical Education: *Acad Med.* 2010;85(5):894-901. doi:10.1097/ACM.0b013e3181d7427c

29. Yao DC, Wright SM. National Survey of Internal Medicine Residency Program Directors Regarding Problem Residents. *JAMA.* 2000;284(9):1099-1104. doi:10.1001/jama.284.9.1099

30. Hauer KE, Ciccone A, Henzel TR, et al. Remediation of the Deficiencies of Physicians Across the Continuum From Medical School to Practice: A Thematic Review of the Literature: *Acad Med.* 2009;84(12):1822-1832. doi:10.1097/ACM.0b013e3181bf3170

31. Ronan-Bentle SE, Avegno J, Hegarty CB, Manthey DE. Dealing with the difficult student in emergency medicine. *Int J Emerg Med.* 2011;4(1):39. doi:10.1186/1865-1380-4-39

32. Weller JM, Misur M, Nicolson S, et al. Can I leave the theatre? A key to more reliable workplace-based assessment. *Br J Anaesth.* 2014;112(6):1083-1091. doi:10.1093/bja/aeu052

33. Saxena V, O'Sullivan PS, Teherani A, Irby DM, Hauer KE. Remediation Techniques for Student Performance Problems After a Comprehensive Clinical Skills Assessment. *Acad Med.* 2009;84(5):669-676. doi:10.1097/ACM.0b013e31819fa832

34. Bearman M, Tai J, Kent F, Edouard V, Nestel D, Molloy E. What should we teach the teachers? Identifying the learning priorities of clinical supervisors. *Adv Health Sci Educ Theory Pract.* 2018;23(1):29-41. doi:10.1007/s10459-017-9772-3

35. Steinert Y. The "problem" learner: whose problem is it? AMEE Guide No. 76. *Med Teach.* 2013;35(4):e1035-1045. doi:10.3109/0142159X.2013.774082

36. Boileau E, St-Onge C, Audétat MC. Is there a way for clinical teachers to assist struggling learners? A synthetic review of the literature. *Adv Med Educ Pract.* 2017;8:89-97. doi:10.2147/AMEP.S123410

37. Schaye V, Guzman B, Burk-Rafel J, et al. Development and Validation of a Machine Learning Model for Automated Assessment of Resident Clinical Reasoning Documentation. *J Gen Intern Med.* 2022;37(9):2230-2238. doi:10.1007/s11606-022-07526-0

38. Burk-Rafel J, Sebok-Syer SS, Santen SA, et al. TRainee Attributable & Automatable Care Evaluations in Real-time (TRACERs): A Scalable Approach for Linking Education to Patient Care. *Perspect Med Educ.* 2023;12(1). doi:10.5334/pme.1013

CHAPTER 8

Targeted Clinical Reasoning Coaching Exercises

ARMED WITH GLOBAL and targeted assessment data, we can now develop an individualized clinical reasoning coaching plan for the struggling learner. The coaching interventions presented in this section align with the micro skills described in the previous chapter: (1) early hypothesis generation, (2) hypothesis-driven data gathering, (3) problem representation, (4) hypothesis refinement, (5) management script activation, and (6) management option selection. Presented in a linear manner, this micro skill approach represents an overly simplified version of the clinical reasoning process for purposes of coaching. In reality, some degree of data gathering must begin the encounter. Furthermore, iterative problem representation and hypothesis generation occur in a cyclical manner as described in Bowen's seminal 2006 article.[1] Our aim is to introduce a framework for coaching that promotes schema development among learners and encourages them to approach each patient encounter systematically. Coaching at the micro skill level facilitates knowledge accumulation and reorganization towards gradual honing and more effective application of content-specific and context-specific pattern recognition. From the coach's perspective, this approach offers targeted points of intervention as well as a defined and generalizable structure for deliberate practice.

As described in detail in chapter 3, while having a strong knowledge base is essential for effective clinical reasoning, the organization of that knowledge is just as important. Knowledge organized in the form of scripts allows for effective and highly efficient pattern recognition. However, most learners struggling with clinical reasoning lack effective pattern recognition. For these learners, schema formation and development are essential. Schemas simultaneously scaffold knowledge acquisition and clinical problem solving.[2] In addition, this process promotes learner development of self-awareness, adaptability, and resilience.[3–5] With the guidance of a coach, learners gain the confidence and capability to approach patient care in a methodical yet flexible manner, laying a foundation for continued development.

The importance of content- and context-specificity cannot be overstated. As discussed in chapter 6, we begin coaching in a simulated environment, usually the coach's office, in which coach and learner co-create the goals of coaching. The coach presents the learner with a range of cases of increasing complexity, using a deliberate practice model that promotes learner reflection. This model, described in chapter 7, approaches clinical reasoning from the perspective of a linearly organized set of micro skills. Ten Cate, Custers, Durning and colleagues provide a wonderful overview of the case-based method for clinical reasoning in their book *Principles and Practice of Case-based Clinical Reasoning Education: A Method for Preclinical Students*,[6] which we highly recommend. In both our experience and the published experience of others, a coaching model employing deliberate practice with targeted feedback improves clinical reasoning among struggling learners.[5–10] Once the learner is comfortable, deliberate practice moves to the clinical environment. We now take the reader step-by-step through our approach.

EARLY HYPOTHESIS GENERATION

Though traditional models of the clinical reasoning process begin with data gathering, we open our framework with early hypothesis generation. In doing so, we emphasize that hypothesis generation begins the moment we encounter a patient or first hear of their story. In fact, almost any cue—the look on a patient's face, a single lab value, or a change in vital signs—prompts our brain to produce potential explanations for what might be going on. Just as we do in our daily interactions with the surrounding environment, we generate hypotheses on first contact.[11] These hypotheses can be general or specific and will evolve over time. In the clinical context, as discussed in chapter 3, diagnostic hypotheses are generated when a match or partial match is made between early cues and illness scripts stored in long-term memory.[12,13] A hypothesis can be held in working memory as a "chunk" to become the focus of subsequent data gathering or cast aside in favor of an alternative hypothesis.[14] By forming a preliminary list of possible diagnoses, the learner begins a structured approach to clinical assessment.

Kostopoulou and colleagues' extensive work on early hypothesis generation among practicing clinicians suggests an improvement in diagnostic accuracy, regardless of the difficulty of the cases and without lengthening the data-gathering process.[15–17] This is consistent with our understanding of diagnostic errors which suggests that many, if not most, errors result from failure to ever consider the diagnosis.[18,19] Sisson and colleagues found that novice learners tend to generate more initial, though less accurate, hypotheses compared to experts, which can be beneficial in broadening their diagnostic considerations early in the reasoning process.[20] This finding aligns with our understanding of dual process theory (DPT) which suggests that novice learners are more reliant on System 2-based deductive reasoning, whereas experts practice System 1-based inductive reasoning using pattern recognition. In this sense, most struggling learners should be considered novice or early learners for purposes of remediation (Figure 8.1). Coderre and colleagues demonstrated that querying initial hypotheses allowed early learners to rectify incorrect diagnoses without harming correct ones when presented with discordant clinical data.[21] Effective hypothesis generation requires flexibility in adapting to patient-specific and contextual factors, guiding subsequent data gathering and refinement.

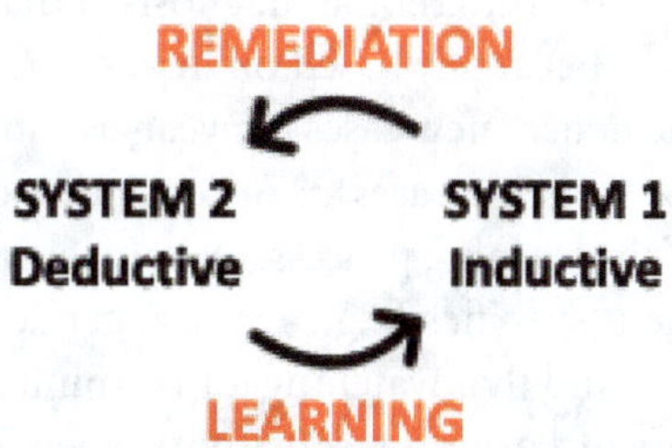

Figure 8.1. The Relationship Between Early Learners and Struggling Learners from the Perspective of Dual Process Theory

Learners struggle with early hypothesis generation primarily due to three reasons. We present targeted coaching exercises to address each.

1. Limitations in knowledge or experience: Learners may lack the germane medical knowledge (or clinical experience) required to generate accurate and relevant hypotheses.[22] It is inevitable that these deficiencies will lead to the development of an overly narrow list of diagnoses or inclusion of unlikely diagnoses. Learners with insufficient medical knowledge and/or experience do not have the breadth and depth of illness scripts necessary for intuitive pattern recognition at this step, especially with limited clinical data. Coaching efforts should focus on providing content-relevant cognitive frameworks for hypothesis generation and specific feedback on the learner's early differential diagnosis. Applying these frameworks repeatedly, across a variety of cases and in a variety of contexts, promotes organization of knowledge towards improved pattern recognition. Coaching that utilizes both System 1 and System 2 reasoning in this way results in greater diagnostic accuracy for early learners.[23] In short, a learner cannot generate a hypothesis that they have never encountered, either through study or clinical experience. For these learners, the knowledge-based frameworks provided in chapter 9 are essential.
2. Premature closure: Learners may struggle to appropriately contextualize clinical information, leading to errors in forming initial hypotheses.[22] In addition, for struggling learners, the deliberate nature of early hypothesis generation can lead them to settle on a diagnosis too early without considering all possibilities.
3. Poor estimation of disease probability: Struggling learners may have difficulty estimating pre-test probability.[24] In fact, clinicians at large struggle with base-rate neglect.[25] Remember from chapter 3 that, despite the importance of classical decision theory, human decision-makers are not rational actors. One benefit of more deliberate early hypothesis generation is that the differential diagnosis at that point in the clinical encounter should be largely based on disease incidence. For purposes of diagnosis, incidence (new cases per year) is a more relevant measure than prevalence (existing cases).[26] Appreciation of incidence data is a critical piece of the learning process. Of course, incidence data must be tailored to patient specifics (e.g., age, sex, gender) and setting. Brush and colleagues found that watching an 18-minute instructional video on the concepts of base rate, sensitivity, specificity, and likelihood

ratios and their implications on the calibration of subjective probability estimates improved diagnostic accuracy among early learners.[27]

Below, we present coaching exercises targeted to address these underlying concerns.

FRAMEWORKS TO COACH EARLY HYPOTHESIS GENERATION[28–31]

The coach encourages the learner to use one or more of these analytic approaches to develop a broad differential diagnosis when approaching a patient encounter. Framework selection is informed by the patient's chief concern, demographic information, and relevant risk factors.

ANATOMY

Consider the organs and surrounding structures in each location and what can go wrong with each. We encourage use of this framework when localization is key to generating an initial differential diagnosis. Examples include pain, redness, swelling, or other signs of inflammation.

Example: For a complaint of chest pain, think of anatomical features in the chest (e.g., skin, muscles, ribs, mediastinum, heart, lungs, spine and associated bony structures) as well as the few instances in which this is potentially confusing because pain may be referred from elsewhere.

PATHOPHYSIOLOGY

Consider the physiological processes of disease leading to the chief complaint. We encourage use of this framework when faced with abnormal vital signs, laboratory values, or imaging findings.

Example: For an abnormally elevated serum creatinine level in outpatient clinic, think of pre-renal, intrinsic, and post-renal causes.

SYSTEMS

Consider disease processes by organ system. We encourage use of systems-based frameworks such as VINDICATE (below) for nonspecific complaints such as fatigue, weight loss, and fever.

Example: For a complaint of unintentional weight loss in a refugee patient

V ascular: ischemic bowel disease
I nfectious/inflammatory: HIV, TB, parasitic infection, endocarditis
N eoplastic: solid tumor (e.g., GI malignancy, lung cancer), lymphoma
D egenerative: advanced COPD, neurodegenerative disease (e.g., Parkinson's Disease)
I atrogenic/intoxication: medication side effects, substance use
C ongenital: cystic fibrosis, hereditary metabolic disorders
A utoimmune: celiac disease, inflammatory bowel disease, connective tissue disease
T raumatic: PTSD and depression
E ndocrine/metabolic: uncontrolled diabetes mellitus, thyroid disease, kidney disease, liver disease

WORST-CASE SCENARIO [32]

Consider specific conditions that can lead to mortality, significant morbidity, or are time urgent. These are cannot-miss diagnoses. We encourage use of this framework for all cases while emphasizing that overemphasis of such diagnoses can, in some cases, lead to overtesting.

Example: For a complaint of acute shortness of breath, consider pulmonary embolism, decompensated heart failure, and myocardial infarction.

PRE-TEST PROBABILITY

As introduced previously, it is important to consider the probability of suspected diseases based on their incidence in a specific population, also referred to as base rate, before any diagnostic tests are conducted. Encourage the learner to routinely familiarize themselves with the epidemiology of their geographic locale and understand how referral filters and recency or availability effects may bias their judgement on what is most likely in a particular clinical setting. We encourage use of this framework for all cases and clinical encounters.

Example: While a chronic cough is usually attributable to post-nasal drip, reactive airway disease, or gastroesophageal reflex, adjustments in prior probability need to be carefully considered, say, during a viral pandemic.

QUALITATIVE BAYES' THEOREM[33]

The learner is asked to verbalize the pre-test probability of each diagnosis categorically using the following framework:

- Very unlikely (less than 10%)
- Unlikely (between 10% and 33%)
- Uncertain (between 34% and 66%)
- Likely (between 67% and 90%)
- Very likely (more likely than 90%)

Next, the coach facilitates a discussion about the need for additional consideration of "very unlikely" and "unlikely" diseases in the context of how risky (i.e., can't miss) each is. Finally, the learner is encouraged to consider the relationship between pre-test and post-test probability. This can be done using an approximation.[33]

DIFFERENTIAL DIAGNOSIS CHECKLISTS

Ely and colleagues created an extensive database of differential diagnosis checklists.[34] The checklists are organized by chief concern, and each diagnosis is marked with an ● for a commonly missed diagnosis and ♠ for a can't-miss diagnosis. The checklists are designed to be printed on two-sided note cards. An example for *cough* is shown below. We suggest that the coach and learner jointly review and discuss the list prior to detailed data gathering. An analysis of the efficacy of this approach with early learners found increased diagnostic accuracy for difficult cases but a decrease in diagnostic accuracy (relative to intuition) for simple cases.[35] This finding again highlights that the ultimate goal of coaching hypothesis generation is development of scripts and schema for effective pattern recognition among struggling learners.

Sore Throat

Viral pharyngitis (adenovirus, rhinovirus, coronavirus, parainfluenza)
Influenza
Group A Streptococcal pharyngitis
Group C/G Streptococcal pharyngitis
● Infectious mononucleosis (Epstein-Barr virus)

(continued)

- Cytomegalovirus pharyngitis
- Herpangina (coxsackievirus)
- ♠ Epiglottitis
- ♠ Peritonsillar abscess
- ♠ Retropharyngeal abscess
- Hand, foot, and mouth disease (coxsackievirus, enterovirus)
- Gonococcal pharyngitis
- Chlamydial pharyngitis
- • Diphtheria
- • HIV acute retroviral syndrome
- Fungal pharyngitis (candida, particularly in immunocompromised patients)
- • Tuberculosis pharyngitis
- ♠ Ludwig's angina
- ♠ Laryngeal diphtheria
- Allergic rhinitis/postnasal drip
- Gastroesophageal reflux disease (GERD)
- • Stevens-Johnson syndrome
- • Behçet's disease
- • Vitamin deficiencies (e.g., iron, B12)
- Irritant exposure (smoke, pollutants, chemical inhalants)
- ♠ Angioedema (allergic/anaphylactic reaction)
- ♠ Malignancy (head/neck cancer, lymphoma)
- Dry air-induced pharyngitis
- Psychogenic throat discomfort

HYPOTHESIS-DRIVEN DATA GATHERING

Early in medical education, most learners are taught to rely on templates to inform history-taking and physical examination. A "full history and physical" has the learner ask the same comprehensive list of questions and conduct a head-to-toe physical exam for all patients.[36] Though memorization and practice of the basics is important, this learning out of context can delay a learner's grasp of defining and discriminating features during history taking and may obscure appreciation of the relevance of abnormal physical exam findings.[37,38] In contrast, hypothesis-driven data gathering (HDDG) is the directed collection of information that informs or challenges initial hypotheses. The goal is for learners who struggle at this step to demonstrate efficiency and focus by asking questions, conducting physical exams, and ordering early testing that narrows the differential diagnosis rather than collecting extraneous data. This targeted approach to data gathering improves diagnostic accuracy and prevents cognitive overload by filtering extraneous information.

For struggling learners who often rely on a set structure, one of the challenges of HDDG is that there is no universal script to follow and no single path that works for every case. Data gathering must be fluid, depending on the hypotheses being considered in the moment. These hypotheses, in turn, are shaped by probabilistic relationships. Uncertainty can be a helpful lens. An expert clinician isn't just collecting information; they are strategically choosing which questions to ask based on which questions are most likely to reduce their diagnostic uncertainty. Some questions have a high diagnostic yield, quickly shifting the probability of one diagnosis over another. Others add little, burning time and cognitive effort without moving the case forward. Diagnostic efficiency hinges on this ability to recognize which data points matter most. Viewing HDDG through the prism of gradually reducing uncertainty can help struggling learners hone this ability.

Hasnain and colleagues identified four behaviors suggestive of HDDG that were associated with improved diagnostic accuracy:[39]

1. Thorough and early exploration of the chief concern (Table 8.1)
2. Asking questions in proximity
3. Asking clarifying questions
4. Summarizing gathered data

A hypothesis-driven approach to data gathering does not obviate the need for a thorough exploration of the patient's chief concern. While the practice of generating an initial differential diagnosis focuses inquiry, it can also lead some learners into confirmation bias, causing them to only ask questions that support the diagnoses they initially thought likely. Instead, learners should collect a sufficiently open-ended initial history (e.g., "tell me more about your *chief concern*") and follow that up with a symptom characterization

(Table 8.1). A common coaching strategy has the struggling learner limit themselves to 3 to 5 clarifying questions during this phase of history-taking, 3 to 5 elements of the physical examination, and so on, depending on the type of data being collected.

After initial exploration of the chief concern, we guide learners to turn their attention to the defining and discriminating features of the case, commonly known as key features or pertinent positives and negatives. Yudkowsky and colleagues found that checklists using clinically discriminating items improved performance relative to thoroughness checklists, highlighting the importance of key features in HDDG.[40] With repeated case exposure and clinical experience, key features can become anchor points in a learner's mind (through the script organization process described previously), allowing them to apply this knowledge to subsequent clinical encounters.[1,41,42] We recommend the coach begin with cases that present typically, so-called "classic" presentations of disease, so that struggling learners can build exemplar scripts.[43,44] This approach establishes a prototype for each diagnosis in the learners mind, allowing for future pattern matching and comparison as learners search for deviations from the typical.[45,46] A prototype is generally defined as a single averaged portrayal of the signs and symptoms that characterize a given disease.[47] We explore the importance of comparing and contrasting illness scripts in more detail when discussing hypothesis refinement.

The initial focus on typical presentations of disease is to acknowledge the developmental nature of reasoning, though one must not downplay the importance of learning atypical presentations of disease. In fact, atypical presentation of common disease is a leading cause of misdiagnosis and malpractice claims.[48] In an excellent paper, "Teaching More About Less: Preparing Clinicians for Practice," Lessing and colleagues advocate for focused teaching on a smaller number of common conditions, emphasizing nuance and variance in clinical presentation rather than covering a broad range of diseases with less depth.[49] This practice should significantly impact our understanding and approach to HDDG because disease presentations (e.g., substernal chest pain in acute myocardial infarction) are rarely specific or sensitive. Kennedy and colleagues analyzed 250 positive and 241 negative likelihood ratios across 67 diagnoses and found that most clinical findings are not diagnostically powerful in isolation (with likelihood ratios close to 1).[50] In addition, positive findings were generally more informative than negative findings, suggesting that we should be cautious before "ruling out" or prematurely closing on a diagnosis, especially based on one pertinent negative finding.[50] For the struggling learner, this further emphasizes the importance of early hypothesis generation with explicit consideration of pre-test probability, namely disease incidence, followed by narrowing of focus to the few history, exam, and other findings that are highly diagnostic.

A list of frameworks and coaching exercises to promote effective HDDG is provided below.

Table 8.1. Cognitive Frameworks for Exploration of the Chief Concern

OPQRST	**COLDERAS**
Onset: When did the symptom start? Was it sudden or gradual? **Provocation/Palliation**: What makes it worse or better? **Quality**: What does it feel like (e.g., sharp, dull, burning)? **Radiation**: Does the pain move to other areas? **Severity**: On a scale of 0 to 10, how severe is it? **Timing**: Is it constant or intermittent? Does it follow a pattern?	**Character**: Describe the symptom. **Onset**: When did it start? **Location**: Where is it? **Duration**: How long does it last? **Exacerbating factors**: What worsens it? **Relieving factors**: What helps? **Associated symptoms**: Any other symptoms? **Severity**: How bad is it?
FARCOLDER	**OLDCARTS**
Frequency: How often do the symptoms occur? **Associated symptoms**: Are there other accompanying symptoms? **Radiation**: Does the symptom spread or move to another area? **Character**: What is the symptom like (e.g., sharp, dull, throbbing)? **Onset**: When did the symptom start? Was it sudden or gradual? **Location**: Where is the symptom located? **Duration**: How long does the symptom last? **Exacerbating factors**: What makes it worse? **Relieving factors**: What makes it better?	**Onset**: When did it begin? **Location**: Where is it located? Does it radiate? **Duration**: How long has it lasted? **Character**: What is the nature of the symptom? **Aggravating factors**: What worsens it? **Relieving factors**: What improves it? **Timing**: Does it occur at specific times? **Severity**: How severe is it?

THE HIGHLIGHTER EXERCISE

This exercise assists the learner in identifying the defining and discriminating features of a case.[28,51] The coach gives the learner an unfamiliar patient note. While reading the note, the learner highlights findings that are pertinent—positive or negative—in one color and highlights irrelevant or less important information in another color. The learner is prompted to think aloud, describing the predictive nature of a given finding and how this iteratively changes their differential diagnosis.

Example:

PATIENT NOTE

CC: "I've had a cough for three weeks."

History of Present Illness:

The patient is a 45-year-old male with a three-week history of a productive cough. He reports yellow-green sputum and occasional streaks of blood. There is no associated chest pain or shortness of breath. The patient denies fever or chills and has had occasional night sweats. He mentions feeling generally tired after work, especially on busy days. His neighbor recently adopted a cat, but he has not been in close contact with it. He also states he recently switched to decaffeinated coffee and isn't sure if that's causing his fatigue. He smokes one pack of cigarettes daily for the past 20 years.

Past Medical History:

- Hypertension
- No history of asthma or chronic obstructive pulmonary disease (COPD)

Medications:

- Lisinopril 10 mg daily
- Over-the-counter antacids as needed

Family History:

- Father with lung cancer diagnosed at age 65

Social History:

- Works as a construction worker
- Reports exposure to asbestos in older buildings

Physical Exam:

- Vital signs: BP 125/85, HR 78, Temp 98.6ºF, SpO2 98% on room air
- Lungs: Crackles in the right lower lobe
- No wheezes or stridor
- Skin: No rashes

EXAMPLE COACHING QUESTIONS

How does the highlighted positive predictive value of "crackles in the right lower lobe" shape your initial working diagnosis?

How does the absence of fever and shortness of breath change your prioritization of potential causes?

THE NEMERGUT-SACCO SQUARE

This exercise calls for deliberate consideration of typical and atypical presentations of disease, both common and uncommon. Learners are given a chief complaint and asked to complete a 2 x 2 table.

CC: 30-year-old female in the emergency department with "trouble catching my breath"

	Typical Presentation	Atypical Presentation
Common Disease	• Asthma • Viral upper respiratory infection (URI) • Pneumonia • Panic attack / Anxiety	• Pregnancy • GERD
Uncommon Disease	• Pulmonary embolism • Pertussis • Anaphylaxis • Vocal cord dysfunction • Pulmonary edema • Anemia • Pneumothorax	• Encephalitis • Glycogen storage disease • Myasthenic crisis • Cardiac tamponade

Coaches can emphasize multiple teaching points:

Green: "Bread and butter" diagnoses for a given CC. Always rule them in or out first.

Blue: High potential for diagnostic error. The condition is common, but the patient does not have the classic constellation of symptoms.

Yellow: These are do-not-miss entities. They may be less prevalent, but if presenting in typical fashion they must be considered.

Red: Rare diagnoses with unusual manifestations. Keep them in mind when nothing else fits or if specific risk factors are present.

SEARCH FOR SCRIPTS [28,30]

Building on our prior discussion, this coaching exercise focuses on prioritization. The coach asks the learner to list two to three history questions and one exam finding relevant to each potential diagnosis. Search for Scripts reinforces the link between hypothesis generation and data gathering, encouraging purposeful data collection. Coach and learner are encouraged to then look up the likelihood ratio for each history and exam finding and reflect on their diagnostic power. The Rational Clinical Examination series and McGee's Evidence Based Physical Exam serve as excellent resources for researching likelihood ratios.[52–54]

PLAYING THE ROLE [28,30]

In this exercise, the learner assumes the role of the patient and practices "convincing" the coach of a specific diagnosis, focusing on presenting relevant clinical information. Playing the Role helps the learner recognize the most pertinent details in supporting or refuting diagnoses. The coach should set a time limit for this exercise (e.g., 30 seconds).

Example: Coach provides the diagnosis of acute heart failure with reduced ejection fraction.

> **Learner**: *I am a 65-year-old male who presents with shortness of breath when I am walking (dyspnea on exertion). I am having trouble just walking to the bathroom after previously being able to walk longer distances. My hands and feet are always cold (cold extremities). I am struggling to sleep as I feel like I'm drowning when I lie flat (orthopnea) and am waking up in the middle of the night gasping for air (paroxysmal nocturnal dyspnea [PND]). My legs are so swollen by the end of the day that I can't put on my shoes (peripheral edema). On exam, I have swollen neck veins (jugular venous distension), crackling sounds in the lungs (pulmonary rales/crackles), and a third-heart sound (S3 gallop).*

HORIZONTAL READING [1,28,30]

This exercise promotes knowledge organization or reorganization in a manner that facilitates retrieval. Struggling learners are asked to research a specific chief concern (rather than a disease or illness) and compare key features of the most common diseases related to that concern. This approach is contrasted with the more traditional assignment of reading about an isolated disease process. Horizontal Reading has the added benefit of combating premature closure and prepares the learner for a greater focus on cross-referencing, discussed later in the hypothesis refinement section. In chapter 9, we consider further application of this symptom-based approach to learning.

Example:

CC: Sore throat

	Diagnosis 1	Diagnosis 2	Diagnosis 3
Risk factors			
Pathophysiology			
Typical symptoms			
Typical signs			

KEY FEATURES[30]

Key features are defined as the "specific and essential elements critical to the resolution of the problem."[55] The coach uses the following script to ask for key features across a range of clinical cases. The strength in this approach lies in the contrast between prototypical cases and variations from the prototype.

1. Select a clinical problem (and an age group).
2. What are the critical steps in the resolution of this problem (for patients in this age group)?"
3. Think of examples—specifically, patients who present in different ways with this same problem.
4. List the key features for these patients, some that will be unique to specific patients, others that will be common across patients.

UNCERTAINTY TRACKING

The coach guides the learner through a clinical case, pausing at key moments to have them assess and articulate their level of diagnostic uncertainty. Before any data is gathered, the coach asks the learner to describe their broad diagnostic considerations and rate their uncertainty on a 1 to 100 scale, with 100 representing maximum uncertainty. As the learner progresses through history-taking, the coach intermittently pauses to ask, "Where are you on the uncertainty scale now? What data have you gathered that moved the number up or down?" With each new piece of information, whether from the physical exam, lab results, or imaging, the coach continues to prompt reflection by asking questions: What's your current uncertainty level? Which diagnoses have gained or lost probability? As they approach a working diagnosis, the learner is challenged to identify the next piece of data that would drive their uncertainty as close to zero as possible. By tracking uncertainty numerically, learners develop a more structured approach to HDDG, prioritizing high-yield questions and avoiding unnecessary information overload.

PROBLEM REPRESENTATION

We now turn our attention to problem representation, commonly defined as the mental characterization of a patient's medical conditions that a clinician develops during the patient encounter.[1,56] The problem representation combines the situational or contextual information about the patient with the clinician's knowledge to create a structured and actionable description of the problem at hand.[38,57] This term is commonly confused with the summary statement, which is the contextualized synthesis of the patient's problem that occurs *after* the patient encounter.[58] Strictly speaking, the problem representation is an unconscious cognitive ability and is therefore difficult to elucidate and teach.[1(p200)] Though the framework we provide in chapters 6 and 7 suggest a linear process, problem representations actually develop iteratively (and quite early in the reasoning process) as data is gathered. When effective, they activate illness scripts, generating new diagnostic hypotheses or comparing and contrasting with previously generated hypotheses.

Connor and Dhaliwal propose a cyclic method of iterative, focused oral presentations and coach feedback based in deliberate practice.[59] One important aspect of this exercise is ensuring that learner and coach understand and employ a basic problem representation structure that includes defining the patient's condition in abstract terms with patient demographics, relevant medical history, syndrome description, and time course. Key to this process is medical vocabulary or learning how to talk like a clinician.[38] More specifically, effective problem representation relies on the learner's ability to convert the patient's words into a conceptualization of the problem using semantic qualifiers, assigning meaning to the case features through temporal and causal relationships.[60] Semantic qualifiers are adjectives or adverbs, usually paired and opposing, that succinctly build this "global sense of the problem."[37] Accordingly, learners struggling with problem representation are commonly described as "missing the big picture" or "not seeing the forest for the trees."

It is critical that the coach understands what makes a good problem representation. Data abstraction and semantic description are key,[61] and an effective problem representation avoids excessive detail, highlighting key features that differentiate among possible diagnoses. When summarized aloud or in written form, the problem representation can facilitate clear communication with other clinicians (e.g., oral presentations, handoffs, calling consults). Research suggests that experts include fewer irrelevant comorbidities and more pertinent examination findings compared to novices.[62] Experts are also more likely to encapsulate clinical data into higher-order terms (e.g., sepsis) rather than listing individual symptoms or findings.[62] While studies on its impact on improving diagnostic accuracy yield mixed results, likely given the confounding nature of other clinical reasoning processes, experts recommend scaffolding the problem representation in a three-part structure (demographics, temporal course, and clinical syndrome) and including temporal semantic qualifiers.[63] Suggested coaching exercises for learners who struggle in this area are provided below.

QUALIFYING OR DESCRIPTIVE SEMANTIC QUALIFIERS?[64]

In this exercise, the coach asks the learner to verbalize their problem representation at various points in the evolution of the case, then provides feedback on the quality of the semantic qualifiers. More specifically, the coach comments on whether the qualifiers transcend description of the problem and assist with distinguishing between diagnostic hypotheses. Table 8.2 reveals commonly used semantic qualifiers.

Table 8.2. Commonly Used Semantic Qualifiers

Category		
Timing	Acute	Chronic
Progression	Worsening	Improving
Location	Proximal	Distal
Laterality	Unilateral	Contralateral
Quality	Sharp	Dull
Associated factors	Post-prandial	Fasting-associated
Color	Pale	Jaundiced
Consistency	Soft	Firm
Bleeding	Bright red	Dark/tarry
Systemic involvement	Localized	Diffuse

SEMANTIC TRANSFORMATION[38]

In this exercise, the learner converts patient language into problem representations with a focus on semantic qualifiers. The coach provides feedback on structure and the quality of semantic transformation. See examples below.

Patient Phrase	Problem Representation
"For the past three days, I've been experiencing fever with chills and sweating that come and go, mostly at night, and I feel extremely fatigued."	Acute onset fever with intermittent chills and night sweats accompanied by severe fatigue
"Whenever I walk up the stairs or carry something heavy, I feel a squeezing pressure in the center of my chest, which lasts a few minutes."	Exertional, episodic substernal chest pressure

(continued)

Patient Phrase	Problem Representation
"I've been coughing constantly, and it feels worse at night. My phlegm is thick, yellowish, and sometimes streaked with blood."	Persistent nocturnal productive cough with blood-tinged sputum
"Every afternoon, around the same time, I develop a throbbing headache that starts behind my eyes and worsens with bright lights or loud noises."	Recurrent retro-orbital throbbing headache with associated photophobia and phonophobia
"I woke up with pain in my lower right abdomen that gets worse when I move or press on it. It feels like a knife. I also feel nauseous and can't eat."	Sudden onset sharp, stabbing abdominal pain exacerbated by movement with associated nausea

WHO, WHAT, AND WHEN?[65,66]

In this exercise, the coach uses the Who, What, and When framework as a scaffold to support the learner's verbalized or documented problem representation and give feedback.

Who: Epidemiology/risk factors for disease
What: Key/differentiating features of the clinical syndrome
When: Time course/pattern/tempo

Example: A 55-year-old male presents to the emergency department with shortness of breath and chest discomfort. He reports occasional knee pain from an old sports injury, had a dental cleaning last week, and feels stressed at work. He denies fever or recent upper respiratory symptoms. His medical history includes hypertension and a remote appendectomy at age 25. He also notes that he smokes one pack per day and recently returned from a long flight.

Learner's Initial Problem Representation:

Who: A 55-year-old male with a history of hypertension, smoking, knee pain, a recent dental cleaning, stress, and a past appendectomy

What: Presents with shortness of breath, chest discomfort, occasional knee pain, and no fever or upper respiratory symptoms

When: Symptoms began suddenly 2 hours ago, after returning from a long flight

Coach Feedback: "Knee pain" and "recent dental cleaning" are unrelated to the acute presentation. "Stress at work" and "past appendectomy" are not pertinent to the current problem. These details dilute the focus on the relevant clinical information. Focus on the relevant demographics and risk factors (55-year-old male, history of smoking, recent long flight). Concentrate on the key clinical features (acute dyspnea, pleuritic chest pain). Emphasize the sudden onset and 2-hour timeframe.

Revised Problem Representation: A 55-year-old male with a history of smoking and recent long flight presenting with acute onset of pleuritic chest pain and dyspnea

A-SOAP[28,67]

This exercise asks the learner to begin their patient presentations with the assessment as opposed to the more traditional SOAP (subjective, objective, assessment, plan) format, priming them to organize and select details that support the big picture. A-SOAP also prompts the coach to provide feedback on the inclusion of relevant data and order in which they are provided.

HYPOTHESIS REFINEMENT

Hypothesis refinement refers to the revision of the differential diagnosis in response to emerging data. This process requires learners to balance flexibility and decisiveness (diagnostic accuracy with efficiency), adapting their reasoning without overreacting to minor changes. Refinement requires critical evaluation of findings to determine their impact on the likelihood of each diagnosis. Given the broad nature of the early differential diagnosis, hypothesis refinement is typically characterized by narrowing and prioritization. The revision process is reliant on the problem representation, as data abstraction allows one to compare and contrast the most pertinent aspects of the patient's presentation with stored illness scripts, iteratively narrowing the number of scripts considered as more data is gathered. It is worth noting that this is not always the case for more complex cases or those with unexpected pivot points. Figure 8.2 highlights the relationship between early components of the clinical reasoning process and displays how the differential diagnosis changes over time from an initially broad list of hypotheses to fewer and fewer options. Of course, hypotheses may also disappear to reappear later in the data gathering process, and new hypotheses may be generated during data gathering.

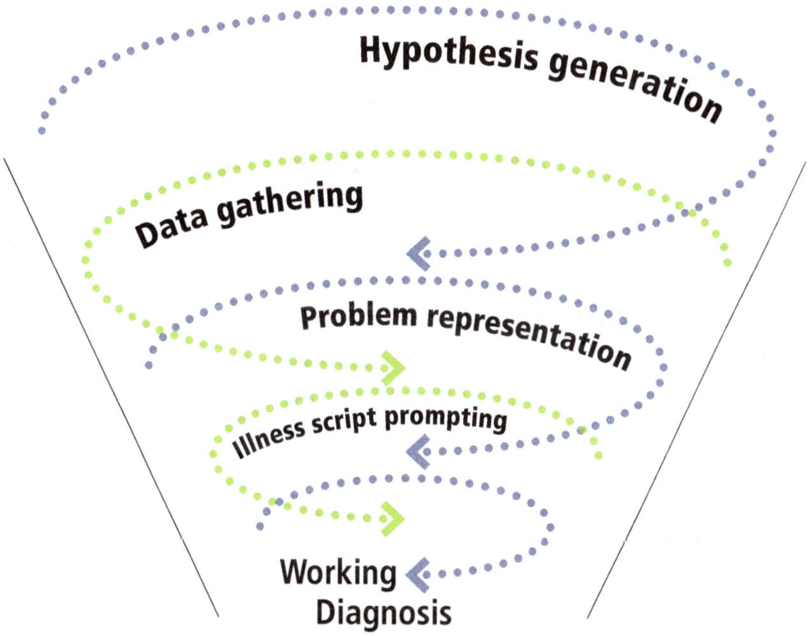

Figure 8.2. The Relationship Between Early Components of the Clinical Reasoning Process and How These Change Over Time

To improve hypothesis refinement, we suggest the coach promote causal reasoning and employ structured reflection. Causal reasoning is the cognitive process of identifying the cause-and-effect relationships between clinical variables.[68] It involves integrating knowledge of pathophysiology to determine how a patient's clinical presentation might be explained by the diagnosis being considered. For example, a patient presenting with dyspnea, orthopnea, and lower extremity edema may trigger recognition of heart failure based on pattern recognition. However, causal reasoning pushes the clinician to ask: What is driving the heart failure? Is it due to longstanding hypertension leading to diastolic dysfunction? Is there an ischemic component? Could it be from an undiagnosed arrhythmia or valvular disease? Remember, we emphasized probabilistic reasoning early in the clinical reasoning process. However, now we are focused on hypothesis refinement; causal reasoning can provide more evidence that our working diagnosis may be correct.[11]

In addition to causal reasoning, deliberate structured reflection is an ideal practice for hypothesis refinement. Mamede and colleagues have published an extensive library of evidence supporting the use of structured reflection to improve diagnostic accuracy.[9,69–73] In the case of hypothesis refinement, structured reflection can promote contrast between diagnostic hypotheses, assessment of fit, and diagnostic verification. Suggested coaching exercises are provided below.

CAUSAL TABLE

Learners complete the table below for each diagnosis being considered. The coach prompts a discussion as to how each condition leads to each clinical finding. What are the physiological or biochemical pathways that support each connection?

	Diagnosis 1	Diagnosis 2	Diagnosis 3
What is the underlying pathophysiologic process that explains these symptoms?			
Does this diagnosis fully explain all clinical findings? If not, what is missing?			
Given your analysis, how likely is this diagnosis compared to the others?			

PIVOT AND CLUSTER STRATEGY[74,75]

This approach promotes the recall of most likely diagnoses in a block, or cluster, to improve pattern recognition, thereby decreasing cognitive load and facilitating more efficient data gathering. After the coach provides the chief concern, the learner places each diagnosis in a cluster led by the "pivot" disease—that is, those diseases that the learner thinks of intuitively using pattern recognition. Taking a pause, the learner identifies a cluster of diagnoses, related by similar clinical manifestations, for each "pivot" diagnosis.

For a more advanced exercise, the coach asks the learner to map each cluster, placing each pivot disease in the center of a circle and spacing cluster diagnoses around the pivot disease based on the degree to which they share key features of the clinical presentation.

Pivot Disease	Cluster Diagnoses	Key Features
Pancreatitis	Gallstone pancreatitis, alcoholic pancreatitis, autoimmune pancreatitis, gastric ulcer, duodenal ulcer, cholecystitis, biliary colic, choledocholithiasis	Epigastric or RUQ pain (can radiate to back or shoulder), nausea, vomiting, lipase/amylase elevation, steatorrhea (chronic cases), Murphy's sign, jaundice and elevated ALP, pain associated with eating
Iron deficiency anemia	Thalassemia, anemia of chronic disease, lead poisoning, vitamin B12 deficiency	Fatigue, pallor, glossitis, pica, low ferritin, microcytic hypochromic RBCs, reactive thrombocytosis
Autoimmune hemolytic anemia	hereditary spherocytosis, paroxysmal nocturnal hemoglobinuria, sickle cell disease, G6PD deficiency	Jaundice, hemoglobinuria, splenomegaly, reticulocytosis, Coombs-positive/negative distinction, extravascular vs intravascular hemolysis features
Myasthenia gravis	Lambert-Eaton syndrome, botulism, Guillain-Barré syndrome, stroke	Fluctuating muscle weakness, ptosis, dysphagia, worsens with exertion (MG) vs improves with use (Lambert-Eaton), negative reflexes (Guillain-Barré), respiratory involvement (botulism)

SCRIPT SORT [28,30]

In this exercise, the coach asks the learner to create a table in which a narrowed list of diagnoses is compared by their overlapping symptoms or signs. For each symptom or sign, the learner places a **+**, **++**, or **+++** depending on the predictiveness of each feature. This allows the learner to analyze each diagnosis in relation to another. See an example below.

Symptom	Pneumonia	Heart Failure	Pulmonary Embolism
Cough	+++	+	+
Shortness of breath (dyspnea)	+	+++	++
Pleuritic chest pain	+++	+	++
Fever	+++	+	+
Productive sputum	+++	+	+

(continued)

(Script Sort continued)

Symptom	Pneumonia	Heart Failure	Pulmonary Embolism
Crackles on lung exam	+++	++	+
Orthopnea	+	+++	+
Paroxysmal nocturnal dyspnea	+	+++	+
Leg swelling (unilateral)	+	+	+++
Hemoptysis	+	+	+++
Tachycardia	+	++	+++
Hypoxia	++	+++	+++
Weight gain/edema	+	+++	+

JUSTIFICATION THINK-ALOUD [67]

Here, the coach asks the learner to briefly summarize the case, then share a prioritized differential diagnosis and commit to the leading diagnosis. The learner articulates their justification for this diagnosis and explains why the alternatives are less likely. As part of the feedback process, the coach role models their process of prioritizing.

COMMON VERSUS CAN'T MISS [67]

This coaching exercise is ideal for the learner who struggles with uncertainty and/or to identify the "can't miss" diagnosis. Though similar to Differential Diagnosis Checklists (introduced earlier to aid in the practice of hypothesis generation) the comparison aspect of this approach is most helpful for hypothesis refinement. For a given chief concern, the coach asks the learner to generate a differential diagnosis that includes a common disease for each "can't miss" disease they are considering. Coaching questions can then prompt the learner to weight the likelihood of each diagnosis based on the gathered data.

Chief Concern: Cough

Can't Miss	Common
Pulmonary embolism	Upper respiratory infection
Tuberculosis	Acute bronchitis

Can't Miss	Common
Lung cancer	Allergic rhinitis
Pneumonia	Postnasal drip
Acute heart failure	Gastroesophageal reflux disease
Severe COVID-19	Viral pneumonitis
Foreign body aspiration	Asthma

ASSESSMENT OF FIT[28]

Here, the coach asks the learner to list clinical data that align with the suspected diagnosis, data that don't fit, and data that are absent but would be expected given the suspected diagnosis. This reflective exercise, which can also be completed for a prioritized list of diagnoses, improves diagnostic accuracy for simple and complex patient presentations.[70]

Diagnosis (minimum 3)	Findings supporting	Findings opposing	Findings that would be expected but not seen
DX1:			
DX2:			
DX3:			
Other DX:			

DIFFERENTIATING VENN DIAGRAM [1,28]

In this exercise, the coach provides a Venn diagram with three diagnoses being considered by the learner. The learner is asked to place relevant signs and symptoms within the circles based on how unique a feature is to a specific illness (key feature) or to a subset of illnesses (differentiating feature). An example is below.

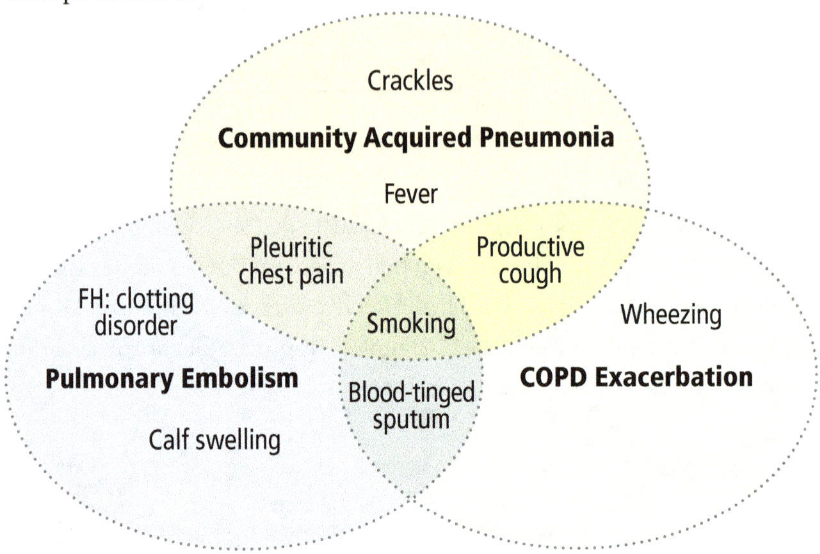

HYPOTHESIS-DRIVEN EXAM

Early learners and struggling learners frequently underutilize physical exam findings, which can be crucial for refining diagnostic hypotheses. Physical exam skills have declined in recent years with increasing reliance on technology and less time spent at the bedside.[76] Hypothesis-Driven Exam emphasizes the examination findings that can alter the likelihood of disease using likelihood ratios.[77] The coach asks the learner to reflect on which examination maneuvers would distinguish or differentiate among the diagnostic possibilities under consideration. The learner provides likelihood ratios to support their claims. We again direct the reader to the Rational Clinical Examination Series and McGee Evidence-Based Physical Diagnosis.[52–54] Thinking of history-taking as the sensitive (rule-out) approach and exam as the specific (confirm or rule-in) approach can be helpful here.[78] As an additional point of emphasis, the physical exam is more than a diagnostic tool; it plays a cultural role in building and maintaining the clinician-patient relationship.[77,79]

MANAGEMENT SCRIPT ACTIVATION

The first step in the management reasoning process (Figure 8.3) is management script activation.[80–82] A definition and introduction to management reasoning is provided in chapter 3. In contrast to diagnostic reasoning, which is inherently a classification task, management reasoning is a process of prioritization, selecting among multiple, usually reasonable, options.[83] For simple cases, management begins after a working diagnosis is identified. However, conceptually, problem representation is the starting point for management, activating a management script just as an illness script is activated in diagnostic reasoning. The management script includes all the possible courses of action a clinician may take (e.g., laboratory tests, imaging, monitoring, medications, procedures, specialty consults, and disposition planning). Management scripts are inherently idiosyncratic, based on a learner or clinician's prior knowledge and experience, and therefore include situational/contextual factors. However, for purposes of coaching, we recommend considering only the illness-specific or diagnosis-specific aspects of management in this first step. Situational and contextual factors are discussed below. In other words, coach and learner should consider the management script as the menu of all possible management options for a given clinical problem.[84,85]

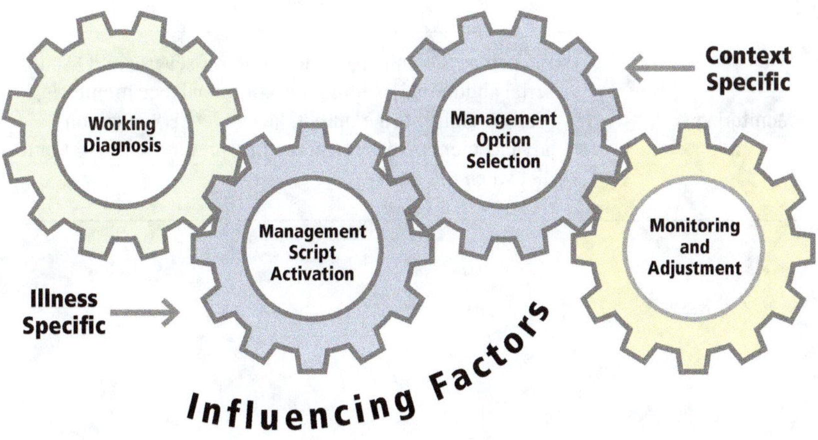

Figure 8.3. A Simplified Management Reasoning Process for Coaching Purposes

Management Script Template, Step 1[180,84]

In this exercise, the coach provides a scaffold for learners to outline management options based on a specific diagnosis (e.g., acute pancreatitis in the example below), including laboratory tests, imaging, procedures, specialists, medications, and monitoring. This scaffold serves as the menu of potential interventions for a given clinical presentation.

Types of Interventions	Script Activation
Laboratory Tests	Complete blood count (CBC), comprehensive metabolic panel (CMP) including liver function tests (LFTs) and electrolytes, serum lipase, serum amylase, C-reactive protein (CRP), serum lactate, arterial blood gas (ABG), serum triglycerides, serum calcium
Imaging	Abdominal ultrasound, computed tomography (CT) of the abdomen and pelvis with contrast, magnetic resonance cholangiopancreatography (MRCP)
Procedures	Endoscopic retrograde cholangiopancreatography (ERCP), paracentesis
Specialist Consultations	Gastroenterology, surgery, nutrition
Medications	Intravenous (IV) fluids (Lactated Ringer's), IV opioids (Fentanyl, Hydromorphone), antiemetics (Ondansetron, Promethazine), antibiotics (Carbapenems, Quinolones + Metronidazole, Piperacillin-Tazobactam), insulin therapy
Monitoring	Intensive care unit (ICU) admission if severe, NPO status, serial abdominal examinations, fluid balance monitoring (daily weights, urine output, lactate levels), nutrition advancement plan (enteral feeding preferred, low-fat oral diet when tolerated)

We suggest that the learner create scenario-based management script templates for commonly encountered clinical presentations. Script templates can be centered on patient chief concerns, abnormal laboratory values, abnormal imaging findings, or any combination thereof. It is helpful to stratify the scenarios based on learner level and clinical setting, prioritizing those most commonly encountered. The following is a representative tiered structure relevant to an inpatient internal medicine service:

Tier 1: Hypotension, hypoxia, tachycardia, chest pain, shortness of breath, fever, altered mental status, syncope/dizziness

Tier 2: AKI, abdominal pain, headache, anemia, hyponatremia, hyperkalemia, metabolic acidosis, nausea/vomiting, GIB (melena, hematochezia), headache, alcohol withdrawal, seizure, agitation, hypertensive emergency

Tier 3: Red/swollen extremity, back pain, cough, hemoptysis, rash, thrombocytopenia, acute liver injury, thrombosis, diarrhea, hyperglycemia, anxiety, fall

Tier 4: Hematuria/dysuria, eosinophilia, thrombocytosis

MANAGEMENT OPTION SELECTION

The second step in management reasoning—and the point at which management reasoning becomes more complex—is management option selection.[81] Because management is based in action and actually requires doing something to the patient, the stakes are now higher. Management reasoning requires explicit consideration of situation and context, prioritizing patient goals and system constraints and affordances.[82,83] For many conditions, clinicians can access practice guidelines or evidence-based recommendations for management. However, learners may struggle when a situation requires deviation from guidelines, which is a frequent occurrence, or when a patient doesn't "fit" the evidence. Management option selection requires consideration of many factors, summarized in Figure 8.4, that influence a learner's threshold to enact a management intervention. The coach is encouraged to use these influencing factors as a springboard for discussions about which management interventions are selected from the learner's initial menu (script) and why. Inherent to this process is a risk/benefit analysis that influences a learner's threshold to test and/or treat.[86,87] Coaching exercises are provided below.

Rapid Evaluation Assessmen

Essential Tasks

Learner Function	Specified Task
Collecting • **Data gathering** *—recognition of urgent or emergent clinical scenario*	• **Collect/Report** history and exam data in hypothesis-directed manner • **Recognize** patient and disease specific factors as potential etiologies of decompensation • **Recognize** severity of clinical problem and contextual signs of urgency or emergency
Interpreting • **Diagnostic reasoning** *—differential diagnosis*	• **Generate** prioritized differential diagnosis of most likely, less likely, unlikely in urgent clinical situations
Management • **Management reasoning** *—initial management option selection* *—response to dynamic information*	• **Direct** evaluation and treatment towards high priority diagnoses • **Initiate** management in patient with urgent decompensation • **Recognize** need to escalate patient care
Communicating • **Patient-centered care** *—communicate care plan and goals of care* *—achieve a shared mental model*	• **Communicate** with health care team members according to role and responsibility to improve task efficiency • **Maintain** focus and two-way communication with patient or surrogate decision-maker in urgent clinical situations
Reflecting • **Metacognition** *—reflection of urgent or emergent clinical scenarios*	• **Demonstrate** the ability to think about one's own thinking (metacognition) in urgent clinical situations • **Mitigate** cognitive tendencies or emotional/situational factors influencing clinical decision making
Overall score _____ /15	

Figure 8.4. Factors Influencing the Selection of Management Options (Graphic created using Markmap https://markmap.js.org/.)

f Clinical Reasoning Tool (REACT)

Assessment of Behaviors

Assessment		
❍ Non-focused history and exam ❍ Included extraneous information ❍ Missed key findings ❍ Did not recognize contextual clues of urgency	❍ History and exam reflect potential diagnoses ❍ Limited recognition of urgent contextual clues ❍ Included limited pertinent positive and negative findings	❍ Logical history and exam for potential diagnoses ❍ Questions assessed likelihood of specific diagnoses ❍ Full recognition of urgency contextual clues ❍ Prioritization on pertinent positive and negative findings
❍ Differential diagnosis missing likely or "can't miss" diagnoses in urgent situations ❍ Includes inappropriate diagnoses	❍ Differential diagnosis included likely and "can't miss" diagnoses in urgent situations but missed key diagnoses ❍ Inappropriate rank-order of diagnoses	❍ Accurately ranked differential diagnosis including key, likely, and "can't miss" diagnoses in urgent situations ❍ Prioritized urgent diagnoses appropriately
❍ Direct evaluation and treatment towards high priority diagnoses ❍ Initiate management in patient with urgent decompensation ❍ Recognize need to escalate patient care	❍ Major focus of evaluation and treatment on likely and urgent diagnoses ❍ Included non-essential testing ❍ Evaluated for response to initial management plan	❍ Efficiently directed management towards most likely and urgent diagnoses ❍ Deferred tests directed towards less likely or less important diagnoses ❍ Evaluated for response to initial interventions
❍ Did not engage health care team members ❍ Did not communicate care plan with patient/family ❍ Did not clarify patient's goals of care	❍ Limited engagement of health care team members to improve task efficiency ❍ Limited effort to communicate with patient/family but used medical jargon or failed to ensure understanding ❍ Limited clarification of patient's goals of care	❍ Fully engaged health care team members according to role and responsibility to improve task efficiency in urgent situation ❍ Effectively communicated care plan with patient/family and ensured understanding ❍ Effective clarification of patient's goals of care
❍ Unaware of cognitive tendencies or emotional/situational factors that may have influenced decision-making ❍ Unable to mitigate cognitive tendencies or emotional/situational factors	❍ Limited awareness of cognitive tendencies or emotional/situational factors that may have influenced decision-making ❍ Limited mitigation of cognitive tendencies or emotional/situational factors	❍ Full awareness of cognitive tendency or emotional/situational factors that may influence decision-making ❍ Effectively mitigates reactions to urgent clinical situations
1 point	2 points	3 points

Management Script Template, Step II[80,84]

In this exercise, the learner builds on the illness-specific management options provided earlier. The learner is asked to justify which management options are selected for the patient at hand. The coach prompts the learner to reference specific influencing factors (from Figure 8.4) in their decision to enact or not enact specific management interventions. The example below continues the acute pancreatitis example.

Types of Interventions	Script Activation	Influencing Factors	Selected Management Option for this Patient
Laboratory Tests	Complete blood count (CBC), comprehensive metabolic panel (CMP), liver function tests (LFTs), electrolytes, serum lipase, serum amylase, C-reactive protein (CRP), serum lactate, arterial blood gas (ABG), serum triglycerides, serum calcium		CBC, CMP, Lipase, LFTs
Imaging	Abdominal ultrasound, computed tomography (CT) abdomen/pelvis with contrast, magnetic resonance cholangiopancreatography (MRCP)		Abdominal Ultrasound
Procedures	Endoscopic retrograde cholangiopancreatography (ERCP), paracentesis		None for now
Specialist Consultations	Gastroenterology consultation, surgery consultation, nutrition consultation		Gastroenterology Consultation
Medications	Intravenous (IV) fluids (Lactated Ringer's), IV opioids (Fentanyl, Hydromorphone), antiemetics (Ondansetron, Promethazine), antibiotics (only if infection suspected), insulin therapy (for triglyceride-induced pancreatitis)		IV fluids, pain control, NPO status
Monitoring and Supportive Care	Intensive care unit (ICU) admission (if severe), serial abdominal examinations, fluid balance monitoring (daily weights, urine output, lactate levels), nutrition advancement plan (enteral feeding preferred)		NPO with planned transition to enteral feeding

MANAGEMENT PAUSE [84,85]

This coaching exercise serves as a reflective tool to assess the quality of proposed management actions with respect to value and shared decision-making and can also be used as a cognitive forcing function to promote analytic reasoning.

1. Why are we choosing this intervention for this patient?
2. What are the potential downsides?
3. What are potential alternatives and why aren't we choosing them?
4. Have we asked the patient for their perspective?

EQUITY REFLECTION[84,85]

Like the Management Pause, this exercise, developed by Dr. Emily Abdoler, encourages reflection on the quality of proposed management actions with respect to equity and can similarly be used as a cognitive forcing function. Equity Reflection asks the learner: Would you choose this management plan for you or your family members if you were in the same situation? If not, what would you want done differently, and why aren't we doing that here? Are there system or patient factors that led to this decision? If so, are there ways you could address these factors?

1. Are we deviating in any way from the standard of care in this situation?
2. If so, in what ways are we deviating? Why are we deviating?
3. Instead of deviating, what could we do differently to ensure we are providing the highest value care?

HIGHLIGHTER, REVISITED[67]

In this exercise, the coach provides the learner with a case accompanied by a management-specific question (e.g., Should this patient be admitted to the hospital or return home to follow-up in clinic? Should this patient be admitted to an acute-care floor or the intensive care unit? Should this patient receive this medication or an alternative medication? Should this patient be placed on telemetry or is an initial ECG sufficient?). The learner highlights key pieces of data that support each decision, then reflects on the most appropriate management decision(s).

HOW CAN AI HELP?

As introduced in chapter 3, generative artificial intelligence (AI) can enhance the targeted coaching of clinical reasoning deficits described in this chapter. Through pattern analysis, AI identifies specific reasoning deficits, such as struggles with HDDG or hypothesis refinement. For example, AI tools can detect when a learner asks irrelevant history questions, overlooks critical diagnostic information, or fails to test hypotheses effectively, thus providing granular feedback that allows both coach and learner to focus on targeted areas for improvement. Importantly, any of the coaching exercises provided in this chapter can be converted into AI prompts, allowing for flexible implementation based on coach and learner needs. AI can then gradually increase case difficulty, acknowledging content specificity and the developmental nature of competency.

Dynamic AI-generated cases can enrich coaching by exposing learners to a range of scenarios, including atypical presentations, while simulating the complexities of real-world clinical environments. For instance, cases can incorporate resource limitations, simulate interprofessional interactions, or introduce unexpected diagnostic findings to challenge and refine learners' reasoning processes. This adaptability can help learners practice applying their reasoning across diverse contexts. Finally, coaches can benefit from AI-generated structured progress reports that summarize performance, highlight specific areas for growth, and recommend actionable next steps.

The coaching exercises introduced in this chapter are summarized in Table 8.3.

Table 8.3. Micro Skills Coaching Exercises

Early hypothesis generation
• Anatomy • Pathophysiology • Systems • Worst-case scenarios • Pretest probability • Qualitative Bayes theorem • Differential diagnosis checklists

Table 8.3. Micro Skills Coaching Exercises *(continued)*

Hypothesis-driven data gathering

- Frameworks to guide learners in focused exploration of the chief concern
  — OPQRST, COLDERAS, FARCOLDER, OLDCARTS
- Highlighter exercise
- Search for scripts
- Playing the role
- Horizontal reading
- Key features
- Uncertainty tracking

Problem representation

- Qualifying or descriptive semantic qualifiers?
- Semantic transformation
- Who, what, and why?
- A-SOAP

Hypothesis refinement

- Causal table
- Pivot and cluster strategy
- Script sort
- Justification think-aloud
- Common vs can't miss
- Assessment of fit
- Differentiating Venn diagram
- Hypothesis-driven exam

Management script activation

- Management script template, Step I

Management option selection

- Management script template, Step II
- Management pause
- Equity reflection
- Highlighter, revisited

SUMMARY

The micro skill coaching framework outlined in this chapter provides a structured approach for addressing clinical reasoning struggles. A granular focus on the cognitive processes of reasoning (early hypothesis generation, hypothesis-driven data gathering, problem representation, hypothesis refinement, and management reasoning) allows coaches to pinpoint the exact area(s) of struggle and thus individualize the intervention. The case-based approach facilitates the development of scripts and schema while the reflective activities ensure that learners can apply reasoning strategies systematically, promoting graduate development and honing of pattern recognition. The exercises in this chapter lend themselves equally well to simulated and authentic clinical environments, and for most, we recommend that coaching begins in a structured, non-clinical setting. Eventually, all clinical reasoning coaching must occur in the authentic clinical environment to capture the challenges of real-time patient care.

References

1. Bowen JL. Educational Strategies to Promote Clinical Diagnostic Reasoning. *N Engl J Med.* 2006;355(21):2217-2225. doi:10.1056/NEJMra054782
2. Cammarata M, Dhaliwal G. Diagnostic Schemas: Form and Function. *J Gen Intern Med.* 2023;38(2):513-516. doi:10.1007/s11606-022-07935-1
3. LeClair RJ, Cleveland JL, Eden K, Binks AP. An integrated pre-clerkship curriculum to build cognitive medical schema: It's not just about the content. *Front Physiol.* 2023;14:1148916. doi:10.3389/fphys.2023.1148916
4. Warburton KM, Goren E, Dine CJ. Comprehensive Assessment of Struggling Learners Referred to a Graduate Medical Education Remediation Program. *J Grad Med Educ.* 2017;9(6):763-767. doi:10.4300/JGME-D-17-00175.1
5. Parsons AS, Dreicer JJ, Martindale JR, Young G, Warburton KM. A Targeted Clinical Reasoning Remediation Program for Residents and Fellows in Need. *J Grad Med Educ.* 2024;16(4):469. doi:10.4300/JGME-D-23-00822.1
6. ten Cate O, Custers EJFM, Durning SJ, eds. *Principles and Practice of Case-Based Clinical Reasoning Education: A Method for Preclinical Students.* Springer; 2018. Accessed January 16, 2025. http://www.ncbi.nlm.nih.gov/books/NBK543760/
7. Moon SH, Myung SJ, Yoon HB, Park JB, Kim JW, Park WB. Deliberate Practice as an Effective Remediation Strategy for Underperforming Medical Students Focused on Clinical Skills: a Prospective Longitudinal Study. *J Korean Med Sci.* 2019;34(11):e84. doi:10.3346/jkms.2019.34.e84

8. Staal J, Waechter J, Allen J, Lee CH, Zwaan L. Deliberate practice of diagnostic clinical reasoning reveals low performance and improvement of diagnostic justification in pre-clerkship students. *BMC Med Educ.* 2023;23(1):684. doi:10.1186/s12909-023-04541-5

9. Mamede S, Schmidt HG. Deliberate reflection and clinical reasoning: Founding ideas and empirical findings. *Med Educ.* 2023;57(1):76-85. doi:10.1111/medu.14863

10. McGaghie WC, Issenberg SB, Cohen ER, Barsuk JH, Wayne DB. Medical Education Featuring Mastery Learning With Deliberate Practice Can Lead to Better Health for Individuals and Populations. *Acad Med.* 2011;86(11):e8. doi:10.1097/ACM.0b013e3182308d37

11. Jerome P. Kassirer. *Learning Clinical Reasoning.* Wolters Kluwer Lippincott Williams & Wilkins Health; 2010. Accessed February 13, 2025. http://archive.org/details/learningclinical00kass

12. Smith ER, DeCoster J. Dual-Process Models in Social and Cognitive Psychology: Conceptual Integration and Links to Underlying Memory Systems. *Personal Soc Psychol Rev.* 2000;4(2):108-131. doi:10.1207/S15327957PSPR0402_01

13. Custers EJFM. Thirty years of illness scripts: Theoretical origins and practical applications. *Med Teach.* 2015;37(5):457-462. doi:10.3109/0142159X.2014.956052

14. Thalmann M, Souza AS, Oberauer K. How does chunking help working memory? *J Exp Psychol Learn Mem Cogn.* 2019;45(1):37-55. doi:10.1037/xlm0000578

15. Kostopoulou O, Lionis C, Angelaki A, Ayis S, Durbaba S, Delaney BC. Early diagnostic suggestions improve accuracy of family physicians: a randomized controlled trial in Greece. *Fam Pract.* 2015;32(3):323-328. doi:10.1093/fampra/cmv012

16. Kostopoulou O, Rosen A, Round T, Wright E, Douiri A, Delaney B. Early diagnostic suggestions improve accuracy of GPs: a randomised controlled trial using computer-simulated patients. *Br J Gen Pract J R Coll Gen Pract.* 2015;65(630):e49-54. doi:10.3399/bjgp15X683161

17. Sirota M, Kostopoulou O, Round T, Samaranayaka S. Prevalence and alternative explanations influence cancer diagnosis: An experimental study with physicians. *Health Psychol Off J Div Health Psychol Am Psychol Assoc.* 2017;36(5):477-485. doi:10.1037/hea0000461

18. Graber ML, Franklin N, Gordon R. Diagnostic error in internal medicine. *Arch Intern Med.* 2005;165(13):1493-1499. doi:10.1001/archinte.165.13.1493

19. Schiff GD, Hasan O, Kim S, et al. Diagnostic error in medicine: analysis of 583 physician-reported errors. *Arch Intern Med.* 2009;169(20):1881-1887. doi:10.1001/archinternmed.2009.333

20. Sisson JC, Donnelly MB, Hess GE, Woolliscroft JO. The characteristics of early diagnostic hypotheses generated by physicians (experts) and students (novices) at one medical school. *Acad Med.* 1991;66(10):607.

21. Coderre S, Wright B, McLaughlin K. To Think Is Good: Querying an Initial Hypothesis Reduces Diagnostic Error in Medical Students. *Acad Med.* 2010;85(7):1125. doi:10.1097/ACM.0b013e3181e1b229

22. Braun LT, Zwaan L, Kiesewetter J, Fischer MR, Schmidmaier R. Diagnostic errors by medical students: results of a prospective qualitative study. *BMC Med Educ.* 2017;17(1):191. doi:10.1186/s12909-017-1044-7

23. Eva KW, Hatala RM, Leblanc VR, Brooks LR. Teaching from the clinical reasoning literature: combined reasoning strategies help novice diagnosticians overcome misleading information. *Med Educ.* 2007;41(12):1152-1158. doi:10.1111/j.1365-2923.2007.02923.x

24. Noguchi Y, Matsui K, Imura H, Kiyota M, Fukui T. Quantitative evaluation of the diagnostic thinking process in medical students. *J Gen Intern Med.* 2002;17(11):839-844. doi:10.1046/j.1525-1497.2002.20139.x

25. Probabilistic reasoning in clinical medicine: Problems and opportunities. In: *Judgment under Uncertainty: Heuristics and Biases.* Cambridge University Press; 1982:249-267. doi:10.1017/CBO9780511809477.019

26. Aberegg SK, Callahan SJ. Common things are common, but what is common? Incorporating probability information into differential diagnosis. *J Eval Clin Pract.* 2022;28(6):1213-1217. doi:10.1111/jep.13636

27. Brush JE, Lee M, Sherbino J, Taylor-Fishwick JC, Norman G. Effect of Teaching Bayesian Methods Using Learning by Concept vs Learning by Example on Medical Students' Ability to Estimate Probability of a Diagnosis. *JAMA Netw Open.* 2019;2(12). doi:10.1001/jamanetworkopen.2019.18023

28. Parsons AS, Clancy CB, Rencic JJ, Warburton KM. Targeted Strategies to Remediate Diagnostic Reasoning Deficits. *Acad Med.* Published online July 27, 2021. doi:10.1097/ACM.0000000000004244

29. Audétat MC, Laurin S, Sanche G, et al. Clinical reasoning difficulties: A taxonomy for clinical teachers. *Med Teach.* 2013;35(3):e984-e989. doi:10.3109/0142159X.2012.733041

30. Stuart E, Blankenburg B, Butani L, Johnstone N, Long M, Marsico N. Thinking about Thinking: Published online 2011:28.

31. Kalet A, Chou CL, eds. *Remediation in Medical Education: A Mid-Course Correction.* Springer International Publishing; 2023. doi:10.1007/978-3-031-32404-8

32. Croskerry P. Achieving quality in clinical decision making: cognitive strategies and detection of bias. *Acad Emerg Med Off J Soc Acad Emerg Med.* 2002;9(11):1184-1204. doi:10.1111/j.1553-2712.2002.tb01574.x

33. Medow MA, Lucey CR. A qualitative approach to Bayes' theorem. *BMJ Evid-Based Med.* 2011;16(6):163-167. doi:10.1136/ebm-2011-0007

34. Ely JW, Graber ML, Croskerry P. Checklists to Reduce Diagnostic Errors. *Acad Med.* 2011;86(3):307. doi:10.1097/ACM.0b013e31820824cd

35. Shimizu T, Matsumoto K, Tokuda Y. Effects of the use of differential diagnosis checklist and general de-biasing checklist on diagnostic performance in comparison to intuitive diagnosis. *Med Teach.* 2013;35(6):e1218-e1229. doi:10.3109/0142159X.2012.742493

36. Downing SM, Yudkowsky R. *Assessment in Health Professions Education.* Routledge; 2009. doi:10.4324/9780203880135

37. Nendaz MR, Bordage G. Promoting diagnostic problem representation. *Med Educ.* 2002;36(8):760-766. doi:10.1046/j.1365-2923.2002.01279.x

38. Bowen JL, ten Cate O. Prerequisites for Learning Clinical Reasoning. In: ten Cate O, Custers EJFM, Durning SJ, eds. *Principles and Practice of Case-Based Clinical Reasoning Education: A Method for Preclinical Students.* Springer; 2018. Accessed January 15, 2025. http://www.ncbi.nlm.nih.gov/books/NBK543761/

39. Hasnain M, Bordage G, Connell KJ, Sinacore JM. History-taking Behaviors Associated with Diagnostic Competence of Clerks: An Exploratory Study. *Acad Med.* 2001;76(10):S14.

40. Yudkowsky R, Park YS, Riddle J, Palladino C, Bordage G. Clinically Discriminating Checklists Versus Thoroughness Checklists: Improving the Validity of Performance Test Scores. *Acad Med.* 2014;89(7):1057. doi:10.1097/ACM.0000000000000235

41. Hatala R, Norman GR, Brooks LR. Impact of a clinical scenario on accuracy of electrocardiogram interpretation. *J Gen Intern Med.* 1999;14(2):126-129. doi:10.1046/j.1525-1497.1999.00298.x

42. Custers EJ, Regehr G, Norman GR. Mental representations of medical diagnostic knowledge: a review. *Acad Med.* 1996;71(10):S55.

43. Levin Michael, Cennimo David, Chen Sophia, Lamba Sangeeta. Teaching Clinical Reasoning to Medical Students: A Case-Based Illness Script Worksheet Approach. *MedEdPORTAL.* 2016;12. doi:10.15766/mep_2374-8265.10445

44. Moghadami M, Amini M, Moghadami M, Dalal B, Charlin B. Teaching clinical reasoning to undergraduate medical students by illness script method: a randomized controlled trial. *BMC Med Educ.* 2021;21(1):87. doi:10.1186/s12909-021-02522-0

45. Pettine WW, Raman DV, Redish AD, Murray JD. Human generalization of internal representations through prototype learning with goal-directed attention. *Nat Hum Behav.* 2023;7(3):442-463. doi:10.1038/s41562-023-01543-7

46. Papa FJ, Li F. Evidence of the preferential use of disease prototypes over case exemplars among early year one medical students prior to and following diagnostic training. *Diagnosis.* 2015;2(4):217-225. doi:10.1515/dx-2015-0024

47. Smith JD, Minda JP. Distinguishing prototype-based and exemplar-based processes in dot-pattern category learning. *J Exp Psychol Learn Mem Cogn.* 2002;28(4):800-811.

48. Phillips RL, Bartholomew LA, Dovey SM, Fryer GE, Miyoshi TJ, Green LA. Learning from malpractice claims about negligent, adverse events in primary care in the United States. *Qual Saf Health Care.* 2004;13(2):121-126. doi:10.1136/qshc.2003.008029

49. Lessing JN, Pierce RG, Dhaliwal G. Teaching More About Less: Preparing Clinicians for Practice. *Am J Med.* 2022;135(6):673-675. doi:10.1016/j.amjmed.2022.01.060

50. Kennedy K. Diagnostic Reasoning and the Accuracy of Findings in the History and Physical Examination. October 22, 2022. Accessed January 18, 2025. https://www.sensible-med.com/p/diagnostic-reasoning-and-the-accuracy?utm_medium=reader2

51. Weinstein A, Gupta S, Pinto-Powell Roshini, et al. Diagnosing and Remediating Clinical Reasoning Difficulties: A Faculty Development Workshop. *MedEdPORTAL.* 13:10650. doi:10.15766/mep_2374-8265.10650

52. McGee S. Simplifying Likelihood Ratios. *J Gen Intern Med.* 2002;17(8):647-650. doi:10.1046/j.1525-1497.2002.10750.x

53. The Rational Clinical Examination. Accessed January 24, 2021. https://jamanetwork.com/collections/6257/the-rational-clinical-examination

54. *Evidence-Based Physical Diagnosis.*; 2021. Accessed February 8, 2025. https://shop.elsevier.com/books/evidence-based-physical-diagnosis/mcgee/978-0-323-75483-5

55. Bordage G, Page G. The key-features approach to assess clinical decisions: validity evidence to date. *Adv Health Sci Educ Theory Pract.* 2018;23(5):1005-1036. doi:10.1007/s10459-018-9830-5

56. Chi MTH, Feltovich PJ, Glaser R. Categorization and Representation of Physics Problems by Experts and Novices. *Cogn Sci.* 1981;5(2):121-152. doi:10.1207/s15516709cog0502_2

57. Barrows HS, Feltovich PJ. The clinical reasoning process. *Med Educ.* 1987;21(2):86-91. doi:10.1111/j.1365-2923.1987.tb00671.x

58. McQuade CN, Bonifacino E. Reasoning on Rounds: Summary Statement or Problem Representation? *J Gen Intern Med.* 2024;39(4):714-714. doi:10.1007/s11606-023-08570-0

59. Connor DM, Dhaliwal G. When less is more for the struggling clinical reasoner. *Diagn Berl Ger.* 2015;2(3):159-162. doi:10.1515/dx-2015-0014

60. Auclair F. Problem formulation by medical students: an observation study. *BMC Med Educ.* 2007;7(1):16. doi:10.1186/1472-6920-7-16

61. Chang RW, Bordage G, Connell KJ. COGNITION, CONFIDENCE, AND CLINICAL SKILLS: The Importance of Early Problem Representation during Case Presentations. *Acad Med.* 1998;73(10):S109.

62. McQuade CN, Simonson MG, Lister J, et al. Characteristics differentiating problem representation synthesis between novices and experts. *J Hosp Med.* 2024;19(6):468-474. doi:10.1002/jhm.13335

63. Braun LT, Zottmann JM, Adolf C, et al. Representation scaffolds improve diagnostic efficiency in medical students. *Med Educ.* 2017;51(11):1118-1126. doi:10.1111/medu.13355

64. Connell KJ, Bordage G, Chang RW, Howard BA, Sinacore J. Measuring the promotion of thinking during precepting encounters in outpatient settings. *Acad Med.* 1999;74(10):S10.

65. Connor DM, Narayan S, Dhaliwal G. A clinical reasoning curriculum for medical students: an interim analysis. *Diagn Berl Ger.* 2021;9(2):265-273. doi:10.1515/dx-2021-0112

66. Bansal A. Problem Representation. The Clinical Problem Solvers. June 12, 2022. Accessed January 20, 2025. https://clinicalproblemsolving.com/2022/06/12/problem-representation/

67. Weinstein Adam, Gupta Shanu, Pinto-Powell Roshini, et al. Diagnosing and Remediating Clinical Reasoning Difficulties: A Faculty Development Workshop. *MedEdPORTAL.* 13. doi:10.15766/mep_2374-8265.10650

68. Bolton JW. Varieties of clinical reasoning. *J Eval Clin Pract.* 2015;21(3):486-489. doi:10.1111/jep.12309

69. Mamede S, Schmidt HG. The structure of reflective practice in medicine. *Med Educ.* 2004;38(12):1302-1308. doi:10.1111/j.1365-2929.2004.01917.x

70. Mamede S, Schmidt H. Reflection in Diagnostic Reasoning: What Really Matters? *Acad Med.* 2014;89(7):959-960. doi:10.1097/ACM.0000000000000306

71. Mamede S, van Gog T, van den Berge K, et al. Effect of availability bias and reflective reasoning on diagnostic accuracy among internal medicine residents. *JAMA.* 2010;304(11):1198-1203. doi:10.1001/jama.2010.1276

72. Mamede S, Splinter TAW, van Gog T, Rikers RMJP, Schmidt HG. Exploring the role of salient distracting clinical features in the emergence of diagnostic errors and the mechanisms through which reflection counteracts mistakes. *BMJ Qual Saf.* 2012;21(4):295-300. doi:10.1136/bmjqs-2011-000518

73. Mamede S, van Gog T, Moura AS, et al. Reflection as a strategy to foster medical students' acquisition of diagnostic competence. *Med Educ.* 2012;46(5):464-472. doi:10.1111/j.1365-2923.2012.04217.x

74. Shimizu T, Tokuda Y. Pivot and cluster strategy: a preventive measure against diagnostic errors. *Int J Gen Med.* 2012;5:917-921. doi:10.2147/IJGM.S38805

75. May JE, Blackburn RJ, Centor RM, Dhaliwal G. Pivot and Cluster: An Exercise in Clinical Reasoning. *J Gen Intern Med.* 2018;33(2):226-230. doi:10.1007/s11606-017-4216-6

76. Uchida T, Park YS, Ovitsh RK, et al. Approaches to Teaching the Physical Exam to Preclerkship Medical Students: Results of a National Survey. *Acad Med.* 2019;94(1):129-134. doi:10.1097/ACM.0000000000002433

77. Garibaldi BT, Olson APJ. The Hypothesis-Driven Physical Examination. *Med Clin North Am.* 2018;102(3):433-442. doi:10.1016/j.mcna.2017.12.005

78. Sibbald M, Cavalcanti RB. The biasing effect of clinical history on physical examination diagnostic accuracy. *Med Educ.* 2011;45(8):827-834. doi:10.1111/j.1365-2923.2011.03997.x

79. Seki SM, DeGeorge KC, Plews-Ogan ML, Parsons AS. Physical exam: where's the evidence? A medical student's experience. *Fam Med Community Health.* 2020;8(1):e000284. doi:10.1136/fmch-2019-000284

80. Parsons AS, Wijesekera TP, Rencic JJ. The Management Script: A Practical Tool for Teaching Management Reasoning. *Acad Med.* 2020;95(8):1179-1185. doi:10.1097/ACM.0000000000003465

81. Wijesekera TP, Parsons AS, Abdoler EA, Trowbridge RL, Durning SJ, Rencic JJ. Management Reasoning: A Toolbox for Educators. *Acad Med.* 2022;97(11):1724. doi:10.1097/ACM.0000000000004796

82. Cook DA, Stephenson CR, Gruppen LD, Durning SJ. Management Reasoning: Empirical Determination of Key Features and a Conceptual Model. *Acad Med.* 2023;98(1):80. doi:10.1097/ACM.0000000000004810

83. Cook DA, Sherbino J, Durning SJ. Management Reasoning: Beyond the Diagnosis. *JAMA*. 2018;319(22):2267-2268. doi:10.1001/jama.2018.4385

84. Abdoler EA, Parsons AS, Wijesekera TP. The future of teaching management reasoning: important questions and potential solutions. *Diagn Berl Ger*. Published online November 23, 2022. doi:10.1515/dx-2022-0048

85. Penner JC, Minter DJ, Abdoler EA, Parsons AS. Reasoning on Rounds Volume 2: a Framework for Teaching Management Reasoning in the Inpatient Setting. *J Gen Intern Med*. Published online December 20, 2024. doi:10.1007/s11606-024-09039-4

86. Pauker SG, Kassirer JP. The threshold approach to clinical decision making. *N Engl J Med*. 1980;302(20):1109-1117. doi:10.1056/NEJM198005153022003

87. Phadke VK, Jagannath AD, Patel AA, Sherman SV. Over the Threshold: an Exercise in Clinical Reasoning. *J Gen Intern Med*. 2022;37(5):1290-1294. doi:10.1007/s11606-021-07206-5

Section 4

Struggle in Context: Targeted Coaching of Behavioral Phenotypes

Section 4 considers clinical reasoning through a slightly different lens and provides an alternative, complementary approach to coaching based on commonly encountered behavioral phenotypes of clinical reasoning struggle.

Situativity theories tell us that cognition is inherently situated in the environment, expanding our view of clinical reasoning from *in the head* to *out in the world.* The phenotypes introduced in chapters 9-15 correspond to elements of performance that are directly observed within the context of patient care as part of the standard assessment of all medical learners. In contrast to the cognitive micro skills described in Section 3, these phenotypes should be familiar to all clinical evaluators. For each phenotype, we explore potential underlying contributors and specific coaching approaches.

CHAPTER 9

Needs to Read More

MEDICAL SCIENCE KNOWLEDGE is a foundational component of medical learning, but simply memorizing content knowledge is not always sufficient for effective clinical reasoning. The ability to organize knowledge into accessible networks such as scripts or schemas is essential for applying that knowledge in practice.[1,2] Accurate assessment of clinical reasoning depends on the learner's content fluency to rule out the confounding effect of a medical knowledge deficiency.[3] In other words, you can't spell if you don't know the alphabet. In the busy clinical environment, and because knowledge and contextual competencies are so closely linked,[4,5] it can be challenging to differentiate between deficits in medical knowledge and clinical reasoning. Medical learners inherently have gaps in knowledge reflective of the variegated nature of clinical exposure during training. Further, there is no clear standard that defines an acceptable fund of medical knowledge in the clinical environment, as knowledge must be case- and context-specific. What matters most is not just the amount of knowledge a learner has but how well it is structured for efficient retrieval and application in specific clinical contexts.[6–8] Clinical reasoning deficits are often mislabeled as isolated problems with knowledge. Most struggling medical learners have an average global fund of knowledge with areas of relative strength and weakness. There are of course exceptions to this.

As we have outlined in chapter 2, a systematic formative assessment process that includes direct observation of the learner, discussion with evaluators, and an interview can be helpful to assess knowledge and reasoning as distinct areas of competency. Clinical reasoning deficits are often uncovered when it becomes apparent that, despite being presented with cases in a familiar area of content, the learner struggles to connect the dots. Connecting the metaphorical dots reflects a combined cognitive and context-based consolidation ability that can require dedicated coaching.[9] This inability to connect the dots often stems from scripts and schemas, which are crucial for synthesizing information and generating accurate problem representations, which are poorly developed.[7] Approximately 10% of graduate medical learners, and a greater percentage of students referred to our remediation programs, have significant deficits in knowledge that globally impact clinical reasoning and require formal intervention. While challenging to address within the time constraints of most training programs, it is possible to simultaneously improve both medical knowledge and clinical reasoning. Targeted coaching exercises provided later in this chapter guide learner organization of knowledge into flexible schemas that enhance both knowledge retrieval and application. Lessons learned from coaching learners with this phenotype of struggle can inform how all learners most effectively acquire, store, and access medical knowledge during medical training.

CASE

Dr. Walker is referred to our centralized remediation program in the early fall of his second year of internal medicine residency with multiple areas of concern. His presentations are disorganized and hard to follow, he struggles to create management plans independently, and his medical knowledge is far behind that expected for his level of training. These concerns have been present since intern year but are more pronounced now that he is leading a team. He has been told to read more. While he is receptive to feedback in general, Dr. Walker has been unsure of where to start. He is reading a textbook and trying to answer standardized test questions when he can, but he is so tired when he returns home from work that he wonders if he is retaining any of the information.

In medical school, Dr. Walker was ranked in the fourth quintile overall. Comments from clinical rotations praised his work ethic and interpersonal skills. He failed one shelf exam on the first attempt, and his USMLE scores were just a few points above passing. Upon reflection about the current and prior struggles, Dr. Walker denies a history of learning or attention disorder but admits that he has never developed effective study strategies, despite putting in a lot of time. He lacks frameworks for efficient data gathering, has never been taught how to formulate a problem representation, and struggles to build and assess the sufficiency of a differential diagnosis. With all but the most straightforward cases, he lacks confidence in his ability to develop a management plan independently. Dr. Walker also has fundamental gaps in medical knowledge as assessed by evaluators in the clinical environment and as evidenced by a critically low score on his residency in-training examination.

HOW DID WE GET HERE? THE DIFFERENTIAL DIAGNOSIS

Some medical learners simply have not put forth a sufficient level of effort to acquire the requisite knowledge base and/or organization for effective clinical reasoning. There are many potential reasons for this. Distractors or stressors impact study schedules, as do coexisting ADHD, depression, anxiety, fatigue, and burnout, combined with myriad other physical and mental health conditions that can impair focus and concentration. Existential anxiety about career choice often manifests as avoidance of work—studying, in this case—as some learners grapple with uncertainty as to whether they wish to continue the current path. Performance anxiety can undermine the ability to initiate and follow a study plan as much as it can affect performance during standardized tests or clinical encounters, in some cases leading to emotional exhaustion and even apathy. Medical learners often develop a compartmentalized, fear-based mindset to cope with the pace and volume of medical content. Experientially, lack of effort means that learners will not reach the integrated learning threshold necessary to build clinical reasoning at a baseline level. This threshold reflects a level of self-awareness at which learners can recognize an imbalance between their skills and the challenges they face.[10]

Others, like Dr. Walker, are putting in at least some effort, but that effort is ineffective. Most medical learners are not explicitly taught how to study and learn.[11] Many cram facts with the goal of performing well on tests and never absorb or integrate information in a way that promotes storage in long-term memory and application to the care of patients. The test-taker mindset may dominate the medical learner's identity, and there is often a tendency to equate contact with content and learning. Effective studying, like clinical reasoning, relies on basic cognitive regulatory processes such as attention, working memory, processing speed, motivation, and inhibitory control as well as the ability to engage in the higher order processes of metacognition and self-regulation. High IQ alone does not predict success at studying, and many medical learners lack self-regulated learning (SRL) skills due to reliance on IQ.[12,13] Ineffective studying may signal the presence of a previously unrecognized learning or cognitive disorder that emerges when the academic and workplace demands begin to outpace the learner's compensatory strategies. Even in the absence of a diagnosis, learners may lack self-awareness. For some, a blind spot exists due to short-sighted identity status adoption, for instance as a test-taker, rather than a future health care provider.[14]

Learners who present with concomitant deficits in medical knowledge and clinical reasoning are often described as "missing the forest for the trees." These difficulties arise from the inability to discriminate between important and less-important information. Many of us have sat next to someone in class who highlights everything in the notes. For highlighting to be an effective learning strategy, the learner must know what needs to be highlighted. The ability to synthesize, prioritize, consolidate, and contextualize a seemingly endless flow of information in medical training is critical for effective learning. This ability is influenced by intelligence, which impacts how efficiently a learner absorbs, understands, and applies material. However, even learners with a high IQ may experience a bottleneck when overwhelmed with the pace and volume of information if they have relative deficiencies in executive functions (EF) such as working memory, processing speed, or cognitive inhibition. From a learning perspective, this bottleneck affects every learner in medical school from the highest performing to the at-risk. Effective studying also depends on the higher order processes of metacognition and self-regulation such that the learner is cognizant of how well they are or are not learning the material and can modify study habits if they are ineffective.[15,16] As we will discuss, these skills are coachable. Table 9.1 provides a list of factors that influence both knowledge accumulation and clinical reasoning.

Table 9.1. Factors that Influence Both Knowledge Accumulation and Clinical Reasoning Medical Learner

1. Insufficient study time

a. Distractors, stressors
b. Co-existing mental or physical health condition
   i. Cognitive disorder (e.g., ADHD), learning disorder
   ii. Anxiety disorder, including performance anxiety
   iii. Mood disorder
   iv. Substance use disorder
c. Burnout or fatigue
d. Existential anxiety

2. Ineffective study time

a. Dominance of test-taker mindset, study for the sake of study
b. Difficulty discriminating important from less-important information
c. Lack of scaffolding
d. Cognitive or learning disorder that impacts IQ, attention, memory, inhibitory control, processing speed, or impulse control
e. Any condition that limits self-awareness

3. Lack of clinical experience

4. Personality or motivational traits

a. Assertiveness, proactivity, curiosity
b. Growth mindset
c. Mastery orientation

In addition to inadequate or unproductive studying, lack of experience predicts this phenotype of struggle. Medical learners may lack the scaffolding to promote acquisition, organization, and retrieval of facts and data in a format that facilitates effective pattern recognition.[17] As discussed in chapter 3, configuration of knowledge in illness and management scripts and schemas is critical for efficient synthesis of data. Scripts and schemas are built through studying and relevant clinical experience.[1] Effective clinical reasoning also requires deliberate practice and, for many, explicit teaching. Table 9.2 provides an illness script template worksheet to assist learners in organizing relevant medical knowledge. Medical learners who lack practical

Table 9.2. An Illness Script Template Exercise

	Content/Guidance
Name of condition	*Insert the disease/condition name (e.g., "appendicitis")*
Definition	*Brief description of the condition (e.g., "inflammation of the appendix due to obstruction of the appendiceal lumen")*
Epidemiology & risk factors	• Epidemiology: prevalence, demographic data • Risk factors: behaviors, exposures, or comorbidities that increase likelihood of disease
Pathophysiology	• Mechanisms that lead to disease • Key pathological processes (e.g., inflammation, autoimmunity, ischemia) • Relevant anatomy/physiology
Clinical presentation (symptoms & signs)	• Typical symptoms (e.g., pain, fatigue, fever) • Common physical exam findings (e.g., tenderness, rash, neurological deficits)
Differential diagnosis	• List conditions with similar presentations • Key distinguishing features to help rule in/out each differential condition
Key clinical pearls	• High-yield take-home messages • Common pitfalls or misconceptions • Helpful memory aids or mnemonics

clinical experience in undergraduate training (e.g., no sub-internship, or a sub-internship in which they functioned as an "extra" with a low census and/or little independent responsibility) may struggle when they get to residency. Learners who trained at a small community residency program may have trouble adapting to the demands of a fellowship program at a large academic medical center with higher census and patient complexity.

Finally, certain personality traits may impact a medical learner's ability to engage as an active participant in their own learning. Learners who do not understand their role, do not ask for help, and do not generally assert themselves in the clinical environment often struggle with both acquisition and application of knowledge in a way that translates to effective patient care. In chapter 7 of *Remediation in Medical Education: A Mid-Course Correction,*[18] Guerrasio, Tran, and Winston point to individual characteristics like growth mindset, grit, and intellectual curiosity that predict adequate and effective studying. They also highlight the importance of guiding the learner to adopt a mastery orientation in which the goal is to understand and apply the material rather than simply to perform well on an examination.

Dr. Walker's struggle in residency is expected based on his performance in medical school and on standardized tests. In addition, he carried a low census of patients on core clinical rotations and did not complete a sub-internship in his chosen area of specialty. He admits that he has never developed effective study strategies despite putting in a lot of effort and does not recall being taught clinical reasoning frameworks in medical school. Dr. Walker describes himself as an introvert who is often shy in social situations, and he acknowledges that he is not always sure of his role on the team.

APPROACH TO SIMULTANEOUSLY COACHING KNOWLEDGE AND REASONING

As in Dr. Walker's case, significant deficits in medical knowledge that limit effective clinical reasoning are often predictable when prior educational experience and performance are considered. It is critical to anticipate these struggles and, when possible, employ preemptive coaching interventions. Provided that underlying conditions are recognized and, when appropriate, intervened upon, coaching learners with these deficits is usually successful—although it takes time.

Others have suggested that multiple performance deficits should be approached sequentially to avoid piling on and creating an excessive amount of demand on the learner, who is often already feeling overwhelmed. Earlier in the arc of training (e.g., in undergraduate medical programs), the knowledge gap can often be addressed first, followed by training and practice employing

Table 9.3. Individual Learning-to-Learn[23] Foundations

Cognitive Task	Content/Guidance	Learning Theory
Elaborate, discriminate, compare between ideas/concepts, find similarities and differences	What do I know? What are the key terms? What are the key concepts? How are they related to each other?	Chunking information[24,25]
Recognize patterns, prioritize information, connect new knowledge to prior understanding	How does this information relate to what I already know? What patterns do I see?	Script and schema development[1,2,26,27]
Synthesize, summarize, integrate across disciplines or contexts	What is the most important takeaway? How can I connect this to clinical practice?	Integration of knowledge via scaffolding[28]
Apply knowledge to novel scenarios or problems	How can I use this knowledge in a real-world scenario? What problem does this solve?	Problem-based learning (PBL)[29] and experiential learning
Monitor progress, identify gaps, and refine study strategies	What am I struggling with? How effective are my study methods?	Self-regulated learning[21] (metacognitive reflection)[30,31]
Evaluate evidence, analyze data critically, and make informed decisions	Is this information reliable? How does it fit with other evidence?	Evidence-based medicine (decision theory, probability theory)[32]
Memorize efficiently and retrieve effectively	How will I remember this information? How can I practice retrieval?	Spaced repetition and retrieval practice[33]

Table 9.4. An Integrative Framework for Metacognitive Questioning

Level	Metacognition Question Type	Description	Application	Examples
1	On the line (literal)	Answers are included directly in the case vignette. Learners practice searching for and identifying literal, concrete information.	Builds learner ability to identify relevant high-yield information within a case presentation	Identification of buzzwords (e.g., pertinent data from the history, physical examination, laboratory and imaging tests, etc) (who, what, when, where, why)
2	Between the line (inferential)	Answers are not directly in the text. Requires learners to draw upon long term memory (LTM) knowledge specific to the case and to make critical judgements related to content and context. Learners search and select key information within the text to associate, discriminate, and prioritize information.	Fosters development of learner trust in their judgements of learning and clinical reasoning. Uses the ability to make critical connections through metacognitive questioning. The questions suppose critical knowledge connections that underlie the facts themselves and the process of working through cases and searching for between the line answers. Challenges errors of commission and errors of omission.	Not only is the answer within the case important but information processing becomes a critical aspect of the clinical reasoning process. This goes beyond the buzzwords that are usually the focus of the initial knowledge intake – learners must now infer.

(continued)

(continued)

Table 9.4. An Integrative Framework for Metacognitive Questioning

Level	Metacognition Question Type	Description	Application	Examples
3	Beyond the line (deductive)	Answers require the learner to connect knowledge to other LTM concepts based on direct experience and prior integration of contextual knowledge	Fosters the integration of facts and application to real-world clinical cases	Identification of knowledge gaps and errors in reasoning inform continued development of clinical reasoning

frameworks for clinical reasoning. However, in graduate medical training programs during which the timeframe is compressed and the competing demands are substantial, this is often not possible. In this chapter, we offer an approach to the simultaneous coaching of both knowledge and reasoning concerns. The guiding principle is to help the learner acquire and retain knowledge in a way that facilitates the development of scripts and schema for effective clinical reasoning. To do this, we suggest an approach incorporating scaffolds and metacognitive reflection.

Scaffolding integrates content and context knowledge, connecting learners with the *why* around learning and promoting engagement in the learning process.[19,20] Practically speaking, this means employing case-based teaching with prompts and questions to guide the learner through the clinical reasoning process, making use of algorithms and frameworks when possible. Effective one-on-one coaching allows the learner to reflect on their learning progression, including self-assessment of the study process and acknowledgement of knowledge gaps.[21,22] Table 9.3 presents learning as the integration of individual cognitive tasks and metacognitive reflection towards organization of clinically relevant information.

Table 9.4 outlines a multi-level integrative framework for metacognitive questioning to facilitate the development and/or reorganization of study strategies with a coach. Level 1, akin to learning the alphabet, represents the foundational acquisition of pertinent knowledge. Level 2 systematically and intentionally opens the door to integration in long-term memory by helping learners to consider and associate knowledge that may be embedded in other concepts. Level 3 facilitates a greater telescopic-to-microscopic consolidative process to connect the learner's knowledge to the larger clinical context. Together, these levels represent the progression from basic data identification to integration and clinical application. Practical case vignettes are provided below the table.

LEVEL 1 (ON the Line)

Vignette: A 45-year-old man presents with chest pain radiating to his left arm, diaphoresis, and nausea. His ECG shows ST-segment elevation in leads II, III, and aVF.

Metacognitive Question: *What are the key findings in the history, physical exam, and diagnostic tests?*

Application: The learner identifies the critical buzzwords in the case such as "ST-segment elevation in leads II, III, and aVF" and "chest pain radiating to the left arm."

Outcome: The learner practices extracting high-yield information directly from the vignette and learns to recognize a classic presentation of an inferior STEMI.

LEVEL 2 (BETWEEN the Line)

Vignette: A 60-year-old woman presents with fatigue and pallor. Her laboratory results show hemoglobin 8.5 g/dL, MCV 110 fL, and elevated homocysteine levels.

Metacognitive Question: *What underlying conditions could explain the patient's macrocytic anemia, and what are the next steps?*

Application: The learner uses long-term memory to recall their differential diagnosis for macrocytic anemia (e.g., B12 deficiency, folate deficiency, myelodysplastic syndrome). They associate elevated homocysteine with B12/folate deficiency and prioritize ordering vitamin levels and a peripheral smear.

Outcome: The learner strengthens their ability to connect case details to foundational knowledge, make logical deductions, and prioritize next steps in diagnosis and management.

LEVEL 3 (BEYOND the Line)

Vignette: A 35-year-old man with a history of intravenous drug use presents with fever, new heart murmur, and Janeway lesions. Blood cultures grow *Staphylococcus aureus.*

Metacognitive Question: *How does this case connect to other scenarios involving systemic infections, and what broader principles can be applied to clinical reasoning in similar cases?*

Application: The learner integrates prior knowledge about infective endocarditis, systemic sepsis, and IV drug use. They connect this case to broader clinical concepts such as the management of bacteremia, cardiac complications, and addressing social determinants of health.

Outcome: The learner develops advanced reasoning by synthesizing clinical, contextual, and experiential knowledge, identifying gaps, and applying these insights to real-world cases.

MOVING FROM TOPIC-BASED TO SYMPTOM-BASED LEARNING

In their highly influential book *Symptom to Diagnosis: An Evidence-Based Guide,*[34] Stern, Cifu, and Altkorn teach the clinical reasoning process beginning with chief concerns instead of diagnoses, providing stepwise algorithms to arrive at likely and alternative hypotheses. This strategy is also effective for the learner who presents with concomitant knowledge and reasoning deficits. In undergraduate medical training, the focus is often on system-based or topic-based learning. During clinical rotations, students are instructed to read about a topic (e.g., gout). They read a chapter or review article about gout, present it to their supervisors the following day, and hopefully memorize a chunk of information labeled in their brain as "gout." If this process is effective, they can later regurgitate the epidemiology, risk factors, natural history, clinical manifestations, laboratory findings, and treatment of gout on command. This type of learning is less relevant for clinicians, whose patients are more likely to seek care for a symptom (e.g., monoarthritis) than a diagnosis (e.g., gout). Medical learners who have stored information exclusively in the form of topics may struggle with clinical reasoning *in vivo.*

In the clinical setting, a more effective strategy is to have the learner refocus their reading with the goal of forming a more intricate and nuanced illness script for monoarthritis, which will include much of the information already retained on gout. This reorganization of information in the brain should be more relevant to the care of patients and facilitate more efficient retrieval of knowledge in real time. A script, or schema, can be formed from a symptom, sign, imaging result, or laboratory value.2 Fortunately, an increasing number of medical schools incorporate problem-based learning into their curricula to help learners contextualize their knowledge in a way that is relevant to the clinical environment. We also highly recommend *The S2D Podcast*[35] as a collection of excellent practical tools for coaching learners as they adapt this approach.

As the learner begins to develop a library of symptom-based scripts, the coach can move on to the standard approach to coaching clinical reasoning outlined in Section 3 and/or proceed to later chapters in Section 4 if there is a clear phenotype of clinical reasoning struggle.

THE IMPORTANCE OF ASKING QUESTIONS

Even with the transition from system-based to symptom-based learning, the learner's success still largely depends on their ability to focus and acquire knowledge and reasoning independently. Consider how most clinicians learn. Few of us simply open a textbook chapter and read it from start to finish. Even fewer of us read even the highest-impact journal from cover to cover. Instead, most experts learn by seeing patients, recognizing the essential gaps in their own knowledge, and assimilating pertinent information from educational resources. However, underperforming learners lack the ability to self-assess and self-regulate.[36] They struggle to decide what of the information they don't know is the most important to know. But this is a skill that can be practiced and coached. It is also a skill that, if properly developed, will have a lasting impact far beyond the coaching period.

In the following simple exercise, learners reflect on gaps in their knowledge while developing high-yield questions in the context of their clinical experience.

Dr. Walker has seven patients on the inpatient general internal medicine service. One of the patients is admitted with hereditary hemochromatosis. Two are admitted with diverticulitis. The coach reviews the patient list with

Dr. Walker to identify patient problems or symptoms that he will likely see repeatedly in training and are therefore important to learn how to manage. Ideally, Dr. Walker recognizes that he will probably see more diverticulitis than hereditary hemochromatosis during residency. The coach can then work with Dr. Walker to formulate a pertinent question about diverticulitis such as, When is surgical management indicated? Many struggling learners initially struggle to focus their inquiry even after identifying an area of interest, and much of the coaching is about helping them to better formulate pertinent questions.

In the aforementioned chapter, Guerrasio, Tran, and Winston emphasize the importance of elaborative interrogation—asking *how* and *why* questions—as a method of deepening understanding of subject material.[18]

ADDITIONAL COACHING EXERCISES

The following exercises, which were designed to be feasible and accessible for all educators, regardless of clinical reasoning expertise, provide structure for subsequent meetings between Dr. Walker and his coach or coaches. They should be easily adaptable to any clinical specialty and/or setting.

Exercise 1

Goal: To help Dr. Walker (1) develop a structured approach to formulating clinical questions, (2) find resources to answer them, and (3) learn how to assimilate and present the information learned

The coach will help Dr. Walker to develop a series of *10 key clinical questions* pertaining to the clinical presentation, differential diagnosis, and management of common clinical scenarios encountered in the in- and out-patient setting in internal medicine. Dr. Walker will be tasked with generating the questions, which will then be submitted to and edited by his coach, who will then provide Dr. Walker with feedback on the quality of his questions. Dr. Walker will develop and document a reading plan for each question. The coach will review and provide feedback to Dr. Walker on his chosen resources. Dr. Walker will then work to build a 15-minute presentation to answer the question which will be delivered in person to his coach during their regular meetings. The coach will assess the quality of the presentation, review his reading plan, and provide feedback to Dr. Walker using the standardized form below.

Coaching sessions are commonly extended by 15 minutes to incorporate a mock oral board experience. The coach can further probe Dr. Walker's knowledge by asking "what if" questions, emphasizing common and "can't miss" diagnoses.

Presentation Feedback
Clinical question
Searches performed
Reading materials
Comment on quality of the presentation

Exercise 2

Goal: To help Dr. Walker apply knowledge gained in Exercise 1 to clinical cases encountered in the context of his clinical rotations, specifically focusing on the development of a differential diagnosis and management plan for common medical conditions encountered in the in- and outpatient setting in internal medicine

Dr. Walker will present 10 patients to his coach over a period of [x] weeks. He should choose cases recently encountered during clinical rotations that, when possible, represent common presenting complaints in either the in- or outpatient setting in internal medicine. In addition to presenting the case, Dr. Walker will outline his approach to diagnosis and treatment of the complaint or complication in question. The coach will assess the clarity and quality of the presentation by completing the following assessment form.

	Case #1	Case #2
Active problem		
Differential diagnosis	1. 2. 3. 4.	1. 2. 3. 4.

	Case #1	Case #2
Management plan	1. 2. 3.	1. 2. 3.
Comment on quality of the presentation		

Exercise 3

Goal: To help improve Dr. Walker's ability to (1) present concisely, including pertinent positives and negatives, (2) prioritize details for follow-up and tasks to complete, and (3) build and assess the sufficiency of a clinical diagnosis, which will help him identify which information to prioritize (and avoid getting lost in detail)

Dr. Walker will bring a recent patient list and signout to the meeting with his coach. The coach will review the list with Dr. Walker, completing the following assessment form. For each patient on the list, Dr. Walker will state concisely the patient's primary issue, the most important clinical and laboratory findings that need to be followed over the next 24 hours, and the tasks on which he will most closely focus. Dr. Walker will provide a one-sentence rationale for all of his choices.

These exercises promote the organization of medical knowledge into illness and management scripts which can be internalized and built upon as schemas as the learner progresses in training and gains experience. Exercise 3 additionally provides a means of practicing the skill of triage, in this case, of the problem list, discussed in more detail in chapter 13.

THE ROLE OF STANDARDIZED TEST QUESTIONS IN THE COACHING PLAN

In her book *Remediation of the Struggling Medical Learner*, Guerrasio provides a detailed list of study skills and strategies for those who struggle with standardized tests.[37] She recommends a minimum of 1500 to 2500 practice questions, stresses the importance of revisiting unfamiliar or difficult material, and suggests that learners try writing their own questions.

When coaching the learner with concomitant knowledge and clinical reasoning deficits, we recommend that the learner complete 10 to 20 standardized practice questions per week from a reliable question bank. These should be contextual—in other words, related to the area of study if the learner is focusing on Exercise 1 or relevant to the current rotation as the learner works through Exercises 2 and 3. It is critical to combine questions with subject matter review, and we often find that struggling learners are doing one without the other and/or not reviewing foundational content prior to testing their knowledge. The learner should review incorrect answers with the coach at their regular meetings.

Patient (initials)	Most active problem (justification)	Three most important clinical and lab findings to follow (justification)	Two most important tasks to complete (justification)
		1. 2. 3.	1. 2.
		1. 2. 3.	1. 2.
		1. 2. 3.	1. 2.
		1. 2. 3.	1. 2.
		1. 2. 3.	1. 2.

Table 9.5. Causes of Incorrect Answers on Standardized Tests

Medical knowledge gap		
Never learned		
Mis-learned		
Knew but could not access (retrieval)		
Clinical reasoning error[38]		
Knew facts but could not apply		
Missed the objective of the question or the question within the question		
Lack of script recognition		
Lack of script specificity		
Premature closure		
Underconfidence		
Inappropriate causal attributions		
Inappropriate adaptive inferences		

Table 9.5. Causes of Incorrect Answers on Standardized Tests

Test-taking issue		
Did not read the entire vignette		
Misread		
Down to 2 answers		
Overthought		
Rushed and made careless error		
Switched right to wrong		
Switched wrong to right		
Ran out of time		

While arriving at the correct answer is not always the goal of clinical reasoning coaching, it is important for learners to understand why they select incorrect answers. As discussed in chapter 2, the wrong answer may reflect insufficient knowledge, difficulty applying knowledge in a testing situation due to poor test-taking strategies (e.g., second-guessing, overthinking, and changing answers), and/or clinical reasoning errors. Table 9.5 provides a categorization system to facilitate reflection on incorrect answers and systematically identify gaps in knowledge when working with a coach. This process should lead the learner to ask effective metacognitive questions and gain insight into the focus of further content review.

Further identification of patterns in missed questions, including whether incorrect answers are clustered at the beginning or end of the test, helps to guide the coaching process. Encouraging the learner to complete timed blocks of standardized questions can help identify issues related to time management and/or underlying issues like anxiety and/or ADHD.

We encourage the coach to directly observe the learner working through a few practice questions at each session to probe their reasoning process. The following tool, developed by investigators at the Uniformed Services University of the Health Sciences, employs a question review form to identify common clinical reasoning errors.[38] Similar to our micro skill assessment described in chapter 7, this tool employs SRL microanalysis.

- Lack of script recognition: learner offers no, or factually incorrect, interpretations of clinical data while reading the question stem
- Lack of script specificity: learner narrows down the answer to two choices by recognizing a general disease category but does not recognize the specific clinical subtype
- Premature closure: learner makes an early decision on the diagnosis; ignores or downplays information inconsistent with the diagnosis
- Underconfidence: learner rates confidence low even when answer is correct; distrusts their own clinical reasoning
- Inappropriate causal attributions: learner provides superficial or incorrect explanations of why the right answer is correct and the wrong answer is incorrect
- Inappropriate adaptive inferences: learner can identify knowledge gaps after answering a practice question but is unable to articulate an effective learning plan

SUMMARY

The knowledge explosion of the modern era necessitates novel coaching and learning strategies. Involving the struggling learner in their own learning is critical, especially as they develop awareness of what they know, don't know, and need to know. The exercises presented in this chapter promote SRL and provide a guide for the clinical reasoning coach. Improving medical knowledge will always strengthen clinical reasoning, making this approach relevant for all learners with clinical reasoning difficulties.

References

1. Custers EJFM. Thirty years of illness scripts: Theoretical origins and practical applications. *Med Teach.* 2015;37(5):457-462. doi:10.3109/0142159X.2014.956052

2. Cammarata M, Dhaliwal G. Diagnostic Schemas: Form and Function. *J Gen Intern Med.* 2023;38(2):513-516. doi:10.1007/s11606-022-07935-1

3. Eva KW, Neville AJ, Norman GR. Exploring the Etiology of Content Specificity: Factors Influencing Analogic Transfer and Problem Solving. *Acad Med.* 1998;73(10):S1.

4. Carraccio C, Burke AE. Beyond Competencies and Milestones: Adding Meaning Through Context. *J Grad Med Educ.* 2010;2(3):419-422. doi:10.4300/JGME-D-10-00127.1

5. Cutrer WB, Atkinson HG, Friedman E, et al. Exploring the characteristics and context that allow Master Adaptive Learners to thrive. *Med Teach.* 2018;40(8):791-796. doi:10.1080/0142159X.2018.1484560

6. Wing EA, Burles F, Ryan JD, Gilboa A. The structure of prior knowledge enhances memory in experts by reducing interference. *Proc Natl Acad Sci U S A.* 2022;119(26):e2204172119. doi:10.1073/pnas.2204172119

7. Schmidt HG, Rikers RMJP. How expertise develops in medicine: knowledge encapsulation and illness script formation. *Med Educ.* 2007;41(12):1133-1139. doi:10.1111/j.1365-2923.2007.02915.x

8. Coderre S, Jenkins D, McLaughlin K. Qualitative differences in knowledge structure are associated with diagnostic performance in medical students. *Adv Health Sci Educ Theory Pract.* 2009;14(5):677-684. doi:10.1007/s10459-008-9149-8

9. Kulasegaram KM, Chaudhary Z, Woods N, Dore K, Neville A, Norman G. Contexts, concepts and cognition: principles for the transfer of basic science knowledge. *Med Educ.* 2017;51(2):184-195. doi:10.1111/medu.13145

10. Watson KM. The Operationalization of Integrated Internal Action Frameworks for Classroom Identity Development and Self-regulating Learners. *Eur J Soc Behav Sci.* 2019;Issue 2. doi:10.15405/ejsbs.257

11. Piza F, Kesselheim JC, Perzhinsky J, et al. Awareness and usage of evidence-based learning strategies among health professions students and faculty. *Med Teach.* 2019;41(12):1411-1418. doi:10.1080/0142159X.2019.1645950

12. Foong CC, Bashir Ghouse NL, Lye AJ, et al. A qualitative study on self-regulated learning among high performing medical students. *BMC Med Educ.* 2021;21(1):320. doi:10.1186/s12909-021-02712-w

13. Boyd T, Besche H, Goldhammer R, Alblooshi A, Coleman BI. First-year medical students' perceptions of a self-regulated learning-informed intervention: an exploratory study. *BMC Med Educ.* 2022;22(1):821. doi:10.1186/s12909-022-03908-4

14. White CB. Smoothing out transitions: how pedagogy influences medical students' achievement of self-regulated learning goals. *Adv Health Sci Educ Theory Pract.* 2007;12(3):279-297. doi:10.1007/s10459-006-9000-z

15. Gandomkar R, Mirzazadeh A, Jalili M, Yazdani K, Fata L, Sandars J. Self-regulated learning processes of medical students during an academic learning task. *Med Educ.* 2016;50(10):1065-1074. doi:10.1111/medu.12975

16. Chang C, Colón-Berlingeri M, Mavis B, Laird-Fick HS, Parker C, Solomon D. Medical Student Progress Examination Performance and Its Relationship With Metacognition, Critical Thinking, and Self-Regulated Learning Strategies. *Acad Med.* 2021;96(2):278. doi:10.1097/ACM.0000000000003766

17. Braun LT, Zottmann JM, Adolf C, et al. Representation scaffolds improve diagnostic efficiency in medical students. *Med Educ.* 2017;51(11):1118-1126. doi:10.1111/medu.13355

18. Kalet A, Chou CL, eds. *Remediation in Medical Education: A Mid-Course Correction.* Springer International Publishing; 2023. doi:10.1007/978-3-031-32404-8

19. Li T, Fan Y, Tan Y, et al. Analytics of self-regulated learning scaffolding: effects on learning processes. *Front Psychol.* 2023;14:1206696. doi:10.3389/fpsyg.2023.1206696

20. Pea RD. The Social and Technological Dimensions of Scaffolding and Related Theoretical Concepts for Learning, Education, and Human Activity. *J Learn Sci.* 2004;13(3):423-451. doi:10.1207/s15327809jls1303_6

21. White CB, Gruppen LD, Fantone JC. Self-regulated learning in medical education. In: *Understanding Medical Education.* John Wiley & Sons, Ltd; 2013:201-211. doi:10.1002/9781118472361.ch15

22. Patel R, Tarrant C, Bonas S, Yates J, Sandars J. The struggling student: a thematic analysis from the self-regulated learning perspective. *Med Educ.* 2015;49(4):417-426. doi:10.1111/medu.12651

23. Cornford IR. Learning-to-learn strategies as a basis for effective lifelong learning. *Int J Lifelong Educ.* 2002;21(4):357-368. doi:10.1080/02601370210141020

24. Thalmann M, Souza AS, Oberauer K. How does chunking help working memory? *J Exp Psychol Learn Mem Cogn.* 2019;45(1):37-55. doi:10.1037/xlm0000578

25. Gobet F, Lane PCR, Croker S, et al. Chunking mechanisms in human learning. *Trends Cogn Sci.* 2001;5(6):236-243. doi:10.1016/s1364-6613(00)01662-4

26. Neisser U. *Cognitive Psychology: Classic Edition.* Psychology Press; 2014. doi:10.4324/9781315736174

27. Neisser U, Becklen R. Selective looking: Attending to visually specified events. *Cognit Psychol.* 1975;7(4):480-494. doi:10.1016/0010-0285(75)90019-5

28. Vygotsky LS. *Mind in Society: Development of Higher Psychological Processes.* Harvard University Press; 1978. doi:10.2307/j.ctvjf9vz4

29. Lu J, Bridges S, Hmelo-Silver CE. Problem-based learning. In: *The Cambridge Handbook of the Learning Sciences, 2nd Ed.* Cambridge handbooks in psychology. Cambridge University Press; 2014:298-318. doi:10.1017/CBO9781139519526.019

30. Flavell JH. Metacognition and cognitive monitoring: A new area of cognitive–developmental inquiry. *Am Psychol.* 1979;34(10):906-911. doi:10.1037/0003-066X.34.10.906

31. Koriat A, Levy-Sadot R. Processes underlying metacognitive judgments: Information-based and experience-based monitoring of one's own knowledge. In: *Dual-Process Theories in Social Psychology.* The Guilford Press; 1999:483-502.

32. Albert DA. Decision Theory in Medicine: A Review and Critique. *Milbank Mem Fund Q Health Soc.* 1978;56(3):362. doi:10.2307/3349653

33. Ausubel DP, Youssef M. The effect of spaced repetition on meaningful retention. *J Gen Psychol.* 1965;73(1):147-150. doi:10.1080/00221309.1965.9711263

34. Stern SDC, Cifu AS, Altkorn D. *Symptom to Diagnosis: An Evidence-Based Guide.*; 2015.

35. S2D: The Symptom to Diagnosis Podcast. Apple Podcasts. Accessed February 11, 2025. https://podcasts.apple.com/us/podcast/s2d-the-symptom-to-diagnosis-podcast/id1548809192

36. Artino ARJ, Hemmer PA, Durning SJ. Using Self-Regulated Learning Theory to Understand the Beliefs, Emotions, and Behaviors of Struggling Medical Students. *Acad Med.* 2011;86(10):S35. doi:10.1097/ACM.0b013e31822a603d

37. Guerrasio J. *Remediation of the Struggling Medical Learner.* 1 edition. Association for Hospital Medical Education; 2013.

38. Andrews MA, Kelly WF, DeZee KJ. Why Does This Learner Perform Poorly on Tests? Using Self-Regulated Learning Theory to Diagnose the Problem and Implement Solutions. *Acad Med.* 2018;93(4):612. doi:10.1097/ACM.0000000000001422

CHAPTER 10

Cannot Tell a Story

CASE

A well-known faculty member enters the office of a remediation coach, looking concerned. "I'm having trouble figuring out some performance issues with one of my nurse practitioner students," they say. The coach, accustomed to these types of conversations, gestures for them to take a seat.

"It's Mr. Ananth—really nice guy, by the way—but he's just so disorganized. I don't mean his workflow. He gets the work done and is great with patients. But when he presents an H&P, the story is all out of whack. The details are out of order and sometimes aren't even relevant. Even some of his SOAP presentations are hard to follow."

The coach nods and asks, "How is his medical knowledge?"

"That's the thing," the faculty member continues. "He is pretty smart. He knows most of the answers to my questions and can generate a 10-item differential for just about anything. But when I asked him to list his top three concerns specifically for our patient with sudden onset dyspnea and metastatic colon cancer, pulmonary embolism (PE) was nowhere on his list. I just don't get it...."

THE IMPORTANCE OF TEAM-BASED COMMUNICATION IN CLINICAL CARE

Over the past decade, the importance of team-based clinical reasoning has gained increasing recognition.[1] This change reflects a shift toward collaborative decision-making that leverages the collective expertise of an interprofessional team.[2,3] Clinicians no longer work in silos when formulating a differential diagnosis or management plan. Reasoning is now a shared responsibility among a team that includes nurses, pharmacists, respiratory therapists, physical therapists, and other allied health professionals.[4] Each of these team members contributes a critical perspective informed by their training and experience, often identifying subtle details or patient-specific concerns that might otherwise go unnoticed. However, for this model to be effective, precise and structured communication between members of the care team is paramount. A medical learner's ability to convey a clear, succinct, and organized clinical story directly influences the team's ability to make timely and well-informed decisions. Patient presentations that are disorganized, incomplete, or fail to prioritize key findings can lead to diagnostic delays or unnecessary interventions. Furthermore, learners must tailor their communication based on the audience and the purpose of the interchange. For example, signout to a night float intern is structured differently from a consult to a specialist or an update to a bedside nurse. Developing this ability early in training not only improves clinical reasoning but also fosters mutual trust, enhances shared situational awareness, and strengthens the overall safety and efficiency of patient care.

Every reader of this book has likely heard at least one, or more likely, several disorganized patient presentations, consult calls to a specialist, or end-of-shift signouts that raised concern about a learner's grasp of the clinical situation. These three forms of communication are central to clinical care and to our assessment of a learner's medical knowledge, clinical reasoning, organization, and communication skills.

The oral case presentation shows us not only what data learners have collected but also how they separate signal from noise and synthesize data to support a coherent narrative. Observing a learner call to a consultant allows us to assess their ability to succinctly convey the relevant features of a clinical case, adapted and framed for the specialist on the other end of the phone. Patient signout allows for a similar assessment, though with the added task of asking the learner to concisely project the short-term clinical course of a patient to a colleague and provide them with a contingency plan. In short, each of these skills requires the learner to tell a story.

THE LEARNER WHO CANNOT TELL A STORY: WHAT COULD BE GOING ON?

Learners who struggle with these skills are often characterized as "disorganized," "lacking the big picture," or "missing the forest for the trees." To tell the patient's story requires relevant medical knowledge, basic clinical reasoning and communication, and effective organizational systems—all of which are central to the craft of clinical medicine. Typically, more than half of learners referred for clinical reasoning remediation have trouble with presentations, calling specialty consults, and/or handoffs of care. Common co-occurring difficulties, which center around drawing conclusions from the patient's story and using those conclusions to make decisions about patient care, include prognosticating (chapter 11), creating independent management plans (chapter 12), triaging tasks (chapter 13), and responding appropriately in urgent situations (chapter 14). Table 10.1 lists the varied ways in which evaluators describe these concerns.

Table 10.1. Common Evaluator Descriptors that Characterize the "Cannot Tell a Story" Phenotype

- Trouble recognizing the central clinical problem, seeing the big picture
- Not connecting the dots
- Struggles to prioritize the problem list, giving equal weight to more/less acute issues
- Limited or narrow differential diagnosis
- Overly expansive or non-specific differential diagnosis
- Anchors, premature closure, rush to judgment
- Struggles to create a plan independently
- Presentations have too much information
- Presentations lack key information
- Information is out of order
- Missing the forest for the trees, gets lost in the weeds
- Lacks confidence
- Appears flustered

Not everyone is a good storyteller. Even when armed with adequate medical knowledge and reasoning abilities, many medical learners are not naturally articulate, fluid, or engaging when they communicate. Some struggle with effective use of nonverbal communication or eye contact. Communication difficulties may reflect a fluency disorder, such as stuttering, that disrupts the normal flow of speech. Conversely, the gift of articulate expression alone does not guarantee an effective presentation. Presenting patients' stories accurately and concisely in the clinical environment requires a great deal of synthesis, prioritization, and editing of information in the moment; it thus relies on intact foundational executive skills such as working memory, attention, inhibitory control, and mental flexibility. Simultaneously, learners must be able to do the following:

- Quickly process incoming and outgoing information and organize their thoughts
- Slow their thoughts down, if needed, to properly structure their presentation
- Keep track of their main line of thinking if interrupted or provided with new data that must be integrated into the clinical picture
- Mentally pivot to integrate new information while also filtering out less important information if questioned or interrupted during the presentation
- Inhibit the tendency to get pulled down a rabbit hole if questioned or interrupted during the presentation

As described in earlier chapters, metacognition and self-regulated learning skills are required for learners to appropriately self-assess and adjust their thinking as needed, while also drawing on past experiences in the moment.[5,6] Learners attempting to communicate patients' stories in the clinical environment must also be able to manage anxiety and/or discomfort (e.g., with public speaking, with uncertainty, and with others' reactions) as they come up. A variety of mental health conditions can impact executive functioning, metacognition, and self-regulation. Learners with anxiety disorders (including performance anxiety) or attention deficit hyperactivity disorder (ADHD) often struggle to tell a story in the clinical setting.[7] Anxiety frequently improves with practice and adoption of frameworks that facilitate organization of thoughts and data. For others, cognitive behavioral therapy and medication are effective adjunctive interventions, especially for performance anxiety. Symptoms of ADHD potentially impact all the areas outlined above and often improve with medication and/or behavior therapy. Learners with autism spectrum disorder or traits may struggle with any of these skills and can be helped with behavior coaching. Such issues require separate attention in accordance with programmatic and institutional policy as they may require external evaluation, treatment, and/or formal accommodations.

APPROACH TO THE LEARNER WHO STRUGGLES TO TELL A STORY

The evaluation of a learner who has difficulty organizing, prioritizing, and/or presenting clinical information begins by considering the following questions:

1. Have they collected the correct data?
2. Have they interpreted the data correctly?
3. Did they have enough time to gather the data?
4. Do they have an effective system for collecting and recording data?
5. Can they put individual data pieces together into bigger ideas?
6. Do they struggle to discriminate between important and unimportant clinical details?
7. Do they use a template for oral presentations? Calling consults? Giving signout?
8. Do they experience subjective feelings of anxiety when communicating patient information (e.g., presentations, calling a consult, signout)?
9. Can they summarize their patients in a "one liner"?
10. Can they create a problem list, ranked by priority?
11. Can they reprioritize the problem list as new data is acquired?
12. Can they create a differential diagnosis, with justification, for the primary clinical problem?
13. Are their written notes disorganized?

Ideally, the answers to these questions are revealed through the combination of an interview with the learner, case review, and direct observation in the clinical environment. As discussed in earlier chapters, the initial formative assessment of any struggling learner should consider performance concerns in their biopsychosocial context, with mindfulness of potential underlying factors. Additionally, it is important to assess these and any clinical reasoning in areas of learner content familiarity to rule out medical knowledge as a confounding deficit.

CASE, CONTINUED

The coach meets with Mr. Ananth to review his system for pre-rounding and determines that Mr. Ananth is doing a reasonable job gathering data in the morning. The coach notices that Mr. Ananth collects a lot of information on each patient; however, he has created impressive templates for organizing this data that seem to work for him, and he is otherwise remarkably efficient. The coach observes Mr. Ananth on rounds two days later. Mr. Ananth does not have any new patients to present that day, but his SOAP presentations reveal certain patterns. His one-liners include the entire past medical history and conclude with a vague list of symptoms and no clear plan. He continues to include unqualified concerns such as "back pain" in the problem list, even when the team has already determined that a retroperitoneal hematoma is the cause of the back pain. As initially noted by the faculty member, his differentials are lengthy, unprioritized, and often disconnected from the patient's most pressing issues.

The coach reviews a collection of Mr. Ananth's H&Ps and progress notes. The same patterns emerge: HPIs that are collections of facts without a clear structure, expansive summary statements listing the entire medical history but failing to highlight the primary issue, and vaguely characterized problems lacking meaningful modifications or contextual details.

THE SIGNIFICANCE OF STRUCTURE AND DISCRIMINATION IN ORGANIZING CLINICAL KNOWLEDGE

The organization of knowledge can be stratified into two levels known as surface structure and deep structure.[8] OPQRST is an example of a *surface structure.* As introduced in chapter 8, OPQRST is a framework commonly used by learners to remember what factors can modify a patient's symptoms: onset, provocation, quality, region/radiation, severity, and timing. Knowledge is characterized by a surface structure when its superficial qualities define how it is organized in the mind. A surface structure also tends to be generic. For example, chronic obstructive pulmonary disease (COPD), congestive heart failure (CHF), pneumonia, pulmonary embolism (PE), pneumothorax, arrhythmia, and acute coronary syndrome (ACS) are all causes of dyspnea. A learner with only superficial knowledge may list all these causes in their differential diagnosis for a patient with dyspnea, in no order, and without regard to patient comorbidities or concomitant symptoms. Conversely, *deep structure* implies organization with purpose and is much more nuanced. Deeply structured medical knowledge reflects appreciation of disease mechanisms and interrelatedness between features of the case and is thus more easily connected with new ideas as they are learned and integrated into memory. When approaching a patient with dyspnea, the learner with deeply structured knowledge can contextualize their reasoning based on the specific patient in front of them, prioritizing causes of dyspnea in relationship to other presenting features of the case. This process lends itself more readily to a prioritized and justified differential diagnosis.

> *Despite having a reasonable grasp of content material, Mr. Ananth's presentations and notes suggest superficially structured knowledge and difficulty discriminating between relevant and irrelevant pieces of information.*

Thus, even when he collects the appropriate data, Mr. Ananth struggles to integrate these data to appreciate the bigger picture. In short, he seems to know the story but not what it means. However, Mr. Ananth's difficulties with assigning significance to pieces of data and linking data to context points us in a helpful direction.

SEMANTIC QUALIFIERS

We understand the meaning of words and phrases based on their context. Consider the word "diet." To a layperson, diet implies restrictive eating and the need to lose weight. To a medical professional, diet is instead a catch-all term referring to what the patient eats and when. The principle of semantics, how words and ideas modify each other in a particular context, is relevant to the meaning we give our patients' stories and informs how we reason through their clinical problems.

Some of the earliest studies examining how clinicians parse clinical cases focused on *semantic qualifiers*. Semantic qualifiers are adjectives or adverbs which translate the patient's own words and clinical presentation into medical terminology, connecting them to our underlying stored knowledge.[9] By distinguishing key features and facilitating pattern recognition, semantic qualifiers guide hypothesis-driven inquiry and help us refine our differential diagnosis. Consider how the differential diagnosis for "acute chest pain" is different from "chronic chest pain." In the original studies by Bordage and colleagues, the greater use of semantic qualifiers by experts was associated with improved diagnostic accuracy.[10–12] For example, a novice might consider a differential diagnosis for "acute knee pain," whereas an expert sees the same patient and characterizes the same issue as "acute monoarticular arthritis in a middle-aged male."[13]

Indiscriminately inserting semantic qualifiers into a patient presentation does not improve diagnostic accuracy.[14–16] This suggests that it is not the mere presence of semantic qualifiers that adds value but the ability to use them to distinguish important from unimportant pieces of information and provide linkage to deeper clinical knowledge.

PROBLEM REPRESENTATION STRUCTURE AND FUNCTION

As introduced in chapters 3 and 7, the problem representation is an internal, mental abstraction of a patient's case which develops early on during the encounter with a patient.[17] Through an iterative process that incorporates the relevant semantic qualifiers, the internal problem representation can be codified into a written or spoken summary statement, often called the "one-liner." The terms problem representation, summary statement, and "one-liner" are commonly confused and inappropriately used as interchangeable phrases.[17] Accuracy and sophistication of the problem representation evolves with expertise. Compared with novice learners, experts include fewer irrelevant details (especially from the past medical history), incorporate more physical examination findings, and synthesize data into higher order concepts (e.g., sepsis and acute hypoxic respiratory failure) in their problem representations.[18] An effective problem representation is composed of three parts: (1) the patient's demographic features and risk factors for disease, (2) the temporal course of the illness, and (3) a description of the clinical syndrome using semantic qualifiers.[13] Diagnostic accuracy has been associated with adherence to this structure and, specifically, inclusion of a rich description of the time course of illness.[18] Interestingly, utilization of this three-part structure also improved the diagnostic accuracy of ChatGPT.[19,20] Problem representations should also be concise. Returning to the knee pain example, a sample summary statement might be: "A 55-year-old man with diabetes presents with the acute onset of right knee arthritis after a night of heavier-than-usual drinking."

Problem representation forms the link between the collected clinical data and the clinician's internal medical knowledge.[21] An effective problem representation informs diagnostic reasoning by prompting retrieval of relevant illness scripts stored in the clinician's long-term memory.[22,23] It informs management reasoning by placing the clinical problem being solved in context through a similar prompting of management scripts.[24–26] A commonality among nearly all learners who exhibit the "cannot tell a story" phenotype of struggle is a lack of comfort, experience, and/or ability in forming an accurate problem representation.

CASE, CONTINUED

The remediation team devises a coaching plan for Mr. Ananth. Since his next block is an elective consult rotation, the coach schedules three one-hour coaching sessions over the next two weeks. Mr. Ananth seems to have a reasonable knowledge base and can generate a differential diagnosis for commonly encountered clinical problems. His organizational systems for pre-rounding and data gathering are adequate. The concepts of problem representation and justification of the differential diagnosis, however, are new to him.

COACHING THE LEARNER WHO STRUGGLES TO TELL A STORY

As is true for all phenotypes of clinical reasoning discussed in this book, the approach to coaching the learner who struggles to tell a story can be considered in phases. Initially, the coach introduces frameworks—in this case, to structure presentations, notes, and the problem representation. Utilizing these tools and frameworks, the learner then engages with the coach in one-on-one, case-based deliberate practice in a simulated setting. Here, variables can be changed, and cognitive flexibility can be developed. Once the coach and learner feel confident in the learner's progress, deliberate practice moves to the clinical environment, in which the learner is observed telling patients' stories in a variety of contexts under direct observation by clinical supervisors.

Fundamentally, coaching the learner who struggles to tell a story centers on teaching them how to access their latent knowledge in a more effective manner, discern signal from noise, and encode data at higher levels of abstraction. For most learners, this begins with formulating an effective problem representation. To that end, we suggest the following initial specific, measurable, and achievable goals of coaching for Mr. Ananth:

1. Identify and richly describe the central patient problem using appropriate semantic qualifiers
2. Construct a succinct problem representation in the form of a summary statement or "one-liner"
3. Generate a refined and prioritized differential diagnosis

While conceptually simple, formulation of an accurate problem representation is often perceived as a high cognitive load task for struggling learners and requires a great deal of practice. We encourage all training programs to incorporate this ability into daily work for all learners, whether on rounds or in teaching conferences.

FRAMEWORKS AND COACHING EXERCISES

Articulated Problem Representation[27,28]

The simplest (and one of the most effective) coaching exercise has learner and coach meet, in the office or after rounds, to review and critique the learner's problem representations for existing patients.[29] Emphasis is given to the risk factors for disease, temporal course of illness, and key features; the learner adjusts accordingly until each problem representation achieves its desired form. Coach and learner can also draw from a case bank to practice creating problem representations using key features and semantic qualifiers.

Differential-Differential Diagnosis

In real-time or in a simulated setting, coaches can employ the "differential-differential diagnosis" exercise. Here, the coach articulates a problem representation for the patient being discussed and modifies one of the details to generate a new problem representation. The coach then asks the learner how this change influences the differential diagnosis. For example, recall our 55-year-old male patient with the acute onset of monoarticular arthritis after a night of heavier-than-usual drinking. Consider, instead, an *18-year-old male* who presents with acute monoarticular arthritis. Instead of gout being at the top of the differential diagnosis, the focus shifts to infectious causes (e.g., disseminated gonococcal disease), reactive arthritis, and other types of rheumatic disease. This strategy emphasizes the importance of an individual patient's risk factors, time course of illness, and other semantic qualifiers in prioritizing and narrowing the set of diagnostic possibilities. The exercise also promotes cognitive flexibility.

The Highlighter Exercise

The highlighter exercise, introduced in chapter 8, is useful for the learner whose presentations and notes miss important details or focus on the wrong details. Here, the learner is provided with written patient notes and asked to identify key features of the case based on possible diagnoses. This promotes more effective discrimination of pertinent information from extraneous information for a problem representation.

For those interested in a structured approach to evaluating the learner's problem representation, we suggest the following scale (Figure 10.1), adapted from the Society to Improve Diagnosis in Medicine's "Assessment of Reasoning Tool."[30]

Learner: **Evaluator:**

Problem Representation	**Assessment**		
	Minimal	**Partial**	**Complete**
Who is the patient? • Demographics • Pertinent Risk factors	• Misidentifies demographics • Fails to include crucial or pertinent risk factors (PMH)	• Proper demographics • Includes all pertinent risk factors, as well as extraneous ones	• Proper demographics • All pertinent risk factors and minimal extraneous • Able to stratify risks to make maintain clarity & conciseness
What is the temporal pattern? • Length (hyperacute, acute, subacute, chronic) • Tempo (stable, progressive, resolving, intermittent, waxing and waning)	• Fails to include the length and/or tempo of the presenting symptom or concern	• Includes both the length tempo in the problem representation	• Includes the length and tempo in the problem representation • Uses semantic qualifiers or clear and specific durations
What is the clinical syndrome? • Key signs, symptoms, and findings	• Fails to identify the key signs, symptoms, and findings pertinent to the case • Includes excessive information that could confuse or trigger inaccurate illness scripts	• Identifies the key signs, symptoms, and findings • Also includes excessive information that could confuse or trigger inaccurate illness scripts	• Identifies the key signs, symptoms, and findings • Minimal to no extraneous information • Leading illness script is clear
Overall Assessment	**Needs Improvement** ☐	**On Target** ☐	**Excellent** ☐
Comments:			

Figure 10.1. Problem Representation Assessment Tool (Adapted with permission from Nicholas Young, MD.)

An additional approach to guide problem representation is to ask the learner to identify the patient's primary clinical problem and then rename that problem using semantic qualifiers. By helping the learner narrow their focus, cognitive load is reduced.[31,32] This exercise also allows the coach to assess how learners prioritize (filter out unimportant information) and synthesize data. The well-defined problem then serves as a natural steppingstone for discussion of the patient's differential diagnosis and management plan. For example, a learner who has offered "dyspnea" as the central clinical problem should be asked to better describe dyspnea using semantic qualifiers (e.g., related to onset, duration, progression, and associated symptoms) and then reflect on how different descriptors impact their differential diagnosis.

Reverse Case Analysis

For this exercise, the coach presents the learner with an established diagnosis and asks them to work backward to construct the patient's problem representation. This focuses the learner's attention on the key defining features of a diagnosis and pushes them to articulate how each finding contributes to the clinical picture. Reverse case analysis encourages deep processing of clinical information by reinforcing the links between symptoms, clinical findings, and disease processes. For example, if the established diagnosis is pneumonia, the learner must work backward to determine the historical details, physical exam findings, and diagnostic test results that support this diagnosis. Reverse case analysis improves the learner's ability to recognize key data they may have initially overlooked or misinterpreted. This approach also allows the coach to highlight areas where the learner may need additional support, such as developing more refined differential diagnoses. For graduate medical learners, this exercise can also be done with management plans. For example, one could begin with a management plan (e.g., ceftriaxone and azithromycin, wean oxygen by nasal canula) and ask the learner to construct a problem representation (e.g., a 65-year-old male presents with acute onset fever, productive cough, shortness of breath, and fatigue).

Table 10.2 provides a sample dialogue between coach and learner as they work together to incorporate these skills.

Table 10.2. Problem Representation Example Coaching Dialogue

Coach	Learner
How would you summarize this patient?	Mrs. Smith is a 60-year-old woman who presented to the emergency department with chest pain and dyspnea.
Good start. Chest pain and dyspnea are the main issues here. Let's focus on the chest pain. Can you describe that with some semantic qualifiers?	Well, it is sharp and located on the right side of the chest. It's also worse with inspiration. Can I call that pleuritic?
Yes, I think you can. Give me your summary statement again, but this time include the semantic qualifiers for location and quality you mentioned. Also, can you try to include the time course for her symptoms?	Oh, you mean how long they've been going on. Sure. This is a 60-year-old woman with acute-onset pleuritic, right-sided chest pain and dyspnea.
That's great. The acute time frame and pleuritic nature of the chest pain are already helping me build my differential for this patient. Don't forget to include findings from your physical examination, though.	I always forget to include the exam. How about this: This is a 60-year-old woman with acute-onset pleuritic, right-sided chest pain and dyspnea who is tachycardic and hypoxemic but has clear lungs on examination.
Excellent. That narrows it down even more for me. Now let's think about her risk factors for different causes of chest pain and dyspnea. Anything stand out to you from her past medical history?	She has COPD and a history of colon cancer from a few years ago. She also has IBS, but I don't think that's related.
I agree the IBS is probably unrelated. Let's put everything together. Say her summary statement one last time.	This is a 60-year-old woman with COPD and treated colon cancer who presents with acute, pleuritic chest pain and dyspnea who is hypoxemic with clear lungs and tachycardic.
Perfect. What's at the top of your differential diagnosis now?	When I say it like that, pulmonary embolism is top of the list.

Abbreviations: COPD, chronic obstructive pulmonary disease; IBS, irritable bowel syndrome. Adapted from Connor and Dhaliwal[29]

As the learner gains proficiency, an effective problem representation becomes the foundation of their continued work on patient presentations and written notes. Several methods exist for structuring these activities.

FRAMEWORKS FOR ORGANIZING THE PATIENT'S STORY

Building on these concepts, Table 10.4 presents a step-by-step framework to guide learners through the relevant clinical reasoning processes as they compile a clinical case presentation. This approach should be generalizable to most clinical settings with necessary attention, of course, to content[33] and context[34] specificity. Early learners, in particular, benefit from explicit coaching focused on the structure of their discussion of a problem. These activities center on prioritization of data and should be undertaken in areas in which the learner has adequate content knowledge.

Table 10.4. 7-Step Approach to Helping a Learner Tell the Patient's Story

Step 1: Learner selects a patient they have seen recently

Step 2: Learner identifies the patient's #1 problem and describes it using 2 to 4 semantic qualifiers
- Emphasize tempo and time course of the illness and modifying conditions (e.g., *sudden-onset severe* dyspnea, *and hypoxemic* with *clear lungs* on auscultation)
- Discuss lumping vs splitting key findings

Step 3: Learner identifies historical items, disease risk factors, physical exam findings, and initial diagnostic testing relevant to the #1 problem

Step 4: Learner synthesizes the results of Steps 2 and 3 into a 1 to 2 sentence problem representation
- Distinguish relevant vs irrelevant details to include in the problem representation
- Model the skill of developing a problem representation by sharing yours

Step 5: Learner uses this problem representation to discuss the three *most likely* (higher base rate) diagnoses and 1 to 2 *cannot miss* (may be less common but would lead to poor outcomes if missed) diagnoses, with justification

Step 6: For the lead diagnosis, learner reflects on what about the case does and does not fit with this diagnosis (structured reflection)*

Step 7: Repeat, using other cases which vary by clinical content area and context (e.g., clinic, hospital admission, discharge, etc) or repeat, modifying details of the case as "what if" scenarios

*Structured Reflection

The exercise outlined in Table 10.4 asks the learner to assess the fit of existing diagnostic hypotheses. Deliberate, structured reflection is one of only a few techniques which have been shown in studies to decrease cognitive biases when reasoning through complex clinical cases.[35] To promote reflection, learners are asked to provide justification for their reasoning, identifying pertinent positives (data for) and pertinent negatives (data against) each item on their differential diagnosis for the primary problem. When the problem representation is effective, its clinical features should directly inform the justification process. The coach can ask learners to answer the following questions for each item on the differential diagnosis: What case factors fit this diagnosis? What doesn't fit with this diagnosis? What details are missing from the case that would help establish this diagnosis?[36–38] In a condensed form of this exercise, the learner reflects solely on their leading diagnosis.

Prioritizing Clinical Data: Case-based Exercise

Goal: To help (1) improve the learner's ability to present concisely, including pertinent positives and negatives; (2) prioritize details for follow-up and tasks to complete; and (3) build and assess the sufficiency of a clinical diagnosis. This will help the learner to identify which information to prioritize and avoid getting lost in detail.

The learner is tasked with bringing a recent patient list and signout to the meeting with their coach. The coach reviews the list with the learner, completing the following assessment form. For each patient on the list, the learner states concisely the patient's primary issue, the most important clinical and laboratory findings that need to be followed over the next 24 hours, and the tasks on which they will most closely focus. The learner provides a one-sentence rationale for all their choices.

Patient (initials)	Most active problem (justification)	Three most important clinical and lab findings to follow (justification)	Two most important tasks to complete (justification)

3R/3W

We have developed the 3R/3W framework as a guide for composing patient presentations and daily progress notes (Figure 10.2), highlighting the importance of regular problem list maintenance as a reflection of learner understanding of "the big picture" and as a springboard for clinical decision-making.[39] Many learners are not explicitly taught to do, or how to do, this. Each day, the learner should Reassess, Rename, and Reprioritize a patient's problem list, based on new data. For each problem, the learner then considers the "What, Why, and What Next?" questions. An example of renaming replaces dyspnea with pneumonia, or pneumonia with pneumococcal pneumonia. The order of problems on the list will change from day to day, reflecting clinical priority and directing activities for the day.

3Rs/3Ws: Guide to Composing Daily Notes

You've finished PRePPING your patient! Before you start your note or give your oral presentation on rounds, think broadly about your patient:

R	**Reassess**	Is the patient better, worse, or the same? Is the current diagnosis still the most likely? Is your current therapeutic plan still effective?
R	**Rename**	Are the problem names as specific as possible, based on TODAY's data? • *Gram-negative rod UTI → Klebsiella UTI* • *SOB → Pneumonia*
R	**Reprioritize**	Is the most active problem listed first? Can you move resolved or chronic problems lower?
W	**What**	Name the problem, with current clinical status (eg Improved, Stable, Worse, New) • *Community Acquired PNA: Improved*
W	**Why**	Describe the differential diagnosis and discuss how the current clinical exam, vitals, labs, and studies support your likely diagnosis.
W	**What Next**	What is the plan for the day? Will you be ready to discharge soon? What do we need to do in order to get the patient to move towards discharge?

Figure 10.2. 3Rs/3Ws: Guide to Composing Daily Notes[39]
(Reprinted with permission from ACGME.)

Structured Case Mapping

Structured case mapping provides a visual framework to connect patient data. Here, the learner is asked to create a diagram that categorizes patient findings into problem domains (e.g., cardiovascular, respiratory, infectious). The coach then guides the learner in narrowing focus by linking information between domains, thus forming a cohesive clinical narrative. Deliberate practice of structured case mapping aids the learner in developing a more systematic approach to synthesizing data and refining their differential diagnoses.

This method is particularly useful for learners who tend to compartmentalize information rather than consider its interrelatedness. By drawing out their thought process, the coach encourages the learner to visualize the relationships between different pieces of data and gain insight into how the data can be integrated into a unified clinical picture. Over time, this exercise encourages learners to develop a more automatic and systematic approach to the organization of clinical data into a story.

Example Case:

A 67-year-old male with a history of hypertension and diabetes presents with shortness of breath, productive cough, and fever for three days.

Step 1: Categorizing the Data
The learner is asked to organize the patient's clinical data into broad categories, such as:

Respiratory: *shortness of breath, productive cough, hypoxia*
Infectious: *fever, leukocytosis, recent sick contacts*
Cardiac: *hypertension, history of heart failure*
Metabolic: *diabetes, recent weight loss*

Step 2: Establishing Links
The coach then guides the learner in drawing connections between these categories. For example, the learner identifies that the respiratory and infectious domains overlap in considering pneumonia as a likely unifying diagnosis. The coach prompts them to connect the cardiac category by discussing how heart failure could present with similar symptoms and how pneumonia could exacerbate the symptoms of underlying cardiac disease.

Step 3: Refining the Problem Representation and Differential Diagnosis
Once the learner has structured their case map, the coach asks them to use it to prioritize the differential diagnosis. Initially, the learner lists several possibilities but struggles to rank them. By revisiting the map, the learner recognizes that pneumonia is the most likely diagnosis, given the fever, productive cough, and radiographic findings.

Refined summary statement:

"A 67-year-old male with hypertension and diabetes presents with three days of productive cough, fever, and shortness of breath."

SNAPPS

Developed in 2003, SNAPPS[40] is best viewed as a practical, workplace-based clinical reasoning teaching and coaching framework that provides structure to the patient presentation.[41,42] Using a think-aloud approach during a clinical encounter, learners are asked to:

S (summarize): summarize the relevant history and physical examination findings
N (narrow): narrow the differential diagnosis to a few possibilities
A (analyze): compare and contrast items on the differential diagnosis
P (probe): pose questions to the teacher/coach about uncertainties or alternative approaches
P (plan): formulate a plan
S (select): select issues for further study

A 2024 systematic review suggests that, especially in residents, SNAPPS may increase the total presentation length as well as the number of differential diagnoses and uncertainties expressed.[43] In short, this tool promotes self-regulated learning by encouraging reflection and providing structure for deliberate practice of diagnostic and management reasoning centered around patient presentations.

IDEA

Using a three-component rating scale, Williams et al assessed the diagnostic reasoning of more than 200 medical students in a series of cases involving standardized patients and found that diagnostic justification performance was inconsistent and often below expectations.[44] Shortly thereafter, Baker and colleagues provided validity evidence for IDEA, a 15-item instrument originally developed in 2003 as a tool to assess medical students' diagnostic reasoning in written admission notes.[45]

- **I** (interpretive summary): similar to what we term problem representation
- **D** (differential diagnosis): with commitment to most likely diagnosis
- **E** (explanation): explanation of reasoning in choosing the most likely diagnosis
- **A** (alternative): alternative diagnoses with pertinent positives and negatives

IDEA is a simple, workplace-based framework that scaffolds formative feedback for learners who are working on improving the structure of presentations or written notes, further highlighting the importance of diagnostic justification.

CRANAPL

CRANAPL (Clinical Reasoning in Admission Note Assessment & Plan) was developed with validity evidence to assess the comprehensiveness of clinical reasoning as documented in the Assessment and Plan sections of admission notes completed by hospital medicine physicians.[46] This 9-item rating scale provides a framework for the formative assessment of diagnostic (specifically problem representation, differential diagnosis with justification), prognostic (length of stay estimation, potential for upgrade in status), and management reasoning in learner patient presentations or written notes.

RENE

Building on the work of these investigators and under the leadership of Dr. Suzanne Boyle, we developed and validated a formative clinical reasoning assessment tool in nephrology fellows known as RENE (Reasoning Evaluation in Nephrology Education).[47] RENE measures three domains of diagnostic reasoning during a written patient encounter as part of a simulated, web-based acute kidney disease consult. Each domain (e.g., problem representation, differential diagnosis with justification, and diagnostic plan with justification), is scored using our novel instrument.

These and other[48] frameworks highlight the importance of oral presentations and written notes and provide a structured approach to providing formative feedback. Their use with struggling learners can inform the coaching of clinical reasoning for all learners.

CASE, CONTINUED

The coach elicits Mr. Ananth's perspective on his presentations and written notes. Upon reflection, Mr. Ananth admits to having problems connecting the dots sometimes. Once he figures out "what is really going on with the patient," he feels comfortable discussing the diagnostic details and management. The coach reviews several options for structuring presentations and notes, and Mr. Ananth ultimately develops an approach that will work for him. Over the next four weeks, Mr. Ananth engages in the exercises outlined in this chapter, both with the coach during coaching sessions and in the clinical environment with his supervising resident. The coach role models diagnostic reasoning such as effective problem representation as they work through cases in subsequent meetings. At the conclusion of the four-week consult block, the coach speaks with Mr. Ananth's supervising attendings, who report that his presentation skills and hypothesis-driven data gathering improved over the course of the rotation. With complex patients, his summary statements were still occasionally laden with irrelevant details, but overall problem lists and differential diagnoses were more focused.

HANDOFFS OF CARE

Transfer of patient responsibility between care providers is a critical transition that, when done well, promotes continuity of care, minimizes error, and ensures patient safety.[49,50] Effective handoffs of care rely on a clinician's clinical reasoning and communication abilities to accurately convey the necessary information. Despite being recognized by the ACGME[51] and the AAMC as a core entrustable professional activity,[52] medical learners may not receive explicit teaching about patient care transitions, and the handoff itself is rarely observed by a supervisor. Learners who struggle with telling a patient's story typically benefit from a structured approach to giving patient signout. I-PASS is a widely recognized example of such an approach that has been validated in many health care settings and shown in a large, multicenter study to reduce preventable adverse events.[49,53]

I (illness severity): stable, unstable, watcher (potentially unstable); include code status

P* (patient summary): succinct description of reason for admission, hospital course, global plan

A (action list): pending tasks and overnight responsibilities (to-do list)

S** (situational awareness): anticipated problems and contingency plans (if/then)

S (synthesis by receiver): receiving provider/team repeats back key points and/or asks questions

*The signout is one of the most practical tests of a medical learner's ability to construct an accurate problem representation.

**Contingency (if/then) planning as an element of prognostic reasoning is discussed in more detail in chapter 11. Situational awareness is defined and discussed in detail in chapter 15.

The I-PASS Study Group, composed of medical educators, health services researchers, and quality improvement and patient safety experts from across North America, has developed accessible curricular materials that provide a standardized, evidence-based approach to teaching and evaluation handoffs of care.[54]

In procedural fields where the handoff of care is unique and often more involved, simulation is an effective teaching and coaching method. In one of many examples in the literature, the anesthesiology simulation Krishnan and colleagues developed in which residents were required to evaluate a complex patient and provide ICU to OR handoff to a peer was viewed by learners as an effective educational tool.[55] The use of simulation as a coaching tool in surgical fields is discussed in more detail in chapter 15.

We encourage coaches to incorporate handoffs of care in the deliberate practice activities of most, if not all, learners who struggle to tell a story.

Table 10.5. Frameworks and Coaching Exercises for the "Cannot Tell a Story" Phenotype

1. **Characterization of the central clinical problem**
   - — Articulate the problem representation
   - — Differential-differential diagnosis
   - — Highlighter exercise
   - — Identify and rename the central clinical problem
   - — Reverse case analysis

(continued)

(Table 10.5 continued)

2. **Organization of the patient's story**
   — 7-Step approach to telling a story
   — Structured reflection
   — Case-based exercise: prioritizing clinical data in diagnostic reasoning
   — 3R/3W
   — Structured case mapping
   — Exercises to promote reorganization of knowledge into scripts (chapter 9)

3. **Teaching, coaching, and formative assessment tools**
   — SNAPPS (presentations – diagnostic and management reasoning)
   — IDEA (notes – diagnostic reasoning)
   — CRANAPL (notes – diagnostic, prognostic, and management reasoning)
   — RENE (notes – diagnostic and management reasoning)
   — I-PASS (handoffs of care – diagnostic, prognostic, and management reasoning)

SUMMARY

In chapter 9 we highlighted the importance of discrimination in medical knowledge acquisition. The ability to prioritize relevant clinical information in a patient encounter is similarly critical to telling a patient's story. Learners who struggle with this ability often come to attention when observed presenting patients, calling subspecialty consults, or providing handoffs of care. Inevitably, written notes are impacted as well. Underlying difficulties with discrimination limit the learner's ability to organize key features of the case into a concise summary. In this chapter, we focus our interventions on characterization of the primary clinical problem and highlight the importance of the problem representation in queuing relevant diagnostic and management scripts. Additionally, we provide several frameworks and coaching tools to guide development. Deliberate practice that incorporates these tools and frameworks across a wide variety of cases and clinical settings improves cognitive flexibility. As learners gain comfort pivoting in the face of changing data, their ability to think on their feet and avoid getting pulled down rabbit holes improves. These approaches can inform the teaching and formative assessment of all learners.

References

1. Graber ML, Rusz D, Jones ML, et al. The new diagnostic team. *Diagn Berl Ger.* 2017;4(4):225-238. doi:10.1515/dx-2017-0022
2. Choi JJ, Contractor JH, Patel VL, Shapiro MF. How team clinical reasoning occurs on ward rounds: Implications for learning. *Clin Teach.* 2023;20(4):e13599. doi:10.1111/tct.13599
3. Olson APJ, Durning SJ, Fernandez Branson C, Sick B, Lane KP, Rencic JJ. Teamwork in clinical reasoning—cooperative or parallel play? *Diagn Berl Ger.* 2020;7(3):307-312. doi:10.1515/dx-2020-0020
4. Olson A, Rencic J, Cosby K, et al. Competencies for improving diagnosis: an interprofessional framework for education and training in health care. *Diagn Berl Ger.* 2019;6(4):335-341. doi:10.1515/dx-2018-0107
5. White CB, Gruppen LD, Fantone JC. Self-regulated learning in medical education. In: *Understanding Medical Education.* John Wiley & Sons, Ltd; 2013:201-211. doi:10.1002/9781118472361.ch15
6. Flavell JH. Metacognition and cognitive monitoring: A new area of cognitive–developmental inquiry. *Am Psychol.* 1979;34(10):906-911. doi:10.1037/0003-066X.34.10.906
7. Warburton KM, Yost JS, Bajo SD, Martindale JR, Parsons AS, Ryan MS. Characteristics of ADHD in Struggling Residents and Fellows. *J Grad Med Educ.* 2024;16(6):730-734. doi:10.4300/JGME-D-24-00449.1
8. Chomsky N. *Aspects of the Theory of Syntax.* 50th ed. The MIT Press; 1965. Accessed February 13, 2025. https://www.jstor.org/stable/j.ctt17kk81z
9. Steward D, Bordage G, Lemieux M. Semantic Structures and Diagnostic Thinking of Experts and Novices. *Acad Med.* 1991;66(9):S70.
10. Bordage G. Why did I miss the diagnosis? Some cognitive explanations and educational implications. *Acad Med.* 1999;74(10):S138.
11. Bordage G, Page G. The key-features approach to assess clinical decisions: validity evidence to date. *Adv Health Sci Educ Theory Pract.* 2018;23(5):1005-1036. doi:10.1007/s10459-018-9830-5
12. Chang RW, Bordage G, Connell KJ. COGNITION, CONFIDENCE, AND CLINICAL SKILLS: The Importance of Early Problem Representation during Case Presentations. *Acad Med.* 1998;73(10):S109.
13. Bowen JL. Educational Strategies to Promote Clinical Diagnostic Reasoning. *N Engl J Med.* 2006;355(21):2217-2225. doi:10.1056/NEJMra054782
14. Young M, Brooks L, Norman G. Found in translation: the impact of familiar symptom descriptions on diagnosis in novices. *Med Educ.* 2007;41(12):1146-1151. doi:10.1111/j.1365-2923.2007.02913.x
15. Eva KW, Wood TJ, Riddle J, Touchie C, Bordage G. How clinical features are presented matters to weaker diagnosticians. *Med Educ.* 2010;44(8):775-785. doi:10.1111/j.1365-2923.2010.03705.x
16. Nendaz MR, Bordage G. Promoting diagnostic problem representation. *Med Educ.* 2002;36(8):760-766. doi:10.1046/j.1365-2923.2002.01279.x

17. McQuade CN, Bonifacino E. Reasoning on Rounds: Summary Statement or Problem Representation? J *Gen Intern Med.* Published online December 12, 2023. doi:10.1007/s11606-023-08570-0

18. McQuade CN, Simonson MG, Lister J, et al. Characteristics differentiating problem representation synthesis between novices and experts. *J Hosp Med.* 2024;19(6):468-474. doi:10.1002/jhm.13335

19. Skittle C, Bonifacino E, McQuade CN. Medical language matters: impact of clinical summary composition on a generative artificial intelligence's diagnostic accuracy. *Diagn Berl Ger.* Published online December 12, 2024. doi:10.1515/dx-2024-0167

20. OpenAI. Accessed February 6, 2025. https://openai.com/

21. Schmidt HG, Rikers RMJP. How expertise develops in medicine: knowledge encapsulation and illness script formation. *Med Educ.* 2007;41(12):1133-1139. doi:10.1111/j.1365-2923.2007.02915.x

22. Custers EJFM. Thirty years of illness scripts: Theoretical origins and practical applications. *Med Teach.* 2015;37(5):457-462. doi:10.3109/0142159X.2014.956052

23. Custers EJ, Regehr G, Norman GR. Mental representations of medical diagnostic knowledge: a review. *Acad Med.* 1996;71(10):S55.

24. Parsons AS, Wijesekera TP, Rencic JJ. The Management Script: A Practical Tool for Teaching Management Reasoning. *Acad Med.* 2020;95(8):1179-1185. doi:10.1097/ACM.0000000000003465

25. Abdoler EA, O'Brien BC, Schwartz BS. Following the Script: An Exploratory Study of the Therapeutic Reasoning Underlying Physicians' Choice of Antimicrobial Therapy. *Acad Med.* 2020;95(8):1238. doi:10.1097/ACM.0000000000003498

26. Cook DA, Stephenson CR, Gruppen LD, Durning SJ. Management reasoning scripts: Qualitative exploration using simulated physician-patient encounters. *Perspect Med Educ.* 2022;11(4):196-206. doi:10.1007/s40037-022-00714-y

27. Parsons AS, Clancy CB, Rencic JJ, Warburton KM. Targeted Strategies to Remediate Diagnostic Reasoning Deficits. *Acad Med.* Published online July 27, 2021. doi:10.1097/ACM.0000000000004244

28. Stuart E, Blankenburg B, Butani L, Johnstone N, Long M, Marsico N. Thinking about Thinking: Published online 2011:28.

29. Connor DM, Dhaliwal G. When less is more for the struggling clinical reasoner. *Diagn Berl Ger.* 2015;2(3):159-162. doi:10.1515/dx-2015-0014

30. Thammasitboon S, Rencic JJ, Trowbridge RL, Olson APJ, Sur M, Dhaliwal G. The Assessment of Reasoning Tool (ART): structuring the conversation between teachers and learners. *Diagn Berl Ger.* 2018;5(4):197-203. doi:10.1515/dx-2018-0052

31. Van Merriënboer JJG, Sweller J. Cognitive load theory in health professional education: design principles and strategies. *Med Educ.* 2010;44(1):85-93. doi:10.1111/j.1365-2923.2009.03498.x

32. Young JQ, Van Merrienboer J, Durning S, Ten Cate O. Cognitive Load Theory: implications for medical education: AMEE Guide No. 86. *Med Teach.* 2014;36(5):371-384. doi:10.3109/0142159X.2014.889290

33. Eva KW, Neville AJ, Norman GR. Exploring the Etiology of Content Specificity: Factors Influencing Analogic Transfer and Problem Solving. *Acad Med.* 1998;73(10):S1.

34. Konopasky A, Artino AR, Battista A, et al. Understanding context specificity: the effect of contextual factors on clinical reasoning. *Diagnosis.* 2020;7(3):257-264. doi:10.1515/dx-2020-0016

35. Mamede S, Schmidt HG. Deliberate reflection and clinical reasoning: Founding ideas and empirical findings. *Med Educ.* 2023;57(1):76-85. doi:10.1111/medu.14863

36. Mamede S, van Gog T, Sampaio AM, de Faria RMD, Maria JP, Schmidt HG. How Can Students' Diagnostic Competence Benefit Most From Practice With Clinical Cases? The Effects of Structured Reflection on Future Diagnosis of the Same and Novel Diseases. *Acad Med.* 2014;89(1):121. doi:10.1097/ACM.0000000000000076

37. Mamede S, van Gog T, Moura AS, et al. Reflection as a strategy to foster medical students' acquisition of diagnostic competence. *Med Educ.* 2012;46(5):464-472. doi:10.1111/j.1365-2923.2012.04217.x

38. Ibiapina C, Mamede S, Moura A, Elói-Santos S, van Gog T. Effects of free, cued and modelled reflection on medical students' diagnostic competence. *Med Educ.* 2014;48(8):796-805. doi:10.1111/medu.12435

39. DeKosky AS, Sedrak MS, Goren E, Dine CJ, Warburton KM. Simple Frameworks for Daily Work: Innovative Strategies to Coach Residents Struggling With Time Management, Organization, and Efficiency. *J Grad Med Educ.* 2018;10(3):325-330. doi:10.4300/JGME-D-17-00756.1

40. Wolpaw TM, Wolpaw DR, Papp KK. SNAPPS: A Learner-centered Model for Outpatient Education. *Acad Med.* 2003;78(9):893.

41. Jain V, Rao S, Jinadani M. Effectiveness of SNAPPS for improving clinical reasoning in postgraduates: randomized controlled trial. *BMC Med Educ.* 2019;19(1):224. doi:10.1186/s12909-019-1670-3

42. Wolpaw T, Papp KK, Bordage G. Using SNAPPS to Facilitate the Expression of Clinical Reasoning and Uncertainties: A Randomized Comparison Group Trial. *Acad Med.* 2009;84(4):517. doi:10.1097/ACM.0b013e31819a8cbf

43. Flores-Cohaila JA, Vizcarra-Jiménez SF, Bermúdez-Peláez MF, Vascones-Román FF, Rivarola-Hidalgo M, Taype-Rondan A. Effects of SNAPPS in clinical reasoning teaching: a systematic review with meta-analysis of randomized controlled trials. *Diagn Berl Ger.* 2024;11(3):220-230. doi:10.1515/dx-2023-0149

44. Williams RG, Klamen DL, Markwell SJ, Cianciolo AT, Colliver JA, Verhulst SJ. Variations in Senior Medical Student Diagnostic Justification Ability. *Acad Med.* 2014;89(5):790. doi:10.1097/ACM.0000000000000215

45. Baker EA, Ledford CH, Fogg L, Way DP, Park YS. The IDEA Assessment Tool: Assessing the Reporting, Diagnostic Reasoning, and Decision-Making Skills Demonstrated in Medical Students' Hospital Admission Notes. *Teach Learn Med.* 2015;27(2):163-173. doi:10.1080/10401334.2015.1011654

46. Kotwal S, Klimpl D, Tackett S, Kauffman R, Wright S. Documentation of Clinical Reasoning in Admission Notes of Hospitalists: Validation of the CRANAPL Assessment Rubric. *J Hosp Med.* 2019;14(12):746-753. doi:10.12788/jhm.3233

47. Boyle SM, Martindale J, Parsons AS, et al. Development and Validation of a Formative Assessment Tool for Nephrology Fellows' Clinical Reasoning. *Clin J Am Soc Nephrol.* 2024;19(1):26. doi:10.2215/CJN.0000000000000315

48. Richardson KM, Cristiano JA, Schafer KR, Shen E, Burns CA. Writing Is Thinking: Implementation and Evaluation of an Internal Medicine Residency Clinical Reasoning and Documentation Curriculum. *Med Sci Educ.* 2022;32(4):773-777. doi:10.1007/s40670-022-01570-5

49. Starmer AJ, Spector ND, Srivastava R, et al. Changes in Medical Errors after Implementation of a Handoff Program. *N Engl J Med.* 2014;371(19):1803-1812. doi:10.1056/NEJMsa1405556

50. Snow V, Beck D, Budnitz T, et al. Transitions of Care Consensus Policy Statement American College of Physicians-Society of General Internal Medicine-Society of Hospital Medicine-American Geriatrics Society-American College of Emergency Physicians-Society of Academic Emergency Medicine. *J Gen Intern Med.* 2009;24(8):971-976. doi:10.1007/s11606-009-0969-x

51. Common Program Requirements. Accessed September 1, 2020. https://www.acgme.org/What-We-Do/Accreditation/Common-Program-Requirements

52. Englander R, Flynn T, Call S, et al. Toward Defining the Foundation of the MD Degree: Core Entrustable Professional Activities for Entering Residency. *Acad Med.* 2016;91(10):1352. doi:10.1097/ACM.0000000000001204

53. Starmer AJ, Spector ND, Srivastava R, et al. I-pass, a mnemonic to standardize verbal handoffs. *Pediatrics.* 2012;129(2):201-204. doi:10.1542/peds.2011-2966

54. Starmer AJ, O'Toole JK, Rosenbluth G, et al. Development, Implementation, and Dissemination of the I-PASS Handoff Curriculum: A Multisite Educational Intervention to Improve Patient Handoffs. *Acad Med.* 2014;89(6):876. doi:10.1097/ACM.0000000000000264

55. Krishnan S, Kumar N, Diaz E, Thornton I, Ghoddoussi F, Ellis TA. Anesthesiology Handoff Simulation Case: A Handoff From Intensive Care Unit to Operating Room for Anesthesiology Learners. *MedEdPORTAL J Teach Learn Resour.* 2020;16:10887. doi:10.15766/mep_2374-8265.10887

CHAPTER 11

Can't Identify Sick vs Not Sick

CASE

Ms. Yang is a physician assistant student preparing to signout her list of patients to the night cover intern. One of her patients, Mr. Smith, a 72-year-old man with a history of chronic obstructive pulmonary disease and heart failure, was admitted earlier in the day for worsening shortness of breath and lower extremity edema. His vitals are currently stable, but he remains on supplemental oxygen at 3L via nasal cannula. Admission labs show a mildly elevated serum creatinine level and an elevated brain-type natriuretic peptide (BNP). His diuretics were increased earlier in the day, with a resultant increase in urine output.

As Ms. Yang organizes her signout, she focuses on contingency planning. She structures her handoff using the following if/then statements to anticipate potential overnight changes in clinical status and provide guidance to the covering intern:

If the oxygen requirement increases, then assess his work of breathing and lung exam. If he shows signs of respiratory distress, order a chest X-ray to assess for worsening pulmonary congestion or pneumonia, and consider escalating to non-invasive ventilation. If he is also tachycardic, you'll want to think about pulmonary embolism and may need a CTPA—but don't forget that his kidney function is not at baseline.

If his urine output drops significantly overnight, then check his oxygen requirement and a repeat creatinine level to help you decide whether to hold or increase the dose of diuretics.

If he becomes hypotensive (SBP < 90 mmHg), then assess for signs of overdiuresis. As long as hypoxia is not worse, consider a fluid challenge and notify the senior resident for further evaluation.

If he develops new confusion, then obtain a blood gas and assess for hypercapnia, as he may be retaining CO2 and could require escalation of respiratory support.

PROGNOSTIC REASONING

It is essential to consider the patient's short-term prognosis in this case because it shapes both immediate management and overnight contingency planning. Ms. Yang isn't just thinking about what is happening now; she is also considering how Mr. Smith's condition could change over the next several hours and what steps the covering intern should take if that happens. The cognitive process underlying this decision-making is known as prognostic reasoning. Our colleagues Dr. Jessica Dreicer and Dr. Thilan Wijesekera define prognostic reasoning as the process of judging the severity of a patient's illness or injury and forecasting their clinical course based on disease-specific knowledge, patient-specific factors, and other relevant data.

As illustrated by this example, prognostic reasoning is not just relevant for long-term predictions. Rather, it is built into almost every decision in patient care. Whether planning ahead for potential overnight issues, making split-second determinations during an emergency, managing a complication in surgery, or helping a patient and family understand what to expect after a new life-limiting diagnosis, prognostic reasoning is about recognizing what is likely to happen next and acting accordingly.

Table 11.1 summarizes common applications of prognostic reasoning in the clinical environment. In routine handoffs of care, a written signout like Ms. Yang's means the covering or accepting provider is not left to react blindly when something changes but is, instead, following a pre-considered plan.

When a patient in the hospital starts to decompensate, decisions need to happen fast. Is this a temporary setback, or is the patient heading toward respiratory failure or shock? The answer to this question impacts all subsequent decisions—whether to initiate supportive measures, whether to escalate to the

ICU, and whether aggressive intervention is even the right call. Making the wrong assumption can lead to delays in appropriate treatment or, conversely, can mean subjecting a patient to interventions that are unlikely to be effective.

The need for immediate prognostication in the operating room is an important part of the skill we term *troubleshooting* in our later chapter on operative clinical reasoning. For example, a sudden drop in blood pressure might be explained by a temporary medication effect or it could indicate a major bleed. The team must intervene immediately, often without the full dataset. As we will discuss, forward planning (i.e., the ability to anticipate) is another critical component of operative reasoning. An expert surgeon is always thinking a few steps ahead: how to stabilize the patient now, what they will need in recovery, and whether events that unfold during the case change the post-operative plan.

Then there are the hardest conversations, those about serious, life-limiting illnesses or end-of-life care. When facing a life-changing diagnosis, patients and their families need honest answers about what the future might look like and how best to prepare.

Table 11.1. Common Applications of Prognostic Reasoning in Clinical Medicine

- Handoffs of care
- Risk stratification and treatment decisions
  - Clinically urgent or emergent situations in a nonoperative setting
  - Troubleshooting in the operating room
  - Procedural risk assessment
  - Decisions regarding hospitalization vs outpatient management, or level of care within an inpatient setting
- Goals of care and advance-care planning
  - Chronic or terminal illness
  - Acute severe illness

In all these examples, communication around the clinician's prognostic reasoning is as important as the reasoning process itself.

CLINICAL REASONING THEORY AND PROGNOSIS

The processes of prognosis, diagnosis, and management are inescapably intertwined. Traditional teaching on prognosis begins with the diagnosis, emphasizing resulting patient outcomes using the 6Ds framework (death, disease, discomfort, disability, dissatisfaction, and destitution).[1] But a patient's prognosis is influenced by more than their diagnosis; rather, a complex mix of biological, clinical, and social factors influence the eventual outcome.[2] Prognostic assessments can be disease specific (e.g., the model to predict survival in patients with end-stage liver disease, i.e., MELD) or symptom specific, occurring before a disease is known (e.g., unexplained weight loss as an indicator of more severe illness before a specific etiology is identified). A patient's severity of illness can inform diagnostic reasoning, and a patient's clinical trajectory greatly influences management decisions (e.g., strongly recommending hip fracture repair in elderly patients based on the increased likelihood of mortality without repair). An important difference between diagnostic and prognostic hypotheses is that, while the former are typically selected from an existing set of possibilities (i.e., clinicians rely on known disease patterns to match a patient's symptoms to a diagnosis), the latter require abduction. In other words, clinicians must generate new explanations to anticipate a patient's future trajectory.[3] By definition, prognostic reasoning is an exercise full of uncertainty.[3] As such, probabilistic models are less reliable.

Consequently, relative to diagnostic and management reasoning, prognostic reasoning, at least in the short-term, is thought to be more reliant on pattern recognition (System 1) than analytical thinking (System 2). Experienced clinicians can often walk into a room and get an immediate sense of how sick a patient is, long before they have reviewed lab results or run risk calculations. They pick up on subtle cues (e.g., how a patient looks, breathes, or responds to questions) that prompt mental shortcuts, built over years of seeing similar cases. This intuitive approach allows them to act quickly. The "eyeball" test, as it is commonly known, is an essential skill for patient triage, resource allocation, and predicting patient disposition (discharge, admission to ward, or ICU).[4] A study of how experienced emergency medicine clinicians make visual assessments to determine whether a patient is critically ill found that the majority of their decisions were rated closer to "knew immediately" rather than "deliberated intently."[4] Another study concluded that prognostic accuracy was similar whether clinical decisions were intuitive or deliberative, suggesting that both modes of thinking can be effective, with pattern recognition having the edge in expediency.[5] As is true with diagnosis and management, prognostic decisions sometimes require toggling between both systems, especially when initial intuition was uncertain. Experience was the key factor; exposure to many clinical cases improved pattern recognition, as did structured reflection.

Determining longer-term prognosis generally requires a more analytical approach, given the inherent complexities of clinical medicine and the multitude of individual factors that impact each decision. To simplify this process for the clinician, multiple prognostic indices have been developed. While valuable in theory and clearly useful in certain clinical situations, these tools are often difficult to apply in routine practice.[6] There are dozens of clinical scoring systems, each designed for different populations and time frames, making it unrealistic for busy clinicians to sift through them all for every clinical decision. Another major issue centers on what these indices leave out. Many do not account for less common but highly morbid conditions, which can drastically impact prognosis.[7] Others fail to incorporate protective factors like strong social support, engagement in the community, or even a history of longevity in close family members. For example, the CURB-65[8] score helps assess pneumonia severity and guides decisions about hospitalization, but it does not capture all the nuanced details of a patient's illness, such as their home support structure or baseline functional status. An experienced clinician integrates these scores with pattern recognition honed over time, learning to anticipate decompensation before it occurs. These contextual factors, as understood by situated cognition, greatly influence prognostic reasoning and cannot be ignored.

CASE, CONTINUED

The intern listens carefully, scrolling through Mr. Smith's past admissions. "Has he needed ICU care before?" they ask.

Ms. Yang glances at the computer. "Not that I recall, but he's had a few admissions for this before."

The intern points to a hospitalization two months ago. "He was admitted for a similar issue—his oxygen requirement jumped to high-flow overnight, and they had to transfer him to the ICU for BiPAP. He was close to being intubated."

Ms. Yang pauses. "That's right, I remember that now. But he's been stable today, so hopefully, we won't see that this time."

The intern nods but still feels uneasy. As they move on to the next patient, the intern makes a mental note to check on Mr. Smith early in the night. They can't shake the feeling that he might already be on the same trajectory as before—and that this time, the team might need to anticipate the deterioration before it fully manifests.

HOW ACCURATE ARE OUR PROGNOSES?

Unfortunately, the available evidence suggests that clinicians are often imprecise in their prognostic estimates. Though underrecognized relative to diagnostic errors in the literature, these prognostic errors, termed *misprognoses*, are common.[9] Morgan and colleagues explored the accuracy of clinicians' probability estimates for common conditions in primary care and found inflated perceptions of disease probability, both before and after diagnostic testing. These inaccuracies may bias prognostic assessments (e.g., overestimating the likelihood of deterioration or the need for aggressive interventions).[10] In a study looking at clinicians' ability to prognosticate in the care of terminally ill patients, only 20% of predictions were accurate, and 63% of predictions were overly optimistic.[11] More experienced clinicians were less likely to make extreme errors, consistent with our understanding of dual process theory. A study of expert neurosurgeons and neurointensivists found wide variations in prognostic predictions for the same patients with traumatic brain injury.[12] These clinicians appropriately adjusted their estimates for well-known prognostic factors like Glasgow Coma Scale (GCS), age, and pupil reactivity but failed to consider other factors such as blood glucose levels and hematoma type. These findings suggest a universal tendency to systematically overlook or undervalue certain data points in prognostic reasoning. In addition, only 15% of clinicians reported using formal prognostic models in practice. Barriers cited included lack of awareness, access, confidence in model predictions, and difficulty obtaining input values. To make matters worse, very little educational time, whether in medical school or residency, is focused on learning how to make accurate prognoses.[13,14]

PHENOTYPES OF PROGNOSTIC REASONING STRUGGLE

The complexity inherent to prognostic reasoning, combined with the reality of its inexactness, leaves many learners in a precarious spot and suggests that we should be more deliberate in our teaching and coaching. Learners rarely struggle with prognostic reasoning in a vacuum. As we demonstrate in subsequent examples, the issues that underlie difficulties with prognostication also impact diagnostic and management reasoning. Common behavioral patterns of prognostic reasoning difficulty are presented in Table 11.2. Though presented distinctly, there is considerable overlap, and many struggling learners exhibit features of more than one phenotype. In chapter 14, we discuss several related phenotypes of struggle centered on management of clinically urgent or emergent situations.

Table 11.2. Behavioral Phenotypes of Learners Struggling with Prognostic Reasoning

Phenotype	Description	Content/Guidance
Overconfident predictor	Overestimates ability to predict prognosis, making broad, definitive statements without sufficient evidence. Some learners feel uncomfortable expressing doubt, so they speak in absolutes to project confidence. Without a mature sense of how variable clinical courses can be, they overvalue their personal intuition or limited past experiences. Once they decide on a prognosis, they focus on data that fits their conclusion and ignore contradictory evidence (i.e., confirmation bias).	• "This patient has no chance of survival" or "They'll be fine by next week." • Diminishes uncertainty in prognostic discussions • Overly confident in predicting mortality based on single factors or limited experience

(continued)

Table 11.2. Behavioral Phenotypes of Learners Struggling with Prognostic Reasoning *(continued)*

Phenotype	Description	Content/Guidance
Generalizer	Assumes all patients with similar presentations will have the same outcome, relying too much on past experiences. These learners are dependent on pattern recognition without the clinical experience required for accuracy. It is simpler to assume a known pattern than to consider each patient's unique complexities. Once a learner anchors on the similarity to a past case, they may overlook key distinguishing features in the current case (i.e., anchoring bias).	• "Last patient I saw with this did well, so this one will too." • Fails to account for individual patient differences and/or contextual factors
Information overloader	Gathers excessive information but struggles to synthesize and prioritize key prognostic indicators. Overlap here with diagnostic and management reasoning struggles. For example, may struggle with hypothesis refinement and may feel overwhelmed by the sheer amount of information, leading to delayed or indecisive clinical actions. This learner struggles to decipher signal from noise.	• Orders multiple tests without integrating results
Avoider	Hesitant to make prognostic estimates or incorporate numerical probability. This learner does not want to make explicit statements about patient outcomes. They worry that giving a numerical risk or any firm stance might lead to criticism if the outcome differs. These learners may find prognostic discussions emotionally charged and prefer to avoid them altogether.	• "It's hard to say what will happen." • Avoids discussing prognosis with patients and families
Concrete thinker	Sees prognosis as strictly good or bad, without appreciating nuances of clinical trajectories. In a system where exam questions often appear dichotomous (e.g., right vs wrong), some learners carry that mindset into clinical reasoning. Without seeing the nuanced trajectories of most patients *in vivo*, it is easy to revert to an overly simple, binary perspective.	• "The patient will either live or die—why assign a number to it?" • Struggles with the concept of probabilistic reasoning

Table 11.2. Behavioral Phenotypes of Learners Struggling with Prognostic Reasoning *(continued)*

Phenotype	Description	Content/Guidance
Emotional decision-maker	Prognostic reasoning is heavily influenced by emotional response to a case rather than objective data. These learners may have had a traumatic past case or personal loss that influences how they perceive current patient trajectories. They may overreact (or underreact) emotionally because they fear causing distress or false hope.	• "I just have a bad feeling about this." • Lets personal attachment to a patient override clinical evidence
Terrible transitioner	Struggles to anticipate clinical trajectory and connect prognosis to management plans, leading to poor signouts and transitions of care. The importance of prognostic reasoning for signout is highlighted in the case that begins this chapter. Without a systematic approach, handoffs of care can become disorganized and miss critical prognostic elements. Some learners focus only on immediate tasks, not recognizing how essential anticipating the more intermediate "next step" is for safe transitions of care. In fast-paced clinical environments, handoffs can be rushed.	• Gives vague or incomplete handoffs: "Just watch them closely." • Misses key clinical inflection points, leading to avoidable deterioration and/or failure to recognize change in clinical status
Crisis delayer	Does not handle urgent or emergent situations well due to difficulty identifying sick versus not sick and anticipating clinical trajectory. Lacking a robust understanding of how quickly certain conditions can worsen, they fail to anticipate the cascade of events leading to decompensation. These learners may worry about appearing alarmist or about "bothering" seniors.	• Fails to recognize when a patient is deteriorating • Delays necessary interventions due to lack of clinical urgency

HOW CAN WE HELP?

As with other clinical reasoning domains described in this book, it is useful to consider the process of prognosis in steps. Prognostic reasoning is thought to occur in two steps: (1) assessment of current illness severity, and (2) prediction of future clinical trajectory. These appraisals help clinicians make timely, informed decisions about needed management and lay the groundwork for communication with the patient about what the next hours, days, months, or years of their illness will look like. However, predicting what will happen next is inherently difficult because clinical scenarios are dynamic, and patient responses to treatment are not always straightforward. Just as in diagnostic and management reasoning, context plays a crucial role in shaping prognostic assessments. There is more to prognostic reasoning than applying formulas; rather, this type of reasoning requires the ability to recognize patterns and adapt them appropriately to each patient's unique circumstances.

Step 1: Assessment of Current Illness Severity

Struggling learners are encouraged to employ a combination of patient-specific, disease-specific, and more general indicators to assess the severity of an illness.[15] Examples of each are included in Table 11.3. This assessment combines elements of intuitive and analytical reasoning.[16,17]

Assessing severity requires balancing data-driven approaches with real-world experience. While experts are particularly reliant on pattern recognition for prognostic reasoning, an early or struggling learner necessarily depends more heavily on objective data. A single lab value or set of vital signs rarely provides a complete picture; rather, trends over time and clinical context matter significantly. Struggling learners often require specific guidance in interpreting and synthesizing data as it informs clinical prognosis.

Step 2: Prediction of Future Clinical Trajectory

When considering how the patient's clinical status will change over time, struggling learners are encouraged to stratify future clinical trajectory by time frame, as summarized in Table 11.4. Predictions about a patient's clinical course rely on assessment of severity and often incorporate predictive tools. However, truly predictive data is difficult to acquire and even harder to apply effectively. Many validated prognostic scores exist, but as

Table 11.3. Factors Influencing Assessment of Current Illness Severity

Factor	Examples
Patient-specific	Age, baseline functional status, medical history, frailty, prior hospitalizations, response to previous treatments, presence of multiple comorbidities, home oxygen use, nutritional status, do-not-resuscitate (DNR) status, cognitive impairment, ability to engage in self-care, recent weight loss, support systems, access to care
Presentation- and disease-specific	End-organ damage in sepsis, extent of pneumonia on imaging, tumor burden in cancer, severity of myocardial infarction on troponins and ECG, presence of new arrhythmias in heart failure, severity of cirrhosis on MELD score, neurological deficits in stroke, inflammatory markers in autoimmune diseases, rate of progression in neurodegenerative disorders
General indicators	Accessory muscle use, altered mental status, hemodynamic instability, escalating oxygen requirement, rising lactate levels, persistent tachycardia, worsening metabolic acidosis, prolonged capillary refill, increased work of breathing, delirium, signs of poor perfusion (cool extremities, mottling), declining urine output, refractory hypotension, inability to protect airway, recurrent fevers despite antibiotics

discussed, their widespread use is limited by practical considerations, lack of generalizability, and failure to capture contextual factors that greatly impact prognosis. Prognostic scores are developed from population-based data, meaning they may not apply perfectly to individual patients. In addition to the aforementioned limitations, these models often rely heavily on laboratory and physiologic data and are static (e.g., validity evidence is for time of admission), failing to account for changes in trajectory—which can be rapid. The biggest challenge in prognostic reasoning is determining how these population-based scores apply to specific patients. Again, experience is key.

Table 11.4. Time Frames for Assessment of Future Clinical Trajectory

Time Frame	Examples
Immediate (seconds to minutes)	Is this a code situation requiring immediate CPR or defibrillation? Should this patient be anticoagulated for a massive pulmonary embolism? Does this patient need urgent chest tube placement for a tension pneumothorax? Is this seizure prolonged, and does it require immediate intervention? Is this patient actively bleeding and in need of rapid transfusion?
Short-term (hours to days)	Is this patient likely to need ICU transfer overnight? Will this patient require escalating oxygen support by morning? Should we anticipate sepsis and begin early broad-spectrum antibiotics? Will this patient develop worsening acute kidney injury and require nephrology consultation? Does this patient need repeat imaging to monitor disease progression?
Medium-term (weeks to months)	Will this patient be able to discharge home or will they need rehab placement? Is this patient at risk for readmission within the next 30 days? How likely is this patient to recover functional independence after a stroke? Will this patient's heart failure worsen despite medication adjustments? Is this patient's cancer prognosis poor enough to begin discussing hospice?
Long-term (months to years)	What is the 5-year survival rate for this cancer diagnosis? Is this patient likely to progress to end-stage renal disease and require dialysis within the next few years? Will this child with congenital heart disease require future surgeries? How likely is this patient with early dementia to need full-time care within a year? Should this patient with cirrhosis be evaluated for liver transplant?

A classic example of assessing immediate trajectory is recognizing a patient in the hospital who "just doesn't look right." Vital signs may be objectively normal, but an experienced clinician will sense imminent deterioration based on factors that aren't easily quantifiable such as a change in mental status, the look of fatigue in their eyes, or an overall sense of fragility. These intuitive assessments, built on exposure to many prior cases, often prove to be more accurate than traditional objective measures.

With this foundational understanding, we suggest the following coaching exercises to support struggling learners. Coaching prognosis generally begins in a simulated environment (e.g., a coach's office or a simulation center) and employs a deliberate practice model. *How* these exercises are carried out will depend on clinical setting and resources. Simulation is ideal for coaching prognostic reasoning because of the unique ability to control the multitude of variables that influence a patient's prognosis. The strength of these exercises lies in their ability to promote learner reflection on decision-making.

COACHING EXERCISES FOCUSED ON IMMEDIATE- OR SHORT-TERM PROGNOSIS

Eyeballing

Step 1: Pattern Recognition

The learner observes a series of patients* for 15 seconds each and is asked to classify each patient as "sick" or "not sick." Recognizing that "sick" and "not sick" is context-specific and will mean different things in different clinical settings, this exercise should be designed to be applicable to the clinical environment in which the learner practices.

*Depending on resource availability, educators can use actual patients in the hospital, standardized patients, or virtual patients to display various phases of acute illness.

Step 2: Analytical Reasoning

For each patient, the coach then provides additional patient information including vital signs, brief history, and lab results. The learner reassesses their initial judgments and verbalizes:

- What changed in their prediction?
- What additional data influenced their new decision?
- Were their initial judgments confirmed or revised?

Step 3: Reflection

The coach provides their own thoughts for comparison and feedback, highlights physiologic signs they use in quick visual assessments, and acknowledges common pitfalls in prognostic intuition. If actual patients are observed, learners are encouraged to track outcomes longitudinally, reviewing charts several days to weeks later.

Uncertainty Calibration

The coach asks the learner to predict the short-term clinical trajectory of several patients. This exercise can be undertaken in a variety of simulated settings, as above, or in the clinical environment with an existing list of patients. Trajectory can be categorized in a manner that applies to the given clinical context. The learner is then asked to rate their confidence in each decision on a 0 to 100 scale. It is helpful if the coach simultaneously engages in the same exercise.

For example, a medical student and their clinical supervisor working in the emergency department predict disposition over the next 24 hours for each of the patients on their service:

- Likely discharge (not sick)
- Likely ward admission (moderate risk)
- Likely ICU admission (high risk)

Subsequent conversations focus on differences and discrepancies in prognostic assessment and confidence level and differentiate disease-specific indicators versus more general warning signs that apply across conditions. This exercise can be varied by adjusting the timeframe for prognosis, as outlined in Table 11.4.

Case Variability

The coach presents multiple hypothetical clinical cases with similar initial presentations but different clinical trajectories and asks the learner to assign a prognostic estimate over one of the time frames outlined in Table 11.4. Coaches can use cases with the same diagnosis. Then, the coach changes one variable at a time (e.g., age, initial vital signs, comorbidities, serum lactate level) and asks the learner to adjust their prognostic estimate accordingly. Coaches guide learners to focus on the following key contextual factors that influence prognosis:

Patient-Specific Factors: Age (e.g., 80-year-old vs 30-year-old with pneumonia), comorbidities (e.g., heart failure, diabetes), prior resilience (e.g., history of quick recovery vs frequent readmissions), baseline functional status, and social determinants of health (e.g., support systems, access to care)

Presentation- and Disease-Specific Factors: Initial vital signs (e.g., BP 90/60 mm Hg vs 130/80 mm Hg in sepsis), lab/imaging findings (e.g., serum lactate level 5 mmol/L vs 2 mmol/L), response to treatment (e.g., rapid improvement vs worsening despite fluid resuscitation), severity at diagnosis (e.g., early vs late sepsis), predictability of disease course (e.g., textbook vs atypical progression)

System-Level Factors: Time of presentation (e.g., weekday afternoon vs 3 AM on a weekend), hospital setting (e.g., tertiary center vs rural hospital), provider variability (e.g., experienced attending vs new learner)

Fork-in-the-Road

This exercise is focused on contingency planning as part of a handoff of care. The coach provides a series of clinical vignettes (real or hypothetical) and asks the learner to develop "if/then" statements to guide the accepting team of clinicians. Each scenario highlights a "fork-in-the-road" where the right contingency plan can prevent a delay in appropriate care. The coach emphasizes the need for precise triggers that prompt immediate action (e.g., oxygen requirement above 6 L/min, heart rate above 130 bpm) rather than vague language. The coach and learner then role play the actual handoff of care, which allows the coach to ask additional "what if" questions and provide feedback on the clarity and accuracy of the signout.

Using Prognosis to Change Management

In this exercise, which is a modification of chart-stimulated recall, the coach and learner review past cases and discuss how changes in prognosis would influence management. The learner reviews admission notes, progress notes, relevant vital signs or lab trends, imaging results, and available discharge summaries. Starting from the initial patient presentation, the learner walks through the clinical course, identifying key decision points (e.g., worsened hypoxia, rise in serum creatinine level). At each decision point, the coach prompts the learner to articulate the original reasoning behind the chosen management (e.g., Why was broad-spectrum antibiotic therapy started at this time?). The coach systematically modifies one or two prognostic variables (e.g., vital signs, lab results, or imaging findings) to create "what-if" scenarios. For example, if the patient's lactate level was only mildly elevated in the real case, the coach might propose, "What if the lactate had been 5.0 mmol/L instead of 2.2 mmol/L?" The learner discusses how these altered prognostic factors would change their interpretation of illness severity and then reevaluates the management plan. The coach highlights how altered prognoses might affect not only acute interventions but also longer-term decisions (e.g., palliative care consultation). After each case, the coach encourages the learner to reflect on the impact of prognostic shifts on management adjustments and highlights areas in which key indicators may have been overlooked.

COACHING EXERCISES FOCUSED ON LONGER TERM PROGNOSIS

How Long to Live?

Although most prognostic models focus on mortality risk, life expectancy is a more useful metric for guiding treatment decisions.[7] In this exercise, the coach describes three clinical vignettes which vary the patient's comorbidities and functional status, such as:

1. 85-year-old with COPD, heart failure, and mild cognitive impairment
2. 72-year-old with diabetes and stage 3 kidney disease
3. 68-year-old with severe frailty and recent fall

The learner classifies life expectancy based on clinical factors and functional status as follows: short (<1 year), intermediate (1 to 5 years), or long (>5 years), and justifies their estimate. The coach then introduces prognostic indices (e.g., ePrognosis[18], frailty scales), asking the learner to recalculate life expectancy and compare results with their initial estimates. We highly recommend ePrognosis, a repository of published geriatric prognostic indices created and maintained by a group from the University of California San Francisco (UCSF).[18] They also provide a "Time to Benefit" tool that allows for estimation of how long it will take a test or treatment to help a given patient and a wide range of modules to improve communication skills.[18]

HOW CAN AI HELP?

AI can assist the coach in enacting these exercises by generating simulated cases and providing structured feedback. Cases generated by AI can be easily modified, allowing learners to see how small changes affect outcomes and thus honing pattern recognition and promoting cognitive flexibility. AI is capable of streamlining literature searches, pointing coach and learner toward the most relevant decision-support tools. Finally, AI can calculate real-time risk estimates using predictive models, helping learners practice assigning probabilities in a way that mirrors prognostic reasoning in the authentic clinical environment.

Example AI Prompt

You are an experienced clinician coach working one-on-one with an advanced learner to improve their uncertainty calibration in short-term prognostic reasoning. Please design a practical, step-by-step exercise that:

1. Introduces 3 to 4 brief patient scenarios in a cyclic manner such that each scenario builds on or varies key contextual factors (e.g., clinical setting, different comorbidities, social supports, or lab abnormalities) so the learner can see how changing one variable affects prognostic confidence
2. Has the learner provide a 0 to 100% confidence rating for each short-term prognostic decision (e.g., "needs ICU now" vs "can stay on the ward"), *immediately* followed by a reflection on why they chose that percentage
3. Includes a concise debrief after each scenario in which you, as the coach, offer feedback on the learner's reasoning, highlight any overlooked data, and compare the learner's confidence rating with your own estimate
4. Outlines a final wrap-up in which the learner identifies patterns in their over- or underconfidence and formulates a plan to adjust their approach for future cases.

Focus on making this a single coaching session with a clear cyclical flow: scenario → confidence rating → brief debrief → new scenario with a varied context. Provide practical tips, scripts, or questions that the coach can use to keep the session engaging and ensure the learner's prognostic reasoning improves by the end.

SUMMARY

Prognostic reasoning is an understudied domain of clinical reasoning. In this chapter, we examine common pitfalls such as overconfidence, avoidance, concrete thinking, and emotional decision-making. Because truly predictive data is difficult to obtain and apply, learners must hone their pattern recognition while synthesizing objective data with contextual factors. The structured coaching exercises provided in this chapter help ensure that learners develop the ability to assess illness severity and predict clinical trajectories.

References

1. Crites G, Stowe J, Murrow L, Gaines J, Richardson WS. Using Evidence to Inform Prognosis Decisions. *MedEdPORTAL.* 11:10280. doi:10.15766/mep_2374-8265.10280
2. Croft P, Altman DG, Deeks JJ, et al. The science of clinical practice: disease diagnosis or patient prognosis? Evidence about "what is likely to happen" should shape clinical practice. *BMC Med.* 2015;13:20. doi:10.1186/s12916-014-0265-4
3. Chiffi D, Zanotti R. Fear of knowledge: Clinical hypotheses in diagnostic and prognostic reasoning. *J Eval Clin Pract.* 2017;23(5):928-934. doi:10.1111/jep.12664
4. Sibbald M, Sherbino J, Preyra I, Coffin-Simpson T, Norman G, Monteiro S. Eyeballing: the use of visual appearance to diagnose 'sick.' *Med Educ.* 2017;51(11):1138-1145. doi:10.1111/medu.13396
5. LoGiudice AB, Sherbino J, Norman G, Monteiro S, Sibbald M. Intuitive and deliberative approaches for diagnosing "well" versus "unwell": evidence from eye tracking, and potential implications for training. *Adv Health Sci Educ Theory Pract.* 2021;26(3):811-825. doi:10.1007/s10459-020-10023-w
6. Hall PA, Going JJ. Predicting the future: a critical appraisal of cancer prognosis studies. *Histopathology.* 1999;35(6):489-494. doi:10.1046/j.1365-2559.1999.00862.x
7. Gill TM. The central role of prognosis in clinical decision making. *JAMA.* 2012;307(2):199-200. doi:10.1001/jama.2011.1992
8. CURB-65 Score for Pneumonia Severity. MDCalc. Accessed February 12, 2025. https://www.mdcalc.com/calc/324/curb-65-score-pneumonia-severity
9. Khullar D, Jena AB. Reducing prognostic errors: a new imperative in quality healthcare. *The BMJ.* 2016;352:i1417. doi:10.1136/bmj.i1417
10. Morgan DJ, Pineles L, Owczarzak J, et al. Accuracy of Practitioner Estimates of Probability of Diagnosis Before and After Testing. *JAMA Intern Med.* 2021;181(6):747-755. doi:10.1001/jamainternmed.2021.0269
11. Christakis NA, Lamont EB. Extent and determinants of error in doctors' prognoses in terminally ill patients: prospective cohort study. *BMJ.* 2000;320(7233):469-472. doi:10.1136/bmj.320.7233.469

12. Turgeon AF, Lauzier F, Burns KEA, et al. Determination of neurologic prognosis and clinical decision making in adult patients with severe traumatic brain injury: a survey of Canadian intensivists, neurosurgeons, and neurologists. *Crit Care Med.* 2013;41(4):1086-1093. doi:10.1097/CCM.0b013e318275d046

13. Christakis NA. *Death Foretold: Prophecy and Prognosis in Medical Care.* University of Chicago Press; 2001. Accessed February 12, 2025. https://press.uchicago.edu/ucp/books/book/chicago/D/bo3641373.html

14. Croft P, Dinant GJ, Coventry P, Barraclough K. Looking to the future: should 'prognosis' be heard as often as 'diagnosis' in medical education? *Educ Prim Care.* 2015;26(6):367-371. doi:10.1080/14739879.2015.1101863

15. Ferrand A, Poleksic J, Racine E. Factors Influencing Physician Prognosis: A Scoping Review. *MDM Policy Pract.* 2022;7(2):23814683221145158. doi:10.1177/23814683221145158

16. Norman G. Dual processing and diagnostic errors. *Adv Health Sci Educ Theory Pract.* 2009;14 Suppl 1:37-49. doi:10.1007/s10459-009-9179-x

17. Croskerry P. A Universal Model of Diagnostic Reasoning. *Acad Med.* 2009;84(8):1022. doi:10.1097/ACM.0b013e3181ace703

18. ePrognosis—About. Accessed February 12, 2025. https://eprognosis.ucsf.edu/about.php

CHAPTER 12

Does Not Have a Plan

DISTINCT FROM DIAGNOSIS and prognosis, management is all about doing. Management is an action-oriented process that carries risk and responsibility. Making a poor decision or missing the window to act can directly harm the patient. Management reasoning (MR) is the cognitive process that informs management actions. As introduced in earlier chapters, MR is defined in the literature as "the process of making decisions about patient management, including choices about treatment, follow-up visits, further testing, and allocation of limited resources."[1,2] While broad in scope, MR is also less well-defined and has been relatively underappreciated in the literature and in clinical teaching. This reflects the somewhat siloed focus on diagnostic error and our common tendency to conflate medical knowledge with management ability—an assumption that overlooks the fact that MR is a distinct cognitive process.[3] Many incorrectly assume that MR boils down to implementing evidence-based guidelines or best-practice protocols, therefore viewing learners' struggles as merely reflecting gaps in knowledge. With a scope far greater than guideline recall, MR demands adaptability to each patient's individual circumstances and requires clinicians to recognize when and how best to apply, deviate from, or supplement standard recommendations.[4,5] This includes the management of patients even when relevant guidelines for evidence-based practice do not exist.

Two notable hallmarks of MR are uncertainty and context specificity.[6] In clinical medicine, there is often no single correct course of action; instead, the clinician must prioritize among many reasonable possibilities. Each choice carries potential risks and benefits to the patient, depending on a broad array of contextual factors. This context specificity means the same problem could be tackled quite differently in two different settings.[7–9] Patient-centered elements such as individual preferences and cultural considerations can dramatically shift management decisions.[10–12] Environmental and system-level components like the availability of diagnostic tests, institutional norms and protocols, and staffing constraints are equally pivotal. Personal biases, prior experiences with the patient or illness, and the learner's stage of professional development color every treatment recommendation a clinician makes.[13,14] Recognizing and balancing these influences is central to MR.

Although MR and diagnostic reasoning (DR) can be separated conceptually, the two often intertwine in clinical practice, and trouble in one area can fuel difficulty in the other.[15] Learners who cling rigidly to protocols without flexibility might also "anchor" on a single diagnosis, missing contextual clues that would shape a more individualized management plan. Learners who agonize over each decision—unsure which route to take—may be similarly hamstrung by diagnostic uncertainty. A minority of struggling learners exhibit an isolated struggle with MR. However, we have observed that, relative to DR difficulties, MR difficulties may be more prominent in specialties in which the number of possible diagnoses are limited and/or DR is less a central part of day-to-day practice. In other words, certain clinical settings are intrinsically more management-focused than others.[16]

In straightforward cases, MR begins with a working diagnosis. More commonly, MR, DR, and prognostic reasoning (chapter 11) occur in a dynamic fashion. Clinically urgent and emergent situations, described in detail in chapter 14, illustrate the non-linear nature. In these situations, treatment must often be initiated before a final diagnosis is established. Shock, for example, cannot wait for diagnostic certainty, so balancing incomplete data with the potential for serious complications becomes both the art and burden of MR.

Given its inherent complexities, it is no surprise that MR is a common area of struggle among learners referred for remediation. Shifting from "figuring out what's wrong" to "deciding what to do about it" can feel to the learner like stepping onto a high-wire. In chapter 8, we characterized two distinct micro skills of MR (management script activation and management option selection) and introduced coaching exercises to guide the learner.[17] Situativity theories tell us that cognition is inherently situated in the environment, expanding our view of MR from in the head to out in the world.[18–21] In this chapter, we outline specific phenotypes of MR struggle in the clinical environment. For each phenotype, we provide a vignette, a short description, and a discussion of coaching strategies.

Analogous to illness scripts, management scripts are high-level, precompiled, conceptual knowledge structures that contain management decisions learned through study and experience.[17,22,23] When a clinician encounters a specific diagnosis or syndrome, the relevant management script is activated, comprising a menu of illness-specific management options such as laboratory studies, imaging, medication, procedures, specialty consults, and monitoring. For instance, for the patient with newly diagnosed hypothyroidism, a basic management script might include initiating levothyroxine, guiding the patient on how to take the medication, and rechecking the thyroid stimulating hormone level in four to six weeks. Clinical decisions in real life are rarely this straightforward. Contextual factors such as patient preference, comorbidities, sociocultural factors, and health system barriers require the clinician to pick and choose from the management script menu.[24,25] This process of choosing the appropriate actions for a specific problem, for a given patient and in a specific context, is termed management option selection.[17]

COMMON SUBPHENOTYPES OF MANAGEMENT REASONING STRUGGLE

1. DRAWS A BLANK

Case

A fourth-year medical student who has always performed well on standardized tests is observed to be hesitant when presenting patients on rounds. She is knowledgeable about her patients' medical conditions, and her presentations are generally well-structured. However, when it comes time to share her assessment and plan, she tends to pause and ask the team a question or look to the senior resident who takes over and outlines the plan for that day. Evaluators have rarely observed her initiating a treatment plan on her own. When asked about this apparent disconnect between medical knowledge and application of that knowledge, the student admits that she has never learned a systematic approach for developing and enacting management plans and often doesn't know where to begin.

Description: The "draws a blank" learner often has a strong knowledge base and can articulate a patient's condition but does not take the next step to propose a management course, thus revealing a gap between their understanding and actual testing and/or treatment actions. Reflecting in part the relative emphasis on DR in the literature and likely in our own training, we rarely provide learners with a systematic approach to crafting a management plan. This may signal a widely held belief that, because management is so context dependent, it is difficult to systematize.[5,26] Unfortunately, the lack of formal teaching means learners tend to abstract their own management scripts from observing the management options selected by supervisors in busy workplace environments. Adding to this challenge is that many supervisors do not share their decision-making process out loud, meaning less experienced learners must infer the reasons behind the management decisions of more experienced clinicians.[27] Many learners fail to learn this by osmosis and require an explicit, organized approach to the creation of a management plan that contains the required elements.

COACHING STRATEGIES

MANAGEMENT SCRIPT TEMPLATE AND THE MANAGEMENT SCRIPT TEMPLATE COMPARISON EXERCISE [17,24,25]

This exercise provides a scaffold for the learner to generate a list of potential management options for an active clinical problem. A typical script might include labs, imaging, procedures, specialty consults, medications, and monitoring. Presenting the learner with the language around these types of interventions allows them to begin identifying their own knowledge gaps in each case and feel more confident suggesting a plan. Learners need to understand why, when, and how each element of a plan might be employed (Table 12.1) and how to make decisions that consider patient preferences, local resource constraints, and the ongoing need to evaluate and adapt the plan over time. A management script template provides the structure to make these fundamental elements of MR more explicit. For all learners, the management script template can be efficiently used in the clinical environment to assess

Table 12.1. A Management Script Template and the Why, When, and How for Each Intervention

Types of Interventions	Why?	When?	How?
Labs	Confirm or rule out a diagnosis, assess disease severity, track therapy response, detect complications, guide adjustments	Immediately vs routine intervals, depending on urgency or clinical evolution. Repeat testing may be needed if results have high impact on management decisions or if the patient's status changes.	Determine which labs are most relevant, ensure proper timing (fasting vs random, time-sensitive draws). Arrange for appropriate follow-up or automated reminders to re-check. Identify thresholds that would prompt a change in therapy (e.g., creatinine for renal function, inflammatory markers for ongoing infection). Balance cost and resource availability.
Imaging	Confirm or exclude suspected diagnoses, localize pathology, assess severity, monitor progression or resolution	Order urgently if a life-threatening condition is suspected (e.g., stroke, PE). Schedule routine imaging for chronic monitoring or less critical findings. Reassess the need for imaging if clinical changes warrant a new look.	Choose an imaging modality (e.g., X-ray, CT, MRI, ultrasound) based on diagnostic yield, patient status (e.g., ability to lie flat, need for sedation), and resource availability. Weigh risks (radiation, contrast use) against potential benefit. Plan how to integrate results into immediate or future management steps (e.g., surgical referral, medication adjustment).

(continued)

Table 12.1. A Management Script Template and the Why, When, and How for Each Intervention *(continued)*

Types of Interventions	Why?	When?	How?
Procedures	Diagnose (biopsy, endoscopy), treat (surgical intervention, drainage), or monitor (catheter placement, device insertion)	Perform urgently if the patient's life or function is at immediate risk (e.g., emergent surgery for acute abdomen). Delay if more conservative options should be tried first, or if medical therapy is still being optimized.	Decide on the setting (bedside, operating room, IR suite). Coordinate with anesthesia or other necessary services. Obtain informed consent and prepare for potential complications. Plan post-procedure monitoring and follow-up; be clear about how the results will impact further management (e.g., pathology findings, success of drainage).
Specialty consults	Seek expertise for diagnostic clarification, procedural assistance, interdisciplinary co-management, or allied health input (nutrition, physical therapy)	Consult immediately if the patient's condition demands urgent expert input (e.g., critical care or urgent cardiology). Schedule routine consultation if comprehensive evaluation or non-urgent specialist involvement is needed.	Identify which specialists (medical, surgical, or allied health) offer the most value. Clarify the question or reason for consult (diagnostic vs management advice). Decide on methods for communication (in-person, phone call, electronic). Establish a follow-up plan that outlines how each specialist's recommendations will be integrated and who ultimately coordinates ongoing care.

Table 12.1. A Management Script Template and the Why, When, and How for Each Intervention *(continued)*

Types of Interventions	Why?	When?	How?
Medications	Treat acute or chronic conditions, alleviate symptoms, prevent complications, optimize existing therapies	Initiate or adjust promptly if patient is hemodynamically unstable, in severe pain, or at high risk for complications. Titrate or discontinue over time based on therapeutic goals, adverse effects, or changes in the patient's clinical course.	Determine whether starting a new medication, restarting a previous one, or discontinuing an unnecessary drug is appropriate. Consider dosing, potential side effects, drug interactions, and required monitoring (labs, vitals). Plan for how to assess adherence and response—when and how often to follow up (e.g., scheduling labs, patient check-ins).
Monitoring	Track response to treatment, detect complications early, ensure patient safety and readiness for escalation/de-escalation of care	Continuous vs intermittent monitoring depends on the acuity of the patient's condition. Increase frequency if the *patient* is deteriorating or if therapy has narrow therapeutic windows. Decrease frequency as stability improves or condition resolves.	Specify which measures to track (vitals, labs, imaging re-check, clinical signs, patient-reported outcomes). Use a schedule or triggers for reassessment. Include family and patient in monitoring plans (e.g., home blood pressure logs). Decide on criteria for treatment modification, discharge, or consulting other services. Integrate monitoring results into ongoing clinical decision-making.

and teach MR. A learner struggling to generate ideas when completing the table may benefit from a different course of action than a learner who can fill in the components but struggles to apply them to individual patients. As part of the real-time feedback process, learners should also compare their management menu to one developed by the coach to reflect on similarities and differences (Table 12.2). Given that knowledge is heavily influenced by context,[28,29] we recommend completing this management script template comparison exercise several times to make sure any differences are not simply due to gaps in the knowledge of or experience with a specific disease and to develop the learner's reasoning as knowledge in the content area improves. For the struggling learner, we recommend deliberate practice of this skill, initially in a simulated environment (e.g., the coach's office) using hypothetical cases, with eventual application in the clinical environment under direct observation with real-time feedback.

Example: A 70-year-old patient on anticoagulation presents with melena, fatigue, and hypotension. Lab tests confirm anemia (Hb 6.2 g/dL), raising concern for an acute GI bleed. Table 12.2 contrasts how an experienced clinician (coach) and a learner might approach management using a management script template.

2. COPY AND PASTE

Case

A second-year psychiatry resident has been praised for efficiency in rounding and writing notes, but concerns arise when multiple attendings notice that he treats virtually every patient with major depressive disorder the same way. He prescribes an SSRI (selective serotonin reuptake inhibitor) at the same starting dose, schedules follow-up in two weeks, and offers generic supportive therapy—regardless of patient history, severity of symptoms, or comorbid conditions. He struggles to adjust his plan if patients deviate from this classic presentation, often explaining, "This worked for my last few patients, so I don't see why it wouldn't work here. I am following the guidelines."

Description: Some learners are overwhelmed by or unaware of the ambiguous nature of MR and prefer to make decisions based solely on

Table 12.2. Example of the Management Script Template Comparison Exercise

Types of Interventions	Potential Management Options (Coach)	Potential Management Options (Learner)
Labs	• Complete blood count (CBC); note that in acute bleeding, the CBC can be falsely normal initially • Type and screen (blood bank preparation) • Prothrombin time (PT) / International Normalized Ratio (INR) • Hepatic function panel (transaminases, bilirubin) • Kidney function tests (blood urea nitrogen [BUN], creatinine [Cr]) • Disseminated intravascular coagulation (DIC) markers (D-dimer, fibrinogen) • Inflammatory markers such as erythrocyte sedimentation rate (ESR), C-reactive protein (CRP), or calprotectin if inflammatory bowel disease (IBD) is suspected • Helicobacter pylori stool antigen or breath test if an upper gastrointestinal source is considered	• Complete blood count (CBC) • Hemoglobin (Hb)
Imaging	• Computed tomography (CT) angiography if bleeding is urgent or massive • Red blood cell (RBC)-labeled (tagged) scan • CT scan of the abdomen if diverticulitis or cancer is suspected	• Kidneys, ureters, and bladder (KUB) X-ray • CT angiography (if endoscopic evaluation by gastroenterology does not identify the source of bleeding)

(continued)

Table 12.2. Example of the Management Script Template Comparison Exercise *(continued)*

Types of Interventions	Potential Management Options (Coach)	Potential Management Options (Learner)
Procedures	• Esophagogastroduodenoscopy (EGD)—timing is critical (urgent vs routine) • Colonoscopy (C-scope), flexible sigmoidoscopy (flex sig) • Push enteroscopy or capsule endoscopy if the bleeding source is difficult to localize • Interventional radiology (IR) embolization if endoscopic methods fail or are not feasible • Surgical correction of hemorrhoids or other bleeding sources if indicated	• Perform endoscopic evaluation (scope) if there is a significant drop in hemoglobin • Place the patient on nil per os (NPO) status and consider bowel preparation prior to the procedure
Specialty consults	• Gastroenterology (GI) for endoscopic diagnosis and intervention • Surgical consultation if endoscopic or IR interventions are insufficient, or if a surgical cause of bleeding is suspected • Interventional radiology (IR) for possible embolization in ongoing bleeding • Intensive care unit (ICU) team if the patient is unstable or requires advanced monitoring	• GI consultation for endoscopy • Hematology (Hem) if bleeding persists, particularly with coagulopathy

Table 12.2. Example of the Management Script Template Comparison Exercise *(continued)*

Types of Interventions	Potential Management Options (Coach)	Potential Management Options (Learner)
Medications	• Erythromycin prior to EGD to improve visualization by clearing gastric contents • Bowel cleanse if lower gastrointestinal bleeding is suspected • Proton pump inhibitor (PPI) administered intravenously (IV) or orally (PO), typically twice a day (BID). High-dose regimens are often used in acute bleeding; H2 blockers have less evidence of benefit • Octreotide if varices are suspected (e.g., in portal hypertension) • Antibiotics if cirrhosis or spontaneous bacterial peritonitis risk is a concern • Helicobacter pylori eradication therapy if H. pylori is detected • Reversal agents for specific anticoagulants if needed (e.g., vitamin K, prothrombin complex concentrate)	• IV PPI plus sucralfate • Transfusion of red blood cells (RBC) or platelets as indicated • Discontinue anticoagulation and antiplatelet agents temporarily if safe to do so

(continued)

Table 12.2. Example of the Management Script Template Comparison Exercise *(continued)*

Types of Interventions	Potential Management Options (Coach)	Potential Management Options (Learner)
Monitoring	• Close observation of vital signs (including orthostatic measurements), mental status, and hemodynamic stability • Maintain at least two large-bore intravenous (IV) lines for possible fluid resuscitation or blood product administration • Continuous telemetry in case of cardiac instability • Administer intravenous fluids (IVF), packed red blood cells (PRBC), or vasopressors if the patient is hypotensive or shows ongoing significant blood loss • Determine triage: step-down unit vs ICU if the patient is unstable • Hold anticoagulants or give fresh frozen plasma (FFP) or desmopressin (DDAVP) for uremia • Protect the airway in cases of upper gastrointestinal bleeding • Consider corticosteroids if an IBD flare is suspected	• Nursing orders to watch for melena or hematochezia (dark or bloody stools) • Frequent checks of blood pressure (BP), hemoglobin (Hb), platelet count, and other vitals • Track any changes in the patient's hemodynamic status and report immediately • Adjust monitoring based on ongoing blood loss or response to treatment

guidelines, protocols, or patterns they have seen effectively applied in similar situations. Patterns can be useful since they automate management decisions and standardize care.[22] However, most management decisions are not entirely algorithmic and require cognitive flexibility. Learners who are overly bound to patterns or protocols often fail to appreciate the contextual nature of these decisions. These learners may struggle to translate generic evidence-based guidelines to specific patient care scenarios and appear to get stuck when consulting the literature. They may struggle to adapt treatment strategies from one patient to another, employing a "copy and paste" management style.

COACHING STRATEGIES

MULTIPLE POSSIBILITIES

Coaching begins with an exploration of the learner's understanding of the relative nature of "right and wrong" management decisions. In the multiple possibilities exercise, the coach provides a case with a working diagnosis and asks the learner to document a plan, then flips the paper over and has the learner consider an alternate course of action. For example, the coach presents a patient admitted with an asthmatic exacerbation who is failing to get better on the usual protocols. In asking the learner for the next steps in management, the coach highlights at least four distinct but acceptable courses of action: escalation of care to the ICU, intravenous bolus of magnesium and continuous albuterol on the floor, three albuterol treatments back-to-back and conversion to intravenous steroids, and addition of a short-acting muscarinic inhaler. Expanding the learner's recognition of diversity in reasonable options highlights the complex and sometimes ambiguous nature of management decisions, even in highly protocolized diseases. This exercise proceeds with the coach helping the learner to appreciate the nuances, including patient preferences, value-based care, side effects, systems-based context, that must be considered while deciding on multiple options.

WORST POSSIBLE IDEA

The coach presents a clinical scenario and asks the learner to describe some of the most inappropriate management options they could imagine a clinician selecting. Being asked to produce "the wrong answer" is often perceived by learners as lower stakes than producing "the right answer" and may more readily stimulate the generation of ideas. The learner may imagine specific situations where there is no "wrong" answer. After they have proposed several "worst possible" management options, the coach asks the learner to imagine a scenario for which these options might be acceptable. This thought exercise encourages the learner to explore the contextual factors they must consider when making management decisions. An example is provided in Figure 12.1.

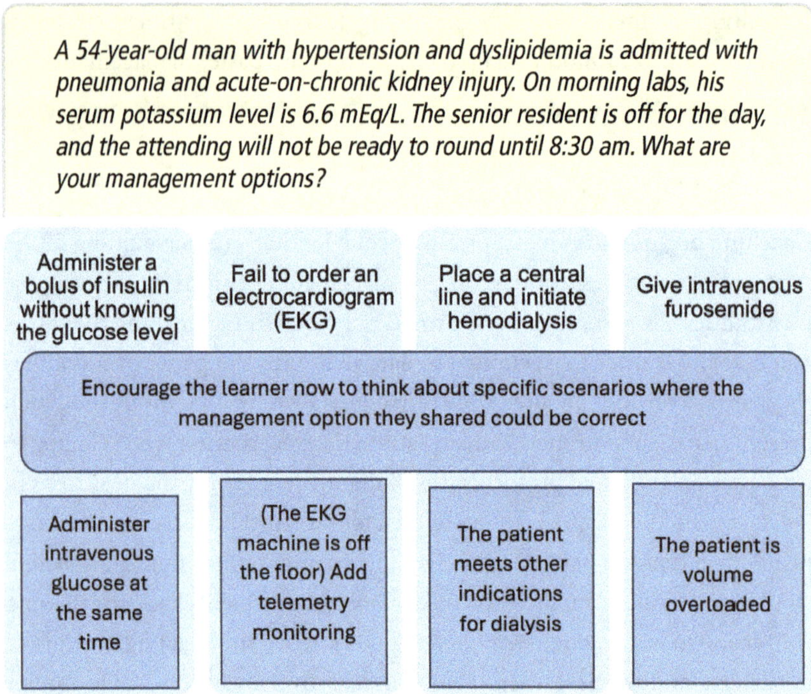

Figure 12.1. The Worst Possible Idea Exercise

PRO/CON OR BENEFIT/HARM LIST

This exercise asks the learner to embrace more than one "right answer" for a given management decision and helps promote recognition that there are potential upsides and downsides to all clinical interventions. The coach asks the learner to complete a list of potential benefits and harms for each element of their management plan. An example is provided in Figure 12.2. This assignment is simple and practical enough for routine practice in the authentic workplace environment.

Imagine a scenario in which the learner is called to the bedside because a patient with cirrhosis is hypotensive. The learner is likely considering many management options such as giving albumin, giving IV fluid bolus, monitoring without intervention, or adding a medication like midodrine to help raise blood pressure.

Giving IV fluid bolus		Adding midodrine		Giving albumin	
Benefit	**Harm**	**Benefit**	**Harm**	**Benefit**	**Harm**
•Volume repletion •Helpful diagnostic intervention •Electrolytes and prevent renal disease	•Cause pulmonary edema •No effect •Fluid now has to be removed •Low sodium	•Improve hypotension •Improve kidney function •Might help with ascites	•Side effects new med •Cardiovascular risks •Dependent or withdrawal •3x daily	•Improve hypotension •Reduce risk of hepato-renal syndrome •Helpful after paracentesis	•Volume overload •Cost and resources •Allergic reactions

Figure 12.2. Creating a Benefit/Harm List for a Proposed Management Plan

MOCK ORAL BOARDS EXERCISE

In addition to helping the learner gain comfort with ambiguity around "right and wrong" choices, the coach can encourage them to practice deviating from the standard course and applying information from one situation to the next. This type of coaching is well-suited to the simulated environment, with the coach presenting a case and asking the learner to develop a management plan. The coach begins by having the learner develop a management script that represents a "standard of care approach" for a specific clinical scenario. The coach then changes elements of the case, posing "what if" scenarios to help the learner develop mental flexibility. It can be useful to work through actual cases with which the learner has struggled as a starting point. Asking questions such as, Why was this intervention appropriate in situation A but not situation B? or Why did this treatment work in patient 1 but led to a complication in patient 2? helps to further the learner's understanding of the role that context plays in management decisions.

3. PARALYSIS BY ANALYSIS

Case

A second-year pediatrics resident is evaluating a 9-year-old child in the emergency department who presents with two days of low-grade fever and abdominal pain. The child's exam is mildly suggestive of appendicitis, but the resident also notes a recent history of viral illness that could explain mesenteric adenitis, and she worries about overlooking other possibilities like constipation or early urinary tract infection. She excelled as an intern when most decisions were made by her seniors, but now, in a supervisory position with heightened autonomy, the sheer number of possible management paths and the weight of each choice feel overwhelming. Rather than deciding on a concrete course of action such as ordering an ultrasound, checking a urinalysis, or consulting surgery, the resident runs through each consideration repeatedly, second-guessing every potential decision. Hours pass without definitive steps taken, and the child remains uncomfortable while the family grows anxious.

Description: Some learners react to uncertainty with a tendency to overthink management decisions, leading to inaction.[30,31] Conversely, intolerance of uncertainty can lead learners to overtreat (e.g., continuing antibiotics for a patient with no clear indication out of fear that they might miss a life-threatening infection).[32] Uncertainty is one of the core principles of MR, given that there is rarely a concrete right or wrong answer in management option selection. When it comes to MR, the answer is almost always "it depends." Ambiguity in medicine can be troublesome and often leads to stress and anxiety. Coaching the learner who is prone to paralysis by analysis in uncertain situations requires reflection on the emotions behind decision making. In the vignette above, the learner may have excelled in roles where she followed orders, but once she was promoted into a supervisory role, the consequences and sheer number of available management options became overwhelming. This highlights the importance of graduated autonomy for learners in their development of effective management reasoning. Granting learners sufficient autonomy to implement their own management plans fosters deeper engagement with the complexities of patient care.[33,34] By "owning" their decisions, they become more attuned to how contextual factors (e.g., patient preferences, resource limitations, and clinical uncertainty) shape each intervention.

Learners who struggle with MR in this manner often describe feeling paralyzed by the fear of making a mistake and worry that errors, whether of omission or commission, could lead to adverse patient outcomes. These learners may also struggle in urgent clinical situations (as we discuss in chapter 14) and/or with decisions involving triage (chapter 13). It is important to ensure that the learner is getting adequate sleep and making time each day to meet their basic physiological needs. Sometimes, the tendency to perseverate or overthink in management situations can reflect underlying attention deficit hyperactivity disorder (ADHD), traits of compulsivity, or an anxiety disorder. Learners who exhibit this type of MR difficulty may also struggle with hypothesis-driven data gathering, not because they can't form hypotheses but because they fear missing something and causing harm to the patient.

In a landmark article published in 1985 titled "The Role of Compulsiveness in the Normal Physician," Gabbard defined a compulsive triad in the personality of physicians characterized by doubt, guilt, and an exaggerated sense of responsibility.[35] Traditionally, we have valued and selected clinicians for these qualities, and yet this triad manifests itself in maladaptive ways as well, causing a predisposition to burnout and error. These characteristics may also lead to difficulties in decision-making which impacts both prognostic and management clinical reasoning.

COACHING STRATEGIES

REFLECT ON CHALLENGING DECISIONS

In this exercise, the coach asks the learner to recall the most challenging management decision they have made and then verbalize what they remember about their decision-making process. The learner recreates the situation and shares, step by step, what was going on inside their mind. The coach should pay special attention to the language used and to the sense of fear, anxiety, stress, or other emotions in the learner's retelling. Helping the learner pause and become more aware of these feelings in moments of decision-making can provide a sense of empowerment which they can apply to future uncertain situations. For the learner unaccustomed to noticing and connecting with feelings in the moment, this can require quite a bit of practice. The coach should validate how difficult it can be to sit with uncertainty.

Excessive doubt or guilt around decision-making may signal that the learner is processing an adverse event or near-miss. Trauma in general can be a catalyst for growth and development of greater self-awareness, tolerance of ambiguity, and understanding of one's own limits. It is important to give the learner space to fully reflect, explore, and process all of the emotions associated with the prior event. Referral to a mental health professional should be considered if there is concern that anxiety, grief, or other cognitive barriers are significantly inhibiting their ability to make decisions.

NORMALIZE UNCERTAINTY

In a wonderful article, Moulder, Harris, and Santhosh explore how uncertainty permeates clinical practice and how educators can take steps to improve their teaching of uncertainty.[36] By explicitly coaching learners to recognize, manage, communicate, and normalize uncertainty, educators can help them craft more patient-aligned management plans. The authors emphasize that structured frameworks (e.g., SNAPPS) and frequent feedback sessions foster transparency around management decisions. They also point out that open acknowledgment of unknowns—whether through open-ended questioning, team discussions, or formal "diagnostic pauses"—builds confidence in tailoring interventions to each patient's unique situation.

COGNITIVE PAUSE

How much clinical information or confidence is required to make a decision? Raising this awareness is valuable; otherwise, learners may endlessly search for more information, continually putting off action until someone else decides for them. Some learners benefit from checklists or scripts to make management decisions. Others find it useful to insert a cognitive pause to increase their confidence that they have all the information available to select a management option. The value of a pause has been demonstrated in a variety of settings, including medicine.[24,25,37–41] Much like professional athletes or musicians who follow a process to warm up and prepare for performance, clinicians can utilize this pause to run through a mental checklist and ensure their process has been systematic and they have explored all angles of a medical decision. We recommend co-creation of such a checklist between the learner and coach (Table 12.3).

Table 12.3. Components of the Cognitive Pause Checklist

1) Have I looked at all the available data?
2) What are my options?
3) What are the main risks and benefits of each option?
4) Am I magnifying the risks of any potential option?
5) Would the perspective of the patient or a colleague be helpful?

By encouraging self-reflection, this exercise moves the learner toward action, thereby launching them out of their paralysis.

REVEAL THE PIECES

Learners who appear to freeze in the face of uncertainty are sometimes struggling to weigh the importance of certain pieces of evidence. Consider, for instance, a patient with acute hypercapnic respiratory failure (pH of 7.2 and pCO2 of 70 mm Hg) who retains a normal mental status. A learner may feel handcuffed in such a situation where one piece of evidence appears contradictory. To help with forward momentum in these circumstances, the coach is encouraged to create a series of low-fidelity case simulations in which attention is drawn to the point at which management decision-making occurs in relationship to the presentation of clinical information. In each case vignette, the coach reveals the pieces of clinical information sequentially, prompting the learner to make a decision after each reveal. This exercise highlights thresholds of certainty and uncertainty in a variety of hypothetical clinical situations.

For example, a 45-year-old female patient with a history of tobacco use, obstructive sleep apnea, asthma, hypertension, and dyslipidemia presents with three days of chest pain. The pain is non-positional, non-reproducible on palpation, and may worsen with exertion. She takes medications for her chronic conditions but rarely attends follow-up appointments. No additional relevant family or social history is reported. Current vital signs show tachycardia and tachypnea, with normal blood pressure and oxygen saturation. She also has mild acute kidney injury. The learner, working a night shift, is considering ordering a CT pulmonary angiogram (CTPA) to evaluate for possible pulmonary embolism. The supervising clinician is at home but can be reached by phone.

The coach reveals the findings shown in Figure 12.3 from left to right, pausing after each disclosure to ask the learner when they would feel confident moving forward with a CTPA. This exercise, for which there is typically no "right" answer, helps the learner gain awareness around the level of certainty required for them to intervene—in this case by ordering a test with multiple inherent risks.

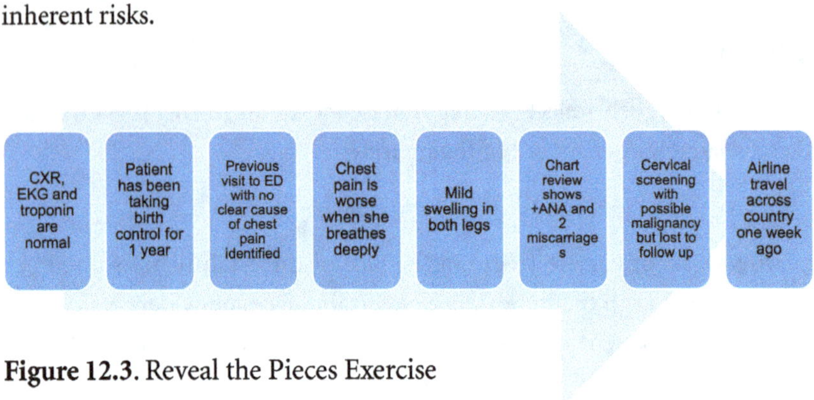

Figure 12.3. Reveal the Pieces Exercise

CONTINGENCY PLANNING

Similar to the pro/con list, this exercise allows the learner to explore different management options and their potential consequences. The coach uses a clinical case (hypothetical or real) to highlight branch points in the learner's management option selection process. For example, an admitted patient with pneumonia is febrile, and the learner must consider what to do with their antibiotic regimen. In a contingency exercise (Figure 12.4), the learner thinks aloud (e.g., What might happen if I switch or do not switch antibiotics?). Proactively exploring a contingency plan is useful in highlighting the best course of action and giving confidence to the learner to move beyond their paralysis by analysis.

Learners who struggle to make decisions in the face of uncertainty are often labeled as underconfident or hesitant and may tend to delegate decisions to other members of the team. Indecision may even be delegated to patients under the guise of shared-decision making. The importance of teaching and modeling assertiveness in medical education is highlighted in chapter 15.

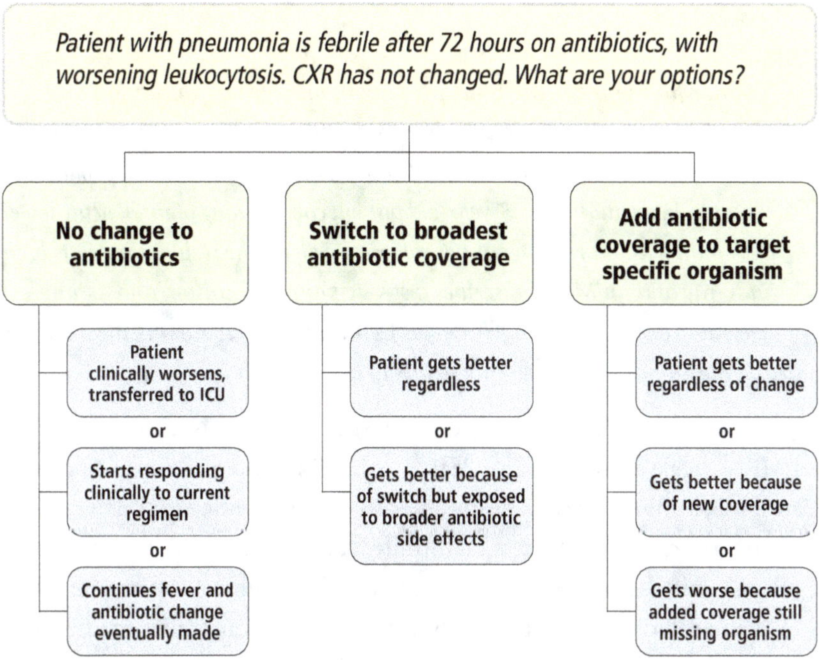

Figure 12.4. Contingency Planning Exercise

Sometimes the intolerance of uncertainty manifests as the tendency to overtreat. Learners can become fixated on the "worst case scenario." A focus on hypothesis refinement, as discussed in chapter 8, is helpful along with these MR exercises. Learners should be encouraged to verbalize the "worst case scenario" in coaching sessions; this often will lessen the anxiety associated with its imagining.

Communication from the coach to supervising faculty should highlight the importance of providing a supportive environment in which the learner can practice with their newfound emotional awareness. Direct observation should focus on encouraging the learner to verbalize the thought process behind their management decisions and, when possible, allow them time to slow down and engage in a cognitive pause on rounds to run through a condensed version of the checklist outlined in Table 12.3.

4. FAILURE TO CALIBRATE

Case

A senior family medicine resident is six months from graduation and has recently garnered attention for his propensity to order extensive labs and imaging when other clinicians would adopt a more conservative approach. For example, in evaluating a 28-year-old patient complaining of mild, acute lower back pain without red flags or neurological deficits, the resident requests both an X-ray and an MRI, prescribes a strong pain medication, and arranges a referral to a spine surgeon. He denies feeling anxious about missing a serious diagnosis and states he simply wants to be thorough.

Description: The tendency to overtest or overtreat is a common form of MR struggle among medical learners.[42,43] This kind of defensive practice can spiral, leading to a cascade of unnecessary interventions.[44–46] High-value care, by contrast, is all about thoughtfully matching tests and treatments to a patient's unique goals and circumstances, while weighing cost and quality.[47] Low-value interventions may offer little to no benefit, can actively cause harm, and run the risk of wasting precious clinical resources.[48] Many professional organizations now publish high-value care guidelines (such as cautioning against routine prealbumin measurement in undernourished patients). Yet not all clinicians routinely apply these recommendations in practice.[49] A learner who consistently overtreats typically does not grasp the implications of high-cost interventions, struggles to interpret diagnostic probabilities correctly, or is driven by an overarching fear of missing something crucial.[50–52]

An often-overlooked reality is that the cost of unnecessary testing goes beyond the dollar amount listed on the clinic or hospital bill. Learners may not consciously consider indirect consequences tied to incidental findings such as unneeded procedures or the anxiety and inconvenience inflicted on patients who endure extra waiting, poking, and prodding.[53,54] While numerous curricula focus on high-value care and emphasize the need to weigh each potential clinical intervention carefully, these broader lessons can only go so far without individualized teaching and coaching in the everyday clinical environment.[55–57] Many struggling learners are unfamiliar with even basic concepts such as likelihood ratios. Coaches and clinical supervisors must model explicit, cost-conscious decision-making and provide targeted feedback on testing and treatment decisions for all learners.

COACHING STRATEGIES

SOAP-V [58,59]

SOAP-V adds value considerations to the common SOAP (subjective-objective-assessment-plan) framework for a learner's presentations and clinical documentation. The SOAP-V model prompts the learner to address the following for a proposed test or treatment:

(1) the evidence that supports a test or treatment
(2) the patient's preferences and values
(3) the financial cost of a test or treatment compared to alternatives

Real-time feedback on these decisions is crucial. Direct review of prior management choices, whether through electronic medical record data or chart audits, allows coach and learner to dissect actual cases and highlight alternative, more value-based strategies.

TOO PRICEY

Shared decision-making (SDM) plays a pivotal role in delivering high-value care by ensuring that clinical decisions align with what matters most to the patient. SDM begins with effective communication: listening to the patient's concerns; breaking down clinical information in understandable terms; and exploring the potential benefits, harms, and costs of each testing or treatment option. Sometimes patients request tests or treatments that feel inappropriate or unnecessary to the clinician. As learners work to navigate the complexities of defining what is "appropriate" and/or "necessary," the TOO PRICEY tool (Figure 12.5) can be used to guide conversations with the patient. TOO PRICEY contains two temporal components: TOO refers to the preparation prior to the conversation, and PRICEY structures the conversation itself. The components of preparation include:

T est/Treatment (know the characteristics of the test or treatment)
O ptions (consider less invasive, lower risk options)
O pen (keep an open mind about patient's concerns and requests).

The conversational elements are:

Perspective (seek patient's perspective)

Reassure (convey confidence that concerning conditions are effectively ruled out)

Incidental/Iatrogenic (discuss risk of incidental findings and adverse effects)

Cost

Empathize

You (return conversation to patient)

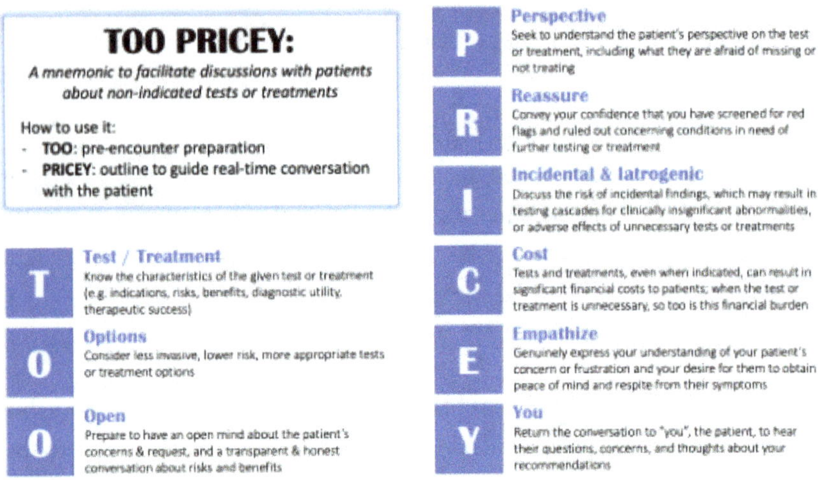

Figure 12.5. TOO PRICEY Mnemonic (Developed by Dr. Rebecca Kowalski.)

TESTING AND TREATMENT THRESHOLDS

Bayesian reasoning refers to the process of incorporating pre-test probabilities and incoming clinical information to calculate post-test probabilities.[60] Germane to almost every decision in clinical practice, the principles of Bayesian reasoning are often not explicitly taught.[61] Figure 12.6 provides a visual aid to clarify this process. We suggest starting with a Fagan nomogram and defining the concept of likelihood ratios (LR).[62] Once the learner is comfortable with these constructs, the coach uses a clinical case to illustrate probability along with testing and treatment thresholds.[63–65] For example, the learner considers a patient with cough, fever, and shortness of breath and is asked to characterize the likelihood of influenza. This step is defined as pretest probability. The learner enters the pretest probability of influenza on one Fagan nomogram and is asked to characterize (1) how confident they would have to be to start treatment for influenza and (2) how confident they would have to be that it is not influenza to skip any further testing. They are then asked to place these numbers on the Fagan nomogram. This process illustrates the concept of thresholds in clinical decision making. The coach then asks the learner to calculate the +LR and -LR for influenza polymerase chain reaction (PCR). The learner is encouraged to reflect on how pretest probability, thresholds, and characteristics of a test can lead to variations in practice patterns.

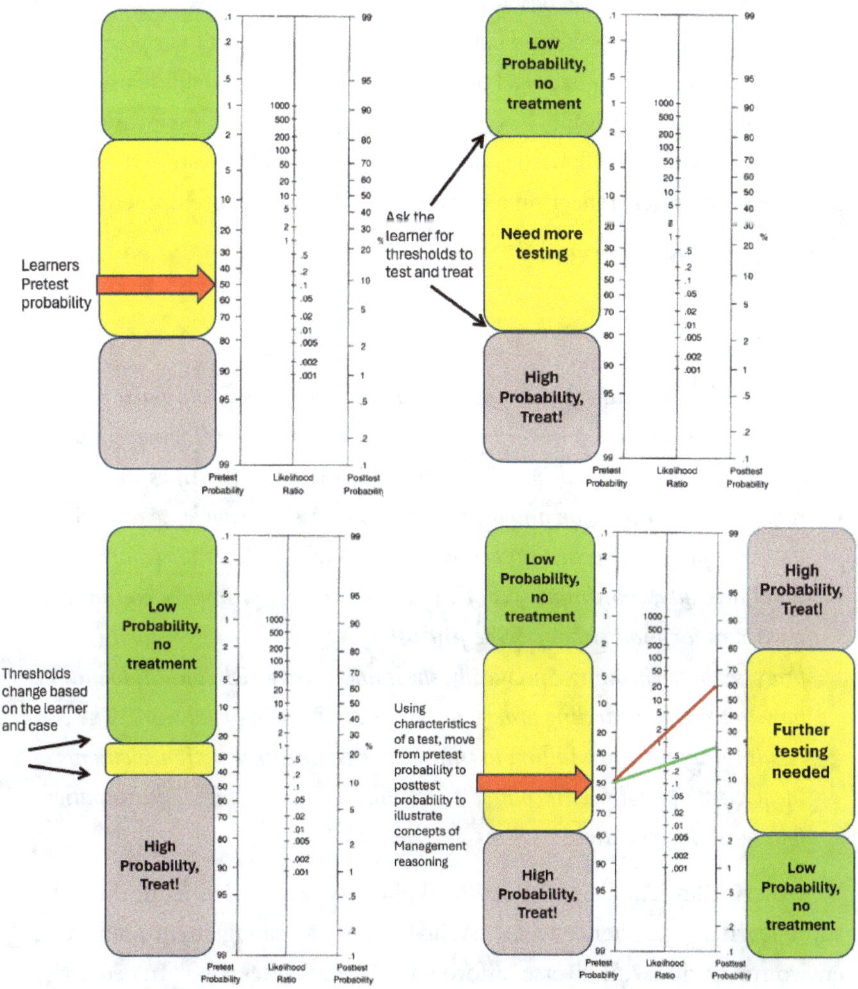

Figure 12.6. Fagan Nomogram for Consideration of Testing and Treatment Thresholds (Adapted with permission from the author.)[66]

Once these concepts are defined and illustrated, the coach guides the learner through additional cases to explore with them how pretest probability and thresholds guide MR decisions. We cannot overstate the importance of helping all learners gain comfort in understanding and utilizing likelihood ratios in their day-to-day practice. In addition, we recommend apps such as EBMcalc,[67] Rx-Bayes,[68] EBM Stats Calc,[69] and DocNomo,[70] to guide these discussions.

Like all clinical reasoning concepts, some learners grasp these ideas intuitively while others require more explicit teaching and dedicated practice. As the learner advances in expertise, they become better equipped to understand their own reasoning process and navigate conversations when their plan differs from that of a supervisor or peer. For instance, it is possible that the learner who consistently overtests simply has a much wider gap between their thresholds to "begin treatment" vs "pursue additional testing." As part of the deliberate practice process, self-reflection guides further study and development.

5. LOST IN THE SYSTEM

Case

A second-year pediatrics resident recognizes a 10-year-old patient with complex care needs: a history of cystic fibrosis, mild developmental delay, and food insecurity. Although the resident expertly identifies the child's respiratory exacerbation and nutritional deficits, she struggles to orchestrate the multiple steps needed to secure follow-up with pulmonology, arrange a swallow study, coordinate with child life services, and involve community resources for food support. She finds the electronic health record (EHR) processes overwhelming. Specifically, she is uncertain which consults to initiate, how to track outstanding orders, and when to involve social work. The end result is that, due to a failure to translate reasoning into action, elements of the patient's plan linger incomplete, delaying both in-hospital and outpatient follow-up interventions.

Description: The "lost in the system" phenotype underscores the difficulty some learners experience when trying to enact a management plan in an environment rich with diverse "affordances" (see chapter 3).[18,71] In pediatrics, as in many other fields, effective management depends on a network of resources that can include the EHR, consultations with specialists, and an interprofessional team composed of nurses, social workers, case managers, pharmacists, dietitians, and more. Ecological psychology suggests that individuals perceive environmental cues, tools, and resources differently based on their own "horizon of observation."[72] A horizon of observation refers to the limits of what a person can perceive, attend to, or interpret within a given context. If a learner is unaware of how to leverage these supports or collaborate with team members such as the social worker or case manager, they may fail to effectively and efficiently implement the management plan.[73]

This challenge also illustrates an application of distributed cognition (introduced in chapter 3) in which tapping into the combined expertise of all team participants and taking advantage of available tools leads to more effective patient care.[74–77] Individual team members' horizons of observation are by definition complementary, reflecting diverse perspectives and revealing additional opportunities or constraints that might otherwise go unnoticed. Advanced technology such as AI-assisted decision tools can contribute meaningfully to this collective cognition and thus ensure that management plans are enacted appropriately. Learners without strategies for pooling these different perspectives and effectively utilizing technology can become overwhelmed, resulting in delayed or incomplete management plans. In chapter 2, we acknowledged the overlap between the ACGME/ABMS[78] competency and AAMC/AACOM/ACGME foundational competency[79] of Systems-Based Practice (SBP) and MR. The following exercises specifically target elements of SBP.

COACHING STRATEGIES

SYSTEM MAPPING

In this exercise, the coach presents a case vignette (real or hypothetical) requiring a multi-faceted management plan. The learner is asked to break down each required element of the plan (e.g., orders, consultations, follow-up tasks) into a clear sequence, noting who is responsible for each step, how tasks are ordered in the EHR, and defining the timeline. The focus is on the practical—*how* to get things done and what barriers may be encountered. The learner should delineate each member of the interprofessional team involved and what their horizon of observation is specific to the case.

REFLECTIVE CASE REVIEW

The learner in this exercise is encouraged to reflect on a recent case in which complex interdisciplinary coordination was required (e.g., a patient with multiple subspecialty needs), highlighting what about the process did/did not go well. To build insight and identify areas for future education and deliberate practice, the coach asks questions such as, Which team members could have been involved earlier? or What step in the EHR workflow was overlooked?

PEER ROLE MODELING

In this exercise, the coach arranges for the learner to shadow or observe a more experienced peer who is adept at navigating both the clinical setting and the EHR. The coach sets clear goals to guide the learner's observation (e.g., communication with the team, documenting tasks, utilization of different elements of the health care system). Learner and coach then reflect specifically on how effectively patients' needs are anticipated and tasks are delegated, and how efficiently the process occurs.

Table 12.3. Frameworks and Coaching Exercises for the "Does Not Have a Plan" Phenotype

1. Draws a blank
a. Management script template b. Management script template comparison exercise
2. Copy and paste
a. Multiple possibilities b. Worst possible idea c. Pro/con or benefit/harm list d. Mock oral boards exercise

(continued)

(Table 12.3 continued)

3. Paralysis by analysis
a. Reflect on challenging decisions b. Normalize uncertainty c. Cognitive pause d. Reveal the pieces e. Contingency planning
4. Failure to calibrate
a. SOAP-V b. TOO PRICEY c. Testing and treatment thresholds
5. Lost in the system
a. System mapping b. Reflective case review c. Peer observation

SUMMARY

MR challenges can span a broad range—from failing to articulate a plan at all to, at the other extreme, piling on unnecessary interventions. For medical learners, much of the observed struggles with MR stem from discomfort with uncertainty and/or a lack of awareness around the boundaries of evidence-based care. The coaching approach described in this chapter encourages the learner to accept and work within the uncertainty that fundamentally characterizes clinical medicine. Using a deliberate practice model, the coach guides the learner through a more intentional process of decision-making around patient management. The case-based approach promotes development of cognitive flexibility and an appreciation of the limitations of guidelines and protocols. We encourage educators to incorporate the use of these frameworks and exercises into the teaching of MR for all learners.

References

1. Cook DA, Sherbino J, Durning SJ. Management Reasoning: Beyond the Diagnosis. *JAMA.* 2018;319(22):2267-2268. doi:10.1001/jama.2018.4385
2. Cook DA, Durning SJ, Sherbino J, Gruppen LD. Management Reasoning: Implications for Health Professions Educators and a Research Agenda. *Acad Med.* 2019;94(9):1310. doi:10.1097/ACM.0000000000002768
3. Committee on Diagnostic Error in Health Care, Board on Health Care Services, Institute of Medicine, The National Academies of Sciences, Engineering, and Medicine. *Improving Diagnosis in Health Care.* (Balogh EP, Miller BT, Ball JR, eds.). National Academies Press (US); 2015. Accessed October 1, 2020. http://www.ncbi.nlm.nih.gov/books/NBK338596/
4. Cook DA, Stephenson CR, Gruppen LD, Durning SJ. Management Reasoning: Empirical Determination of Key Features and a Conceptual Model. *Acad Med.* 2023;98(1):80. doi:10.1097/ACM.0000000000004810
5. Boyle JG, Walters MR, Burton FM, et al. On context specificity and management reasoning: moving beyond diagnosis. *Diagn Berl Ger.* Published online January 8, 2025. doi:10.1515/dx-2024-0122
6. Wijesekera TP, Parsons AS, Abdoler EA, Trowbridge RL, Durning SJ, Rencic JJ. Management Reasoning: A Toolbox for Educators. *Acad Med.* 2022;97(11):1724. doi:10.1097/ACM.0000000000004796
7. Konopasky A, Artino AR, Battista A, et al. Understanding context specificity: the effect of contextual factors on clinical reasoning. *Diagnosis.* 2020;7(3):257-264. doi:10.1515/dx-2020-0016
8. Durning SJ, Artino AR, Pangaro LN, Van Der Vleuten C, Schuwirth L. Perspective: Redefining Context in the Clinical Encounter: Implications for Research and Training in Medical Education: *Acad Med.* 2010;85(5):894-901. doi:10.1097/ACM.0b013e3181d7427c
9. Durning SJ, Artino AR, Boulet JR, Dorrance K, van der Vleuten C, Schuwirth L. The impact of selected contextual factors on experts' clinical reasoning performance (does context impact clinical reasoning performance in experts?). *Adv Health Sci Educ Theory Pract.* 2012;17(1):65-79. doi:10.1007/s10459-011-9294-3
10. Leidner C, Vennedey V, Hillen H, et al. Implementation of patient-centred care: which system-level determinants matter from a decision maker's perspective? Results from a qualitative interview study across various health and social care organisations. *BMJ Open.* 2021;11(9):e050054. doi:10.1136/bmjopen-2021-050054
11. Scholl I, LaRussa A, Hahlweg P, Kobrin S, Elwyn G. Organizational- and system-level characteristics that influence implementation of shared decision-making and strategies to address them - a scoping review. *Implement Sci IS.* 2018;13(1):40. doi:10.1186/s13012-018-0731-z
12. Hower KI, Vennedey V, Hillen HA, et al. Implementation of patient-centred care: which organisational determinants matter from decision maker's perspective? Results from a qualitative interview study across various health and social care organisations. *BMJ Open.* 2019;9(4):e027591. doi:10.1136/bmjopen-2018-027591

13. Croskerry P. Adaptive expertise in medical decision making. *Med Teach.* 2018;40(8):803-808. doi:10.1080/0142159X.2018.1484898

14. Norman GR, Monteiro SD, Sherbino J, Ilgen JS, Schmidt HG, Mamede S. The Causes of Errors in Clinical Reasoning: Cognitive Biases, Knowledge Deficits, and Dual Process Thinking. *Acad Med.* 2017;92(1):23-30. doi:10.1097/ACM.0000000000001421

15. Ilgen JS, Eva KW, Regehr G. What's in a Label? Is Diagnosis the Start or the End of Clinical Reasoning? *J Gen Intern Med.* 2016;31(4):435-437. doi:10.1007/s11606-016-3592-7

16. Choi JJ, Contractor JH, Patel VL, Shapiro MF. How team clinical reasoning occurs on ward rounds: Implications for learning. *Clin Teach.* 2023;20(4):e13599. doi:10.1111/tct.13599

17. Parsons AS, Wijesekera TP, Rencic JJ. The Management Script: A Practical Tool for Teaching Management Reasoning. *Acad Med.* 2020;95(8):1179-1185. doi:10.1097/ACM.0000000000003465

18. Parsons AS, Wijesekera TP, Olson APJ, Torre D, Durning SJ, Daniel M. Beyond thinking fast and slow: Implications of a transtheoretical model of clinical reasoning and error on teaching, assessment, and research. *Med Teach.* Published online June 5, 2024:1-12. doi:10.1080/0142159X.2024.2359963

19. Torre D, Durning SJ, Rencic J, Lang V, Holmboe E, Daniel M. Widening the lens on teaching and assessing clinical reasoning: from "in the head" to "out in the world." *Diagn Berl Ger.* 2020;7(3):181-190. doi:10.1515/dx-2019-0098

20. Durning SJ, Artino AR. Situativity theory: a perspective on how participants and the environment can interact: AMEE Guide no. 52. *Med Teach.* 2011;33(3):188-199. doi:10.3109/0142159X.2011.550965

21. Merkebu J, Battistone M, McMains K, et al. Situativity: a family of social cognitive theories for understanding clinical reasoning and diagnostic error. *Diagn Berl Ger.* 2020;7(3):169-176. doi:10.1515/dx-2019-0100

22. Cook DA, Stephenson CR, Gruppen LD, Durning SJ. Management reasoning scripts: Qualitative exploration using simulated physician-patient encounters. *Perspect Med Educ.* 2022;11(4):196-206. doi:10.1007/s40037-022-00714-y

23. Abdoler EA, O'Brien BC, Schwartz BS. Following the Script: An Exploratory Study of the Therapeutic Reasoning Underlying Physicians' Choice of Antimicrobial Therapy. *Acad Med.* 2020;95(8):1238. doi:10.1097/ACM.0000000000003498

24. Abdoler EA, Parsons AS, Wijesekera TP. The future of teaching management reasoning: important questions and potential solutions. *Diagn Berl Ger.* Published online November 23, 2022. doi:10.1515/dx-2022-0048

25. Penner JC, Minter DJ, Abdoler EA, Parsons AS. Reasoning on Rounds Volume 2: a Framework for Teaching Management Reasoning in the Inpatient Setting. *J Gen Intern Med.* Published online December 20, 2024. doi:10.1007/s11606-024-09039-4

26. Cook DA, Durning SJ, Stephenson CR, Gruppen LD, Lineberry M. Assessment of management reasoning: Design considerations drawn from analysis of simulated outpatient encounters. *Med Teach.* 2025;47(2):218-232. doi:10.1080/0142159X.2024.2337251

27. Jagannath AD, Dreicer JJ, Penner JC, Dhaliwal G. The cognitive apprenticeship: advancing reasoning education by thinking aloud. *Diagn Berl Ger.* Published online December 1, 2022. doi:10.1515/dx-2022-0043

28. Daniel M, Durning SJ, Wilson E, Abdoler E, Torre D. Situated cognition: clinical reasoning and error are context dependent. *Diagnosis.* 2020;7(3):341-342. doi:10.1515/dx-2020-0011

29. Rencic J, Schuwirth LWT, Gruppen LD, Durning SJ. A situated cognition model for clinical reasoning performance assessment: a narrative review. *Diagn Berl Ger.* 2020;7(3):227-240. doi:10.1515/dx-2019-0106

30. Farnan JM, Johnson JK, Meltzer DO, Humphrey HJ, Arora VM. Resident uncertainty in clinical decision making and impact on patient care: a qualitative study. *Qual Saf Health Care.* 2008;17(2):122-126. doi:10.1136/qshc.2007.023184

31. Han PKJ, Klein WMP, Arora NK. Varieties of uncertainty in health care: a conceptual taxonomy. *Med Decis Mak Int J Soc Med Decis Mak.* 2011;31(6):828-838. doi:10.1177/0272989x11393976

32. Brun C, Zerhouni O, Akinyemi A, Houtin L, Monvoisin R, Pinsault N. Impact of uncertainty intolerance on clinical reasoning: A scoping review of the 21st-century literature. *J Eval Clin Pract.* 2023;29(3):539-553. doi:10.1111/jep.13756

33. Ilgen JS, de Bruin ABH, Teunissen PW, Sherbino J, Regehr G. Supported Independence: The Role of Supervision to Help Trainees Manage Uncertainty. *Acad Med.* 2021;96(11S):S81. doi:10.1097/ACM.0000000000004308

34. Crockett C, Joshi C, Rosenbaum M, Suneja M. Learning to drive: resident physicians' perceptions of how attending physicians promote and undermine autonomy. *BMC Med Educ.* 2019;19(1):293. doi:10.1186/s12909-019-1732-6

35. Gabbard GO. The role of compulsiveness in the normal physician. *JAMA.* 1985;254(20):2926-2929.

36. Moulder G, Harris E, Santhosh L. Teaching the science of uncertainty. *Diagn Berl Ger.* 2023;10(1):13-18. doi:10.1515/dx-2022-0045

37. Lee JY, Szulewski A, Young JQ, Donkers J, Jarodzka H, van Merriënboer JJG. The medical pause: Importance, processes and training. *Med Educ.* 2021;55(10):1152-1160. doi:10.1111/medu.14529

38. Cornell EG, Harris E, McCune E, et al. Scaling up a diagnostic pause at the ICU-to-ward transition: an exploration of barriers and facilitators to implementation of the ICU-PAUSE handoff tool. *Diagn Berl Ger.* 2023;10(4):417-423. doi:10.1515/dx-2023-0046

39. Gupta A, Quinn M, Greene MT, Fowler KE, Chopra V. Implementation of a bundle to improve diagnosis in hospitalized patients: lessons learned. *Diagn Berl Ger.* 2025;12(1):68-73. doi:10.1515/dx-2024-0099

40. Huang GC, Kriegel G, Wheaton C, et al. Implementation of diagnostic pauses in the ambulatory setting. *BMJ Qual Saf.* 2018;27(6):492-497. doi:10.1136/bmjqs-2017-007192

41. Martin BJ, Plews-Ogan M, Parsons AS. Ethical Pause as a Framework for High-Value Care of Hospitalized Covid-19 Patients. *Clin Ethics.* 2022;17(1):1-4. doi:10.1177/14777509211011434

42. Lyu H, Xu T, Brotman D, et al. Overtreatment in the United States. *PloS One.* 2017;12(9):e0181970. doi:10.1371/journal.pone.0181970

43. Brownlee S, Chalkidou K, Doust J, et al. Evidence for overuse of medical services around the world. *Lancet Lond Engl.* 2017;390(10090):156-168. doi:10.1016/S0140-6736(16)32585-5

44. Niess MA, Prochazka A. Preoperative Chest X-rays: A Teachable Moment. *JAMA Intern Med.* 2014;174(1):12. doi:10.1001/jamainternmed.2013.10531

45. Eaton KP, Levy K, Soong C, et al. Evidence-Based Guidelines to Eliminate Repetitive Laboratory Testing. *JAMA Intern Med.* 2017;177(12):1833-1839. doi:10.1001/jamainternmed.2017.5152

46. Mold JW, Stein HF. The Cascade Effect in the Clinical Care of Patients. *N Engl J Med.* 1986;314(8):512-514. doi:10.1056/NEJM198602203140809

47. Shah N, Arora V, Moriates C. *Understanding Value Based Healthcare.* McGraw-Hill Education; 2015.

48. Shrank WH, Rogstad TL, Parekh N. Waste in the US Health Care System: Estimated Costs and Potential for Savings. *JAMA.* 2019;322(15):1501-1509. doi:10.1001/jama.2019.13978

49. Kerr EA, Kullgren JT, Saini SD. Choosing Wisely: How To Fulfill The Promise In The Next 5 Years. *Health Aff (Millwood).* 2017;36(11):2012-2018. doi:10.1377/hlthaff.2017.0953

50. Korenstein D. Medical Overuse as a Physician Cognitive Error: Looking Under the Hood. *JAMA Intern Med.* 2019;179(1):26-27. doi:10.1001/jamainternmed.2018.5136

51. Korenstein D, Chimonas S, Barrow B, Keyhani S, Troy A, Lipitz-Snyderman A. Development of a Conceptual Map of Negative Consequences for Patients of Overuse of Medical Tests and Treatments. *JAMA Intern Med.* 2018;178(10):1401-1407. doi:10.1001/jamainternmed.2018.3573

52. Scott IA, Soon J, Elshaug AG, Lindner R. Countering cognitive biases in minimising low value care. *Med J Aust.* 2017;206(9):407-411. doi:10.5694/mja16.00999

53. Grady D, Redberg RF. Less is more: how less health care can result in better health. *Arch Intern Med.* 2010;170(9):749-750. doi:10.1001/archinternmed.2010.90

54. Hicks LK. Reframing overuse in health care: time to focus on the harms. *J Oncol Pract.* 2015;11(3):168-170. doi:10.1200/JOP.2015.004283

55. Cayea D, Tartaglia K, Pahwa A, Harrell H, Shaheen A, Lang VJ. Current and Optimal Training in High-Value Care in the Internal Medicine Clerkship: A National Curricular Needs Assessment. *Acad Med.* 2018;93(10):1511-1516. doi:10.1097/ACM.0000000000002192

56. Ford V, Frischtak H, Wiencek JR, Parsons AS. A High-Value Care Curriculum Using Individual and Group Structured Reflection. *South Med J.* 2021;114(12):797-800. doi:10.14423/SMJ.0000000000001325

57. Niranjan-Azadi A, Moulder G, Gusic ME, Hoke G, Pahwa A, Parsons AS. A novel virtual course to teach medical students high-value decision-making. *Clin Teach.* 2023;20(4):e13597. doi:10.1111/tct.13597

58. Moser EM, Huang GC, Packer CD, et al. SOAP-V: Introducing a method to empower medical students to be change agents in bending the cost curve. *J Hosp Med.* 2016;11(3):217-220. doi:10.1002/jhm.2489

59. Moser EM, Fazio SB, Packer CD, et al. SOAP to SOAP-V: A New Paradigm for Teaching Students High Value Care. *Am J Med.* 2017;130(11):1331-1336.e2. doi:10.1016/j.amjmed.2017.07.014

60. Mazur DJ. A history of evidence in medical decisions: from the diagnostic sign to Bayesian inference. *Med Decis Mak Int J Soc Med Decis Mak.* 2012;32(2):227-231. doi:10.1177/0272989X11434739

61. Brush JE, Lee M, Sherbino J, Taylor-Fishwick JC, Norman G. Effect of Teaching Bayesian Methods Using Learning by Concept vs Learning by Example on Medical Students' Ability to Estimate Probability of a Diagnosis. *JAMA Netw Open.* 2019;2(12). doi:10.1001/jamanetworkopen.2019.18023

62. McGee S. Simplifying Likelihood Ratios. *J Gen Intern Med.* 2002;17(8):647-650. doi:10.1046/j.1525-1497.2002.10750.x

63. Pauker SG, Kassirer JP. The threshold approach to clinical decision making. *N Engl J Med.* 1980;302(20):1109-1117. doi:10.1056/NEJM198005153022003

64. Phadke VK, Jagannath AD, Patel AA, Sherman SV. Over the Threshold: an Exercise in Clinical Reasoning. *J Gen Intern Med.* 2022;37(5):1290-1294. doi:10.1007/s11606-021-07206-5

65. Stojan JN, Daniel M, Morgan HK, Whitman L, Gruppen LD. A Randomized Cohort Study of Diagnostic and Therapeutic Thresholds in Medical Student Clinical Reasoning. *Acad Med.* 2017;92(11S):S43. doi:10.1097/ACM.0000000000001909

66. Kinnear B, Hagedorn PA, Kelleher M, Ohlinger C, Tolentino J. Integrating Bayesian reasoning into medical education using smartphone apps. *Diagn Berl Ger.* 2019;6(2):85-89. doi:10.1515/dx-2018-0065

67. LLC FIS LLC, DBA EBMcalc, LLC FIS. EBMalc Medical calculators, Calculated Medicine, equations, clinical criteria sets, decision trees, and data coverters. EBMcalc. Accessed February 21, 2025. https://EBMcalc.com/

68. Welcome to Rx-Bayes - The BEST App for Clinical Bayesian Reasoning. Accessed February 21, 2025. http://rxbayes.com

69. EBM Calculators. EBM Calculators. Accessed February 21, 2025. https://ebm-tools.knowledgetranslation.net/calculator

70. DocNomo on the App Store. Accessed February 21, 2025. https://apps.apple.com/us/app/docnomo/id901279945

71. Daniel M, Torre D, Durning SJ, Wilson E, Rencic JJ. Ecological psychology: diagnosing and treating patients in complex environments. *Diagn Berl Ger.* 2020;7(3):339-340. doi:10.1515/dx-2020-0008

72. Perceiving, Acting and Knowing: Toward an Ecological Psychology. Routledge & CRC Press. Accessed November 24, 2023. https://www.routledge.com/Perceiving-Acting-and-Knowing-Toward-an-Ecological-Psychology/Shaw-Bransford/p/book/9781138205055

73. Olson A, Rencic J, Cosby K, et al. Competencies for improving diagnosis: an interprofessional framework for education and training in health care. *Diagn Berl Ger.* 2019;6(4):335-341. doi:10.1515/dx-2018-0107

74. Boyle JG, Walters MR, Jamieson S, Durning SJ. Distributed cognition: Theoretical insights and practical applications to health professions education: AMEE Guide No. 159. *Med Teach.* Published online April 12, 2023:1-11. doi:10.1080/0142159X.2023.2190479

75. Boyle JG, Walters MR, Jamieson S, Durning SJ. Reframing context specificity in team diagnosis using the theory of distributed cognition. *Diagn Berl Ger.* 2023;10(3):235-241. doi:10.1515/dx-2022-0100

76. Wilson E, Daniel M, Rao A, et al. A scoping review of distributed cognition in acute care clinical decision-making. *Diagn Berl Ger.* 2023;10(2):68-88. doi:10.1515/dx-2022-0095

77. Wilson E, Seifert C, Durning SJ, Torre D, Daniel M. Distributed cognition: interactions between individuals and artifacts. *Diagnosis.* 2020;7(3):343-344. doi:10.1515/dx-2020-0012

78. ACGME Home. Accessed January 22, 2025. https://www.acgme.org/

79. UME Competencies AAMC | AACOM | ACGME. Accessed January 22, 2025. https://engage.aamc.org/UME-Competencies-AAMC-ACGME-AACOM

CHAPTER 13

Struggles to Triage

TASK PRIORITIZATION AND TRIAGE IN MEDICAL TRAINING

LEARNERS FACE MANY competing demands during their education and training, both within the clinical environment and in the process of integrating clinical work with nonclinical work-related tasks and non-work life. Trainees are expected to take safe and efficient care of their patients and care for themselves, all while furthering their own education. The time required to achieve these goals often exceeds the available amount of time in the day. Our mentor, Dr. John Schorling, teaches that time is the ultimate zero-sum game. Every moment spent on task A is time taken away from task B. The clinical environment is by nature unpredictable and characterized by frequent interruptions, variable expectations and resources, intrinsic system shortfalls, and the pressure to think on one's feet in high-stakes situations. Thus, clinicians in general are in the position of perpetually triaging tasks, much like military health care providers deciding whom to treat first in a chaotic wartime setting. The process of triage involves complex, in-the-moment analysis that considers the consequences of choosing one patient or task over another. It is more than simply prioritizing assignments. Triage implies a restriction of resources—in this case, time—in which failure to act may lead to immediate adverse outcome. Triage suggests urgency and a reactive stance, whereas prioritization may occur in calmer times and allow for more planning and proactivity. Both are important skills for medical learners, regardless of specialty.

Table 13.1. Examples of Triaging Tasks in the Clinical Environment

- Structuring time when time is limited
  - Prioritizing the daily task list
  - Pre-rounding
  - Prioritizing simultaneous clinical encounters
- Managing time-sensitive interruptions
  - Responding to an urgent request (e.g., critical test result, patient with change in clinical status) while working on a less-urgent task (e.g., handling a routine patient admission, seeing a patient in clinic, reading nonurgent radiology scans, performing a nonurgent procedure)
  - Reacting to a change in clinical status while performing a procedure
  - Integrating new data and re-prioritizing existing task list based on this new data

BE EFFICIENT! STRUCTURING TIME WHEN TIME IS LIMITED

All medical learners encounter pressure to manage their time efficiently. In certain specialties, clinicians are evaluated based on how many tasks they accomplish in a given time interval. In others, days are split into chunks, with specific expectations based on time of day. If trainees are unable to structure these limited blocks of time deliberately, their care plans will be incomplete or disorganized, they will appear flustered and overwhelmed, work may not be completed on time or at all, and they will ultimately require more supervision. When inefficient use of time leads to longer days, risk of stress and burnout increases with many potential downstream consequences. In many specialties, trainees are faced with multiple patients at once and must decide whom to see first. If they prioritize incorrectly, patient care can be delayed, leading to adverse outcomes.

In general, structuring time when time is limited requires effective systems such as templates, checklists, and facility with the electronic medical record to maximize efficiency. Experts rely on medical knowledge and clinical reasoning that signal which data, tasks, and clinical situations are important and/or urgent. As learners progress, this knowledge can become organized and automated in the form of mental schemas.[1]

BE AVAILABLE! MULTITASK! DEALING WITH INTERRUPTIONS

Interruptions are a part of life for the medical learner, as is the demand to multitask. Interruptions, which threaten even the most dependable organizational systems, typically introduce new tasks. They require that one rapidly shift gears, assess the urgency and importance of the new task in relation to the existing tasks, and make decisions about timing and potential delegation of the new task. Ultimately, one then needs to return to the original task. Psychologists maintain that our brains are not capable of multitasking, that we cannot focus on more than one thing at once.[2] When we feel we are multitasking, we are actually switching back and forth between tasks or performing two or more tasks in rapid succession, often without awareness. It follows that efficacy in "multitasking" reflects one's ability to cope with interruption and effective task shifting. The ACGME[3] lists multitasking as a core competency in several medical specialties.[4] In emergency medicine, task shifting is considered a fundamental skill that reflects both the patient care and systems-based practice competencies. The Emergency Medicine Milestones provide a framework for evaluation of this skill which is also evaluated formally on standardized examinations.[5–7] For all medical learners, the cognitive load generated from interruptions and task shifting is impacted by the complexity and familiarity of the tasks as well as the environment and type of interruption.[8–11] Potential costs include errors and burnout.

TASK TRIAGE AS CLINICAL REASONING OF THE HIGHEST ORDER

Timely completion of important and urgent clinical responsibilities in medical training implies proficiency across multiple competencies, including, in our framework, medical knowledge, clinical reasoning, and organization and efficiency. The learner must possess enough knowledge about each situation to interpret data, to recognize acuity, and to identify which tasks are important and urgent. They must implement effective systems for organizing data and tasks. In chapter 4, we presented clinical reasoning as related to a hierarchy that incorporates executive function, metacognition, and self-regulation. In this framework, triaging tasks in the clinical environment exists at the top of the pyramid as an example of the highest order skillset, requiring basic intellectual, cognitive, and social-emotional capacity as well as the ability to self-reflect.

Imagine that, while placing admission orders for a patient they just interviewed, a learner is paged with a critical laboratory value on a different patient. The learner must rapidly shift gears and decide if the new task requires immediate attention. This requires that they understand the task and its importance and urgency, both in the absolute sense and relative to the task in which they are currently engaged. They must be aware of and manage their own emotional response to being interrupted and faced with a potential emergency—and potentially the emotions of others. Eventually, they will need to return to the original task. To do this well requires adequate working memory, processing speed, attention skills, and the ability to suppress additional distractions. Of particular importance is cognitive flexibility, or adaptability, which refers to the learner's ability to integrate information in the moment and change course rapidly in the face of shifting clinical circumstances. The social-emotional and metacognitive elements of the pyramid discussed in chapter 4 are particularly important in situations that call for task triage under pressure.[12–15] Specifically, the learner must be able to reflect upon their own thinking process (i.e., metacognitive awareness) with cognizance of how and why they are making decisions.[12] Learners faced with multiple competing demands in high pressure situations often describe feeling overwhelmed and frustrated.

Prioritizing tasks during a busy clinical day is fundamentally a management reasoning activity.[16,17] Timely completion of daily work is facilitated by the learner's ability to recognize concerning and less concerning patterns (System 1) in the data. This pattern recognition, as in the case of diagnostic reasoning, is guided by the relevant knowledge and experience with the task and situation. Until the learner develops this experience, we can provide frameworks for training tasks supported by coaching. The need for situational experience acknowledges the importance of context when triaging tasks, as understood by situated cognition.[18–20] Therefore, assessment and coaching must eventually be done in the authentic clinical environment. Triaging clinical tasks requires knowledge of the tasks and implications for doing or not doing each task with consideration of context-specific variables such as the patient's current condition (e.g., diagnosis, acuity, urgency), the patient's goals and values, the interprofessional care team needed to complete the tasks, and system utilization requirements and/or barriers. Management reasoning is discussed in more detail in chapter 12.

The clinical environment, with all its potential instability, inefficiencies, and high emotion, can expose relative limitations in any of these foundational skills among medical learners. Many learners can triage tasks in situations with lower patient census or acuity but struggle when these demands increase because their compensatory strategy in the former is time. When that resource is cut short, they run into difficulty. There are often bottlenecks around processing speed, attention, adaptability, and emotion regulation. And thus, we see that even intelligent and typically well-organized learners may struggle to make these critical decisions *in vivo*. Many learners have trouble integrating information quickly or pivoting in the face of new information, and these issues are magnified in situations of high volume and acuity. For those who rely on a slower pace with fewer distractions to put their thoughts together and create a management plan, the clinical environment can be challenging. Even with the requisite knowledge, organizational systems, and basic executive functioning and self-regulation learning skills, not everyone is innately skillful at triaging tasks under pressure.

INEFFECTIVE TASK TRIAGE: WHAT COULD BE GOING ON?

Learners who have trouble prioritizing tasks in the clinical environment often struggle with other aspects of clinical performance. Common coexisting issues include timely completion of tasks in general, disorganized presentations, and a variety of clinical reasoning deficits. Any condition that impairs executive functioning, including physical and mental health conditions, can affect the ability to handle interruptions and structure time when time is limited. Table 13.2 lists conditions that may underlie difficulties with triage.

Table 13.2. Mental Health Conditions that May Underlie Difficulty with Triaging Tasks

- Anxiety disorders
  - — Generalized anxiety disorder (GAD)
  - — Obsessive compulsive disorder (OCD)
  - — Performance anxiety
- Attention deficit hyperactivity disorder (ADHD)
- Autism spectrum disorder (ASD) or traits
- Depressive disorders
- Stress and fatigue
- Substance use disorders
- Personality disorders or traits

As discussed in chapter 2, we recommend screening all struggling medical learners for underlying mental health conditions. We also urge programs to provide a means for confidential, expedited evaluation and treatment of these and other conditions, as they are common and impact performance and well-being in myriad ways. We discuss specific scenarios below.

COMMON SUBPHENOTYPES OF STRUGGLE WITH TRIAGE: DESCRIPTIONS AND COACHING STRATEGIES

Learners who have difficulty triaging tasks typically come to attention following an error (often of omission, e.g., something is missed) or when it becomes apparent that work is not being completed in a timely manner. In this section, we review common phenotypes of struggle, possible underlying issues, and suggestions for coaching that can be carried out in a variety of settings. These approaches work best when circumstances permit the development of a longitudinal and trusted relationship between learner and coach.

1. DERAILED BY INTERRUPTIONS

Case

A radiology resident is reading routine radiographic studies and is interrupted mid-study with a telephone call about an urgent consult. She recognizes that the consult now takes priority and completes this task. She returns to the former task and cannot remember where she was. She is so afraid to miss something that she goes back and re-reads the entire scan. There are several subsequent interruptions, and by the end of the day she is significantly behind and must stay late to finish her work. In an alternate scenario, the interrupted radiology resident returns to the former task, rushes through it, and misses an important finding. Task shifting due to interruptions in the clinical environment can lead to inefficiencies and errors. Both can lead to stress, emotional exhaustion, and reduced self-efficacy.

Description: While anyone can become flustered in the face of an interruption, we see more consistent patterns of this type of struggle in learners with anxiety and/or ADHD who rely on routines to manage their symptoms. Disruption in the routine leads to exacerbation of symptoms and may lead to duplication of work or careless errors. The likelihood of disruptions increases with patient load and complexity and especially when trainees are asked to operate simultaneously in different clinical environments (e.g., inpatient and outpatient settings). Given the limits of working memory, all clinicians are prone to cognitive overload when shifting tasks or juggling patients at different points in their care process.

COACHING STRATEGIES

To coach a learner who becomes derailed with interruptions, we recommend the following:

a. Assist the learner in the development of dependable systems for completion of core primary tasks that are likely to be interrupted. If possible, the resident should adhere to a template when reviewing studies and work through the template in order.
b. When possible, learners should minimize interruptions in advance, particularly during tasks that require high cognitive load. Learners are encouraged to create strategies for preemptively delegating interruptions (e.g., to a peer: "Can you hold my pager for one hour while I complete this task?") or deferring them (e.g., to the nursing staff: "Can you hold all non-emergent calls for one hour while I complete this task?").
c. Interruption management once engaged in a task. Work with the learner to:

i. Decide which tasks cannot be interrupted under any circumstance (e.g., performing a procedure)

ii. Determine whether the interruption needs to be handled immediately or can be delegated or deferred until later

   a) If it can be deferred, ensure that the learner has an effective system for recording and prioritizing the deferred task(s) in relation to other tasks

   b) For interruptions that can be delegated or deferred, have the learner practice saying "No" or "I will do this later." Create scenarios in which these responses are met with resistance to help the learner practice and hone the skill of assertive communication.

iii. Develop an external cueing system to facilitate resuming the original task accurately and efficiently while minimizing tax on the working memory. This system must be straightforward, quick, and meaningful to the learner. Examples include:

   a) Note to self to serve as a reminder of where the learner was in the task (e.g., a post-it note stating "I stopped here" when reading a scan). Alternatively, the learner who was interrupted while moving through their to-do list might draw a circle around the task that they were planning to complete next.

   b) Utilization of technology when possible. This learner could create a smart phrase if recording her interpretation in the electronic health record that allows her to reorient seamlessly and avoid losing her place after being interrupted.

   c) Enlist someone, at the time of the interruption, to check in with the learner as a reminder at a certain time.

d. Create context-relevant simulated exercises in which the learner is interrupted while performing a task. Allowing the learner to reason aloud while the coach poses "what if" questions as clinical variables are altered serves as an effective form of deliberate practice when accompanied by immediate feedback and an opportunity for reflection on the learner's reasoning process. In situations where the original task involves clinical reasoning, learners may be tempted to fall back on heuristics if feeling rushed or flustered after an interruption. To avoid the associated biases and minimize the risk of error, the coach should remind the learner to be mindful of slowing down upon immediate return to the original task and checking their thought process, avoiding the tendency to rush.

e. Provide a supportive space for learners to discuss the feelings that come up when they are interrupted. Ask the learner to reflect on prior experiences, then normalize that handling disruptions can be challenging and that many clinicians feel anxious, frustrated, or even angry when they are interrupted. Raising awareness of these feelings, learning to name them in the moment, and pausing to take a breath when they realize they have been triggered can guide them toward more thoughtful decision-making and potentially less distress when interrupted in the future.

If the learner or the coach is concerned that the difficulty caused by interruptions is severe or may signal an underlying diagnosis such as an anxiety disorder or ADHD, it is appropriate to refer to a mental health professional in accordance with programmatic and institutional policy.

2. RESISTANT TO INTERRUPTIONS

Case

A surgical resident on call in the hospital is making his way through a long to-do list. He is bright, with reasonable organizational systems for keeping track of his tasks. After completing item one on the list, a postoperative wound check, he moves on to item two, obtaining consent for a procedure. As he begins to gather the consent forms, he is called from the lab with a serum potassium value of 6.3 mEq/L on a cross-cover patient. "Check post-operative K" was item number six on the list. Frustrated by the interruption, he jots down the lab value and continues with the consent process. He will get to it in order, when it is time for number six.

Description: Some medical learners display apparent rigidity when approaching their task list and are particularly resistant to the idea of reprioritizing a to-do list, even in the face of new data that they interpret correctly. In this case, the resident knows that the lab value is abnormal and potentially urgent, and he knows how to treat hyperkalemia; however, he is resistant to being interrupted or the idea of approaching tasks out of order.

As discussed, we observe a spectrum of discomfort with interruptions, and not all learners who struggle with interruptions have an underlying diagnosis. A lengthy to-do list can feel overwhelming for anyone, and being asked to skip a task or move through tasks out of order may exacerbate feelings of being out of control or fear of missing something. Inability to pivot and display mental flexibility in clinical situations when presented with new information can be associated with perfectionistic traits, anxiety disorders (including OCD), ADHD, and autism spectrum disorder or traits in which routines, including approaching all tasks from start to finish in order, are part of a person's emotional self-regulation and symptom management. For different reasons in each of these situations, deviating from the routine creates discomfort, and learners may initially appear unwilling to compromise on what they consider the only way to get things done.

COACHING STRATEGIES

To coach a learner who is resistant to interruptions, we recommend the following:

a. Ensure that the learner has a reliable system (e.g., a checklist) for keeping track of and prioritizing tasks.
b. Normalize that it can be hard to deviate from routine. Explore with the learner what routine means to them and what they worry will happen if the original sequence of events is disrupted. Provide a supportive space for them to share feelings like anxiety, anger, frustration, or powerlessness that arise when interruptions require reprioritization of tasks. Validate that it is hard to be interrupted. Reassure that development of systems and practicing being interrupted will ultimately help them feel more in control.
c. As in the "derailed by interruptions" example, assist the learner in developing an external cueing system to keep track of where they were when they were interrupted, what they have/have not done, and what needs to be done next so that they feel more comfortable moving out of order.
d. Create simulated cases in which the learner is provided with a task list and then interrupted in different ways to practice these skills and improve mental flexibility.
e. In the clinical environment, using an existing task list, ask the learner to create a top five to-do list every three hours, ordered by priority. Assign prearranged times (e.g., 8 AM, 11 AM, etc) and have them set alarms if necessary. The focus should be on re-prioritizing tasks as

issues arise throughout the day. The learner should review these selections with their coach (in real time if the coach is working with them, or later if not), share their reasoning, and receive feedback on their assignment of priority. If the learner is meeting with the coach at a different time, they can jot down notes and/or take photos of their lists at different times to jog their memory later. The learner should also be given the opportunity to reflect on what was challenging about the exercise and what types of feelings arose when forced to stop and deviate from the original plan.

Referral to a mental health professional should be considered if the coach or learner is concerned about an underlying diagnosis or if the rigidity around interruptions is resistant to coaching efforts.

3. CAN'T FIGURE OUT WHAT TASK IS MOST IMPORTANT

Case

A medical student is struggling on her sub-internship in which she is expected to act as an intern equivalent. She received a grade of Honors in most of her core clerkships, where her census was 1 to 3 patients. She has excellent medical knowledge, is a hard worker, and is noted to be thorough. With higher patient census and complexity, she becomes overwhelmed, gets behind, and requires a lot of supervision. When tasks are equally pressing, despite a good understanding of what is going on with her patients, she is unsure of what to do first.

Description: It is common for learners, particularly early in their training, to experience uncertainty when prioritizing tasks or patients. This skill is often not explicitly taught. As discussed, effective prioritization of tasks in a busy clinical environment is fundamentally a management reasoning activity that also requires medical knowledge, effective systems for data gathering and task completion, and management scripts/schema. Certain specialties and clinical environments rely on the clinician's ability to triage more than others. High demands such as bigger patient census, higher patient acuity or complexity, and greater time constraints may expose relative weaknesses in the basic cognitive abilities required for this skill (e.g., processing speed, attention, adaptability) and may limit the capacity for metacognition and self-regulation.

COACHING STRATEGIES

In her book *Remediation of the Struggling Medical Learner*,[21] Guerrasio recommends that learners develop a system for identifying tasks of highest priority (using time constraints) and emphasizes the importance of role modeling and frequent feedback. Coaching this skill can begin in a simulated environment (e.g., the coach's office) which may feel less overwhelming and allows the coach more time to assess the learner's reasoning and provide real-time feedback. Eventually, the skill must be practiced, with oversight, in the clinical environment. We recommend the following:

a. Urge the learner to be deliberate and specific about prioritizing tasks as follows:

   1 - High priority for completion immediately following rounds
   2 - Intermediate priority (can be completed later in the day as time allows)
   3 - Low priority for completion only by day's end
   4 - Very low priority (can be delayed until the following day or later)

   Encourage learners to be mindful of how long they spend on each activity and, for those who struggle with getting behind, to impose time limits on certain tasks. To help systematize this process, we have previously developed and published tools to structure the processes of admitting a patient, pre-rounding, and composing daily notes and presentations.[22] These instruments, discussed in more detail later in this chapter, break down the components of each task into specific, observable steps. For some learners, we also employ tracking spreadsheets that time steps and can be used to facilitate reflection and review in later coaching sessions. Subsequent interventions may be tailored to address specific inefficiencies.

b. An exercise that can be completed in the clinical environment with a peer, near peer, or faculty coach requires the learner to rate the urgency of calls received from nurses and other care providers in a defined period of time. The rating system will depend on learner level and clinical setting. For example:

   We give the intern or medical student rotating on an inpatient service a 1-8 scale for cross-cover calls overnight:

   1- Just an FYI
   2- No need for action overnight, relay to morning team

3- Order placed or decision made; discuss with resident whenever next meet
4- Order placed or decision made; text resident now to discuss
5- Consult with resident before decision made or order placed
6- Text resident to join you in seeing patient to help with decision or order
7- Call resident and rapid response team
8- Call code

In a similar exercise, learners can apply a level of urgency (1 to 5) to all tasks during the day, then present this list to a coach at the end of the day and receive feedback on their assignments while exploring the reasoning behind their decisions. The goal is to introduce a more objective way of assessing the learner's recognition of urgency and ability to triage. The learner should review the rankings with the coach and reflect on their reasoning with feedback from the coach. Ultimately, they can practice this exercise in real time with their supervisor to further develop these skills in the clinical environment.

c. Exercise 3 from chapter 9 encourages the learner to prioritize clinical information and clinical tasks in the context of managing patients in the clinical environment. The learner is instructed to bring a recent patient list and signout to the meeting with their coach. For each patient on the list, the learner is asked to identify the most important clinical and laboratory findings that need to be followed over the next 24 hours. The learner is encouraged to provide a brief rationale for all of their choices. An evaluation form to guide observation and feedback is included.

4. GOES DOWN RABBIT HOLES, CHASES ZEBRAS

Case

A pediatrics resident returns to the workroom after seeing a teenage patient for an annual sports physical. He reports that the patient is a football player with normally well-controlled asthma whose symptoms have recently become harder to manage after a presumed viral infection with prolonged cough. The resident spent most of his time in the clinical encounter gathering information about the settings of the patient's football practice—specifically, the grasses on the field and any "unusual plants" in the area—and suggested a consult to the immunology team to work up allergy symptoms. Upon further probing, the resident has not obtained a detailed history of the recent virus, asked about smoking, or inquired about the patient's immunization status and ease of acquiring and using his current asthma medications.

Description: This learner displays a characteristic form of struggle with triaging of clinical tasks and clinical information that is often described as "missing the forest for the trees." Their presentations and written notes often do not convey a grasp of the "big picture" with patients. These learners invariably have trouble structuring their time, get behind, and appear disorganized. They become frequently distracted with objectively less-important issues that can lead to delays in addressing items of higher priority. They may perseverate on unimportant, traditionally straightforward tasks and self-describe "falling down rabbit holes." This can occur during history-taking, completing straightforward tasks such as electrolyte repletion or following up on imaging studies, and during pre-rounding. Similarly, learners who exhibit this phenotype of triage difficulty may focus on "zebras" to the exclusion of considering more common diagnoses ("horses") when constructing a differential diagnosis. Even when in possession of sufficient medical knowledge to prioritize a problem or task list in theory, these learners struggle to apply this knowledge to practice. There is considerable overlap between this phenotype of triage difficulty and the learner discussed in chapter 9 with concomitant medical knowledge and clinical reasoning deficits. Learners who "miss the forest for the trees" often do so in multiple different environments with multiple different skills.

Learners who display these behaviors often describe underlying perfectionist tendencies and the need to execute tasks perfectly. Compulsivity that is initially adaptive may become maladaptive in some learners and lead to an inability to complete their work. The "compulsive triad" in physicians is characterized by self-doubt, guilt, and an exaggerated sense of responsibility.[23] Some learners experience such crippling self-doubt that they focus on tasks of low importance, with which they are confident, to the exclusion of tasks of high importance, with which they are less confident.

Not everyone who displays these characteristics has an underlying diagnosis, but common co-existing issues include ADHD, anxiety disorders, and traits of autism spectrum disorder (ASD). Learners with anxiety are often compelled to fixate on certain tasks by the fear of missing something. In contrast, learners with ADHD may be easily distracted by tasks on which they choose to hyperfocus, even if they are unimportant. In both cases, the learner may be resistant to switching tasks once they have fallen down the rabbit hole, causing them to ultimately run out of time. Learners with ASD traits may perseverate intensely on a topic or task of interest and lose sight of other, more urgent or important responsibilities.

COACHING STRATEGIES

To coach the learner who falls down rabbit holes or chases zebras, we recommend the following:

a. Help the learner develop greater self-awareness around their tendency to become distracted with less-important tasks or information. Using specific examples, either self-identified by the learner or pulled from evaluations, coaching should provide ample opportunity for the learner to reflect upon their experience. At what point do they recognize they are being pulled off course? What is motivating them to go down the rabbit hole or chase the zebra? Sometimes there is a pull toward something more interesting; other times there is a push away from something mundane, unfamiliar, or uncomfortable for some other reason. Have the learner think about how these behaviors are adaptive and maladaptive. It is important to validate that, for all clinicians, some tasks feel tedious or are less interesting. When provided with this supportive space, many learners can identify when they become distracted and learn to insert an in-the-moment pause and resist the temptation. Once they are motivated to change (usually after they begin to see that the current behaviors are maladaptive) and with practice, they can often begin to redirect their attention to stay on task. Other learners may be compelled to deviate from the course by the fear of missing something. Learners with this fear can be encouraged to reflect on the worst-case scenario or what they are worried about missing.
b. Encourage the learner to develop systems for keeping themselves on track.
    i. Learners should create written templates or frameworks for common tasks such as admitting new patients, seeing a patient in the clinic, writing notes, and pre-rounding (discussed later in this chapter). Learners prone to distraction often benefit from breaking these tasks into timed steps, setting alarms if

necessary, to keep themselves on track until their awareness improves. Naming the steps of processes that many of us perform unconsciously can be helpful to draw attention to areas where the learner is getting stuck or pulled off course. We developed the TRIAGE tool (Figure 13.1) to help learners who struggle to complete a patient admission efficiently.[22,24] The ordering of specific tasks can also be customized to the institution's specific clinical services or electronic health record system.

In the clinical environment, a separate tracking spreadsheet can be used to track time spent on each step and indicate interruptions or difficulties sticking to the template. The 3R/3W tool (discussed in chapter 10) provides a framework for organizing daily patient notes and emphasizes the process of reassessing, renaming, and reprioritizing the patient's problems.

Tools like these which can be adapted based on specialty or clinical setting can be used in three ways:

1. To set expectations with the learner ahead of time (e.g., how long each step should take)
2. To promote learner self-awareness during the task completion itself (e.g., how long each step took, places where they became "stuck")
3. To facilitate reflection with the coach after the fact. During the debrief, the coach can review areas where the learner got stuck or became distracted. The coach can then take the learner through "what if" scenarios, adding theoretical interruptions as the learner works through the exercise.

    i. Ensure the learner has a reliable system of checklists that outline the tasks that must be completed. The top 5 to-do list introduced earlier in this chapter can be helpful here in that it encourages the learner to be deliberate about running their to-do list at set intervals throughout the day. In this case, the work is in keeping them on task and regularly assessing priority, then reflecting later with the coach about what was challenging about the exercise. Practicing this skill, that is, being deliberate about how they are spending their time and why, can help with focus. The coach should review with the learner how they structure their day and consider timing them as they complete various tasks and providing real-time feedback on their time management. For learners who struggle with distractions due to fear of missing something, the coach can encourage the learner to create a can't miss checklist, then provide feedback on their choices.

Triage an H&P*

T	**Triage**	**Obtain most recent objective data** • Vital signs / chief concern / ED or clinic notes • Quick scan of labs/microscopy data • Quick scan of current imaging
R	**Review**	**Chart biopsy/more in depth clinical review EHR** • Trend vital signs • Trend labs (compare to baseline values) • Review PMH/medications/allergies • Review last outpatient progress note • Review last discharge summary/signout • Review pertinent prior imaging
I	**Investigate/ Inquire**	**Review hospital course thus far** • Medications given (antibiotics, fluids, etc) • ED work-up • ED clinician HPI and assessment **Handoff of care from ED/clinic provider**
A	**Admission orders**	**Place initial admission orders** **Compose draft problem list in signout document** • Acute problems (i.e., neutropenic fever) • Chronic problems (i.e., AML, HTN, DM)
G	**Go see the patient**	**See the patient (problem-based, focused H&P)**
E	**Evaluate orders**	**Place detailed orders** • Interventions • Medication reconciliation • Diagnostic tests
An	**Assess, formulate plan**	**Formulate assessment & plan (complete signout)** • Prioritize acute problem list • Each problem should include 3 Ws: — What, Why, What next? • What else? Chronic problem list
H & P	**Write it in the chart**	**Complete H&P and place in chart**

*H&P: history and physical examination, ED: emergency department, EHR: electronic health record, PMH: past medical history, AML: acute myelogenous leukemia, HTN: hypertension, DM: diabetes mellitus

Figure 13.1. TRIAGE an H&P: Guide for Structuring Patient Admissions[22] (Adapted with permission from *JGME.*)

Because this phenotype of struggle with task triage is often associated with underlying neurodevelopmental or mental health issues, we recommend having a low threshold for referral to a mental health professional if the behaviors continue despite coaching or if the learner conveys distress in trying to change behavior. Even with coaching, it can be difficult for learners with untreated ADHD and/or anxiety or ASD traits to resist falling down rabbit holes or chasing zebras.

PUTTING THESE SKILLS TOGETHER

Case

Dr. Shah (he/him/his) is a first-year nephrology fellow who is struggling to manage a busy patient list. He has trouble prioritizing tasks in the face of what feels like a constant influx of new consults and changing data. There have been some near misses, and he requires a lot of oversight to make sure patients get the appropriate care in a timely fashion. To help Dr. Shah better identify which questions to ask and what information to gather to make decisions about triage, his coach created the following exercise.

COACHING STRATEGY

The coach presented Dr. Shah with the following hypothetical list of nine patients on the general nephrology consult service. The list includes basic information about the age and sex of the patient, the reason for consultation, clinical history, and overnight events included in the sign-out from peers.

	Age/Sex	Consult for	History
1	54M	**HD**	Chronic dialysis patient who missed 3 sessions of hemodialysis (HD). On presentation to the emergency department, his BP was 200/100 mm Hg, and he required bilevel positive airway pressure (BiPAP). After hemodialysis overnight, SBP is 140 mm Hg and he is on room air.
2	42M	**CRRT**	Patient developed cardiogenic shock after an influenza infection and now has cardiorenal acute kidney

(continued)

	Age/ Sex	Consult for	History
			injury (AKI). He has been tolerating continuous renal replacement therapy (CRRT) for several days with 200 cc/hr net ultrafiltration (UF).
3	**48F**	**CRRT**	Recent transfer from an outside hospital for AKI after an episode of acute pancreatitis. She was on continuous CRRT prior to transfer and is now anuric on two pressors. Ventilator requirements are unchanged (FiO2 is 40%). K on the morning of transfer is 5.2 mEq/L.
4	**60M**	**Hyponatremia**	Patient admitted for chemotherapy and transferred to the CCU for volume overload requiring diuretics. Nephrology is consulted for hyponatremia. Na was 135 mEq/L on admission, 133 mEq/L two days later, 131 mEq/L today.
5	**61M**	**CRRT**	Patient admitted for ST-elevation myocardial infarction (STEMI) with subsequent cardiac arrest during cardiac catheterization. A left ventricular support system was placed, and he was put on extracorporeal membrane oxygenation (ECMO) overnight. His CRRT is running well.
6	**64F**	**HD**	Chronic dialysis patient who missed 3 sessions of HD. Potassium is 8.2 weak peaked T-waves and a wide QRS on EKG.
7	**89M**	**Acute on chronic kidney injury**	Patient admitted with abdominal pain. He received IV contrast in the emergency department and was admitted to the SICU for monitoring of bowel obstruction. Nephrology was called on hospital day 3 rising creatinine (baseline 2 mg/dL, now 2.3 mg/dL). The patient is not on vasopressors and he is making urine. Creatinine is stable today.
8	**48F**	**Plasmapheresis**	Patient with Guillain-Barre syndrome who is scheduled for her 4th pheresis treatment today.
9	**46F**	**Plasmapheresis**	Patient with myasthenia gravis who had 3rd pheresis yesterday. She is intubated and hemodynamically stable.

The coach began by asking:

1. What initial additional information do you need to assess acuity level and begin to prioritize your task list?

Together, the coach and learner created an additional column to the right on the spreadsheet, entitled "To Do."

	Age/ Sex	Consult for	To Do
1	54M	**HD**	Assess for additional HD
2	42M	**CRRT**	Check on CRRT machine and make sure going okay
3	48F	**CRRT**	See to perform initial consult, consent family, and start CRRT
4	60M	**Hyponatremia**	See to perform initial consult on a non-urgent basis
5	61M	**CRRT**	Check on CRRT machine and make sure things are going okay
6	64F	**HD**	Initiate emergent temporizing therapies, notify HD staff, consent, orders, and HD
7	89M	**Acute on chronic kidney injury**	Check on volume status and electrolytes
8	48F	**Plasmapheresis**	See non-urgently. Assess plans for additional therapy and/or line management.
9	46F	**Plasmapheresis**	See non-urgently. Pheresis orders for tomorrow

With this information, the coach then asked Dr. Shah to:

2. Identify and rank the four sickest patients on this list who (1) need to be seen/addressed first, (2) any patients whose care can, at least temporarily, be deferred, and (3) any patients for whom you need more information to make your next decisions.

Dr. Shah correctly identified patients 6, 5, 3, and 2, in order of descending acuity, who needed to be addressed urgently. Patients 1, 4, and 7 required more information. Based on available information, patients 8 and 9 could wait.

	Priority	Consult for	To Do
1	More info	**HD**	Assess for additional HD
2	#4	**CRRT**	Check on CRRT machine and make sure going okay
3	#3	**CRRT**	See to perform initial consult, consent family, and start CRRT
4	More info	**Hyponatremia**	See to perform initial consult on a non-urgent basis
5	#2	**CRRT**	Check on CRRT machine and make sure things are going okay
6	#1	**HD**	Initiate emergent temporizing therapies, notify HD staff, consent, orders, and HD
7	More info	**Acute on chronic kidney injury**	Check on volume status and electrolytes
8	Defer	**Plasmapheresis**	See non-urgently. Assess plans for additional therapy and/or line management.
9	Defer	**Plasmapheresis**	See non-urgently. Pheresis orders for tomorrow

Next, the coach provided some updates on Dr. Shah's patients as follows:

	Priority	Update	Action
1	More info	The patient appeared volume overloaded on exam, K 5.5	You decided to do an additional HD session with UF, and the patient did well
2	#4	During the morning, his machine clotted	You adjusted the filtration fraction (FF) and now it is running well after rebuild
3	#3	You started her on CRRT	She is doing fine, CRRT is running
4	More info	The patient appeared well, hyponatremia was chronic and asymptomatic and in the setting of volume overload	You recommended continued diuresis
5	#2	Over the course of the day, pressor requirements increased, and you asked for repeat labs	You await repeat labs
6	#1	You performed HD, which she tolerated, and you asked for repeat labs	You await repeat labs
7	More info	The patient looked good, still making urine, labs are okay	You recommend supportive care
8	Defer	The nurse called to tell you that the patient just started on pheresis, and things are going well	Needs to be seen on routine pheresis
9	Defer	No events	Needs to be seen non-urgently. Pheresis orders for tomorrow

While the coach was providing updates, Dr. Shah received a theoretical page for another pheresis consult. The patient is a 70-year-old female admitted to the MICU with AKI and hemoptysis. She was just intubated and underwent bronchoscopy which revealed diffuse alveolar hemorrhage (DAH). A second call came in one minute later from the unit caring for patient 5 whose K is now 6 mEq/L with a lactate of 8 mmol/L.

3. Based on these updates, Dr. Shah was asked to reprioritize his task list.

Dr. Shah correctly identified that he should now prioritize patient 5 and the new consult. He should call the dialysis nurses to inform them about a likely new plasmapheresis treatment, then assess patient 5 at the bedside, adjust the CRRT orders accordingly, and talk to the primary team. He should then go immediately to the MICU to assess the new consult with DAH.

This is a realistic, and somewhat fun, exercise that simulates real clinical life in a low-stakes, risk-free setting and allows learners to practice clinical reasoning pertaining to triage. This exercise also allows learners to consider task triage in situations of resource constraints and allows them to role-play assertive communication. Recognizing and responding to urgent situations is discussed in more detail in chapter 14.

5. UNPREPARED FOR ROUNDS

Case

A medical student on the internal medicine clerkship is habitually unprepared for attending rounds. She comes in earlier than her peers and seems to be working hard, but she has rarely seen all of her patients before rounds. Patient presentations omit key pieces of data, and she often appears flustered. Her standardized test scores are slightly above average, and she is able to correctly answer most fact-based questions on rounds.

Description: Pre-rounding is a complex endeavor that typically occurs first thing in the morning and involves data collection and synthesis in preparation for scheduled work such as attending rounds or reporting to the clinic or operating room. The process of data-gathering must be deliberate and hypothesis-driven, as learners are required to sift through copious amounts of information, some of it irrelevant. The fundamentals of hypothesis-driven data collection are taught through case-based learning during the pre-clinical years of medical school, during which students learn to take histories and perform physical examinations that align with differential diagnoses. However, pre-rounding itself is rarely directly observed or explicitly taught and nearly always occurs within a constricted timeframe. Medical learners that struggle with pre-rounding spend disproportionate amounts of time in the electronic health record (EHR) and are often perceived as disorganized or inefficient. Lost in the EHR labyrinth, they may fail to complete tasks or appear underprepared for rounds, despite excelling in the classroom.

Like history-taking, pre-rounding is dependent on several faculties, including clinical reasoning, medical knowledge, and EHR navigation. Several theories of information gathering shed light on this multifaceted skill. Signal detection theory (SDT) posits that information gatherers classify data as signal or noise at varying thresholds.[25–27] Novices are often conservative signal detectors, disproportionally classifying information as meaningful; consequently, they become overwhelmed by abnormal, though irrelevant, data.[25,28,29] Only with years of experience do data-gathers develop more nuanced signal detection, filtering out noise while identifying atypical signals.[25,30] In the clinical setting, signal detection is molded by repositories of illness scripts and feedback on data relevance gained through practice.[30–32] Information foraging theory (IFT) provides a framework for studying navigational characteristics of information gathering.[33] IFT, developed in the dawn of the internet age, divides information gathering into components.[33,34] As with SDT, clinical experience influences information foraging through a process called hypothesis-driven search.[35] In the case of pre-rounding, experienced clinicians may read a history of present illness and generate clinical questions that guide a search for specific diagnostic studies. Furthermore, experienced clinicians can discern the value of information sources, deciding whether they are worth the read before wasting precious time. While pre-rounding improves naturally through experience, certain learners are "stuck in the weeds," impacting task follow-through and, ultimately, patient care.

At our institution, we sought to create an environment where pre-rounding could be observed without compromising protected health information or clinical duties. Several internal medicine attending physicians collaborated to create complex and realistic cases that were later built into an Epic TM training environment populated with both pertinent and non-pertinent clinical information in the form of notes, laboratory values, and imaging studies. These cases are used in one-on-one coaching settings to observe and provide guidance for learners on EHR navigation, note-taking methods, and the integration of clinical reasoning into data collection. In addition to observed pre-rounding, learners are asked to present the fictitious case, allowing the coach to observe how data-collection may influence presentation quality. When observing simulated and real-world pre-rounding, learners encounter the following pitfalls (Table 13.2):

Table 13.2. Pre-Rounding Pitfalls

Order of operations	**Redundancy**	Notes and labs are viewed in redundant ways due to the multiple options for objective data review offered by EHRs.
	Lack of customization	Learners often have not customized the EHR to fit their current rotation and must sort through scarcely used tabs that are not constructed in SOAP format.
Distractors	**Overvaluation of notes**	Learners take long-form notes on historical information rather than prioritizing the history they personally obtain. They have yet to develop a sense of "note value," spending time reading notes that contain irrelevant auto-populated data.
	Clinical significance of objective findings	Learners are challenged by objective data that falls outside of references ranges that may be otherwise insignificant.
Omissions	**Medication administration review**	Learners frequently skip this step entirely.
	Nuanced objective data	More specific objective data, such as the number of bowel movements for a patient with hepatic encephalopathy, are missed because of inexperience.
Note taking	**Auto-populated data**	Automatically generated rounding sheets, which provide summaries of 24-hour vital signs and labs, are appealing as time-savers. Such templates, however, often result in learners not analyzing the data themselves.
	Non-structured template	Lost in historical/subjective data review, learners often run out of note-taking space. Consequently, notes may be disorderly and nonlinear.

Many skills rooted in signal detection, such as lab interpretation, may improve naturally with clinical experience. However, some of the challenges faced by learners are organizational in nature, creating an opportunity for teaching best practices. In concert with the one-on-one coaching settings we held with learners, we observed the simulated pre-rounding of experienced internal medicine hospitalists. Through the lens of educational theories like IFT, SDT, and schema theory, we performed a thematic analysis to answer the following question: What organizational strategies do experienced clinicians employ while pre-rounding that can be taught to early learners? We have identified several themes which guide the content of pre-rounding coaching with medical learners (Table 13.3).

Table 13.3. Expert Strategies in Pre-Rounding

Order of operations	**EHR customization**	Tabs are ordered in a conventional structure of objective data (SOAP* format), incorporating specialized tabs that compare clinically relevant trends or filter out unwanted noise (i.e., diuretic overview tab which overlays diuretic use with serum creatine level and urine output).
	Prioritization of objective data	Initial investigation prioritizes assessment of clinical acuity through review of recent vital signs and labs. Starting with objective data also decreases bias from other providers' assessment/plans.
	Distinct phases	Initial navigation patterns are consistent and predictable, with objective data review occurring in a relatively fixed order. Later in the process, data review becomes problem focused, and navigation patterns correspond to the unique problems in each case.
Note taking	**Condensed**	Notes contain trends and "to do" items. Historical information is scarcely written down, beyond basic one-liners.
Diagnostic reflection	**Problem spotting**	Diagnostic labels are assigned during data review during which, for instance, "acute kidney injury" may be added to a problem list the moment an increasing serum creatinine level is detected.

*SOAP: subjective, objective, assessment, plan

COACHING STRATEGIES

To coach the learner who struggles with pre-rounding, we recommend the following:

a. General pre-rounding strategies
    i. Epic customization to reflect SOAP format
    ii. Prioritization of early objective data review
c. Development of concise note-taking habits that incorporate active problem spotting. Because every learner is different, tailor learning objectives to a particular learner's tendencies. Similarly, because pre-rounding is more of an art than a science, as a final assignment encourage learners to create their own pre-rounding templates and order of operations that can be later tested and refined in the training environment.
b. Our PRePPING the Patient tool (Figure 13.2) is a pre-rounding guide which outlines the specific tasks involved in managing an active list of patients prior to attending rounds.[22,24] Ideally, the process begins before arrival at the hospital and includes conscious preparation and mindfulness. Better time allocation for each task helps learners to overcome logistical barriers, and specific expectations outline what must be accomplished during each patient interaction.

"PRePPING" the Patients: Guide to Pre-Rounding		
P	**Plan** the day	**On the way to work, think about:** • Planned discharges vs ongoing care plans • Current patient plans for the day
Re	**Review** signout	**Obtain written and verbal signout, review overnight events**
P	**Prioritize**	**Make game plan:** • Assess the need for urgent/emergent interventions based on signout. Do you need to contact the supervising resident? • Decide on rounding order based on acuity, geography, and discharge planning
P	**Prepare**	**Scan vital signs, talk to nursing staff, review overnight events**

(continued)

(Figure 13.2 continued)

I	**Inside** the room	**Perform focused ROS* and physical exam to answer these key questions:** • Is the primary reason for hospitalization/primary complaint better, worse, or same? • Are the relevant physical exam findings better, worse or same? • Is the patient ready for discharge? Have you achieved all medical goals? Are they eating, drinking, going to the bathroom, walking, and have a place to go?
N	**Note** your findings	**Complete subjective and objective sections of note**
G	**ReGroup**	**After you have seen all patients:** • Check labs • Replete electrolytes, transfuse blood • Place other routine orders • ***Reassess, rename and reprioritize*** each problem • Within each problem, **compose *the What, the Why, and the What Next***?

*ROS: review of systems

Figure 13.2. PRePPING the Patients: Guide to Pre-Rounding[22] (Adapted with permission from *JGME*.)

GENERAL COACHING AND TIME-MANAGEMENT STRATEGIES

All medical learners should be encouraged to develop a system for organizing their clinical tasks. We agree with Dr. Guerrasio that there is no one right way to do this and have observed that different people use different systems effectively. Templates and master lists with checkboxes are common strategies for structuring tasks and blocks of time. Because triaging tasks accurately and efficiently requires deliberate practice, it is critical that all learners be directly observed performing this skill in the workplace with frequent, real-time feedback. Peers or near peers are often the best role models of efficiency practices and are more likely to be available during pivot points throughout the day to perform direct observation and provide feedback.

General time management strategies for maximizing efficiency and minimizing exhaustion and error include chunking or monotasking, in which work is approached in focused chunks (e.g., emptying the electronic inbox) with a defined start and stop time. As much as possible, interruptions should be minimized during these blocks of time. Particularly for learners with ADHD or who are prone to distraction, finding a quiet place to perform work during these blocks of time is critical. For medical learners in the clinical setting, one might accomplish this by letting the nurses know that, for the next 20 minutes, you will be reviewing slides with the pathologist or performing a procedure, and if possible, pages and calls should be held until the end of the 20 minutes—at which point you will reach out to them. Alternatively, pages or calls can be delegated to a peer during this period. Learners can help each other to protect time for uninterrupted work during a shift. It is also important to take breaks after focused periods of activity.

Learners should be reminded to prioritize basic physiologic needs such as adequate sleep, exercise, and nutrition. Self-care is necessary to ensure the energy, focus, and mental clarity that is necessary to effectively triage tasks in the clinical environment.

Table 13.4. Strategies for Coaching the Learner Who Struggles with Triage

1. Development of effective organizational and time management systems
    a. Templates for completing basic tasks
    b. Checklists for tracking tasks, prioritizing tasks
    c. Efforts to minimize interruptions
        i. Delegate and/or defer tasks when possible
    d. System for managing interruptions
        i. External cueing systems for returning to original task
        ii. Practice assertive communication
    e. Scheduled time for important and nonurgent activities
2. Creating a safe and supportive space
    a. Raising awareness of, and normalizing, thoughts and feelings that arise during struggles with triage
    b. Normalize that it can be hard to be interrupted and to deviate from routine, reflect on the meaning and benefits of routine
    c. Increase self-awareness that the learner is going down rabbit holes or getting distracted by zebras, explore fear of missing something, distractibility

(continued)

(Table 13.4 continued)

3. Exercises to promote deliberate practice of triage skills
    a. Practice being interrupted, improve adaptability
    b. Practice prioritizing tasks and being interrupted and reprioritizing
    c. Rate the urgency of calls
    d. Top 5 to do list every 3 hours (reprioritization exercise)
    e. Articulated PR
    f. Base rates
    g. TRIAGE H&P Guide to Admitting a Patient
    h. PRePPing the Patients Guide to Pre-rounding
4. Referral for mental health support if underlying cause suspected or significant distress despite coaching efforts

THE ROLE OF SIMULATION IN ASSESSING AND COACHING TASK TRIAGE

Table 13.4 summarizes our coaching approach for medical learners who struggle with triage and prioritization. Exercises 3.a. through 3.h. can be taught and/or practiced in the clinical environment. Likewise, they present an opportunity to utilize simulation to promote deliberate practice of skills like managing interruptions, prioritizing tasks, communicating assertively, and structuring blocks of time. In this book, we define simulation-based medical education broadly to include any teaching method that uses hypothetical clinical scenarios to teach and practice clinical reasoning under direct observation. Most of the examples provided in this chapter do not require a simulation center or other advanced technology, but rather lean on the coach's creativity in the design of, or modification of existing, clinical cases through which to develop and hone skills and systems.

For those with the relevant resources and capability, the skills introduced in this chapter lend themselves to a wide range of simulation-based educational modalities that can be employed for teaching, assessment, and/or coaching. Several creative examples exist in the literature. Mohan and colleagues developed adventure-based and puzzle-based video game training interventions to teach clinical reasoning around trauma triage.[36] Simulation has been used to replicate a busy emergency medicine environment in which learners can practice simultaneous management of multiple patients with varying levels of acuity[37] and to expose internal medicine residents to multiple simultaneous critical events with the opportunity for post-event debriefing.[38] Huang and colleagues created and validated an assessment tool and scoring system for emergency medicine trainees engaged in simulated "multitasking" scenarios of varying levels of difficulty.[39] Finally, Chan and colleagues designed GridlockED, a collaborative strategy game to teach and practice the skills of triage in a simulated emergency department setting.[40]

SUMMARY

Struggles with triage underlie a variety of clinical performance concerns and are often underrecognized and/or mislabeled. Medical learners typically do not receive specific training on the skills highlighted in this chapter. While many structure time and triage tasks effectively without conscious thought, others require explicit instruction and benefit from being more deliberate in their approach. It is critical for supervisors to directly observe these skills and recognize problems early to minimize what can, for those who struggle, become toppling dominoes of performance anxiety, a sense of reduced self-efficacy, and patient error. While we have grouped these phenotypes by behavior, it is important to recognize the diversity of conditions and thought processes that underlie each pattern of behavior. Coaching difficulties with task triage requires an individualized approach. Because of the central role of context and the environment in the ability to handle interruptions and triage tasks, coaching of these skills must ultimately occur within the clinical environment. In this chapter, we have provided several examples of practical exercises for use by all educators in a variety of clinical settings. Most of the exercises center around the development of systems (e.g., templates, checklists, cueing routines) that facilitate managing interruptions, structuring time, prioritizing information, and staying on track. Learners who struggle with triage benefit from a longitudinal relationship with a coach.

Acknowledgement: Thank you to Amanda Renaghan, MD, nephrologist and medical educator, for creating the nephrology case presented in this chapter. Thank you to Joanna Yost, PhD, clinical psychologist, for her input and guidance on the mental health aspects of this chapter.

References

1. Cammarata M, Dhaliwal G. Diagnostic Schemas: Form and Function. *J Gen Intern Med.* 2023;38(2):513-516. doi:10.1007/s11606-022-07935-1
2. Multitasking: Switching costs. https://www.apa.org. Accessed February 4, 2025. https://www.apa.org/topics/research/multitasking
3. ACGME Home. Accessed January 22, 2025. https://www.acgme.org/
4. Adams TN, Rho JC. Multitasking simulation: Present application and future directions. *Med Teach.* 2017;39(2):120-122. doi:10.1080/0142159X.2016.1230666
5. Heng KW. Teaching and evaluating multitasking ability in emergency medicine residents - what is the best practice? *Int J Emerg Med.* 2014;7(1):41. doi:10.1186/s12245-014-0041-4
6. Wang EE, Dyne PL, Du H. Systems-based practice: Summary of the 2010 Council of Emergency Medicine Residency Directors Academic Assembly Consensus Workgroup--teaching and evaluating the difficult-to-teach competencies. *Acad Emerg Med Off J Soc Acad Emerg Med.* 2011;18 Suppl 2:S110-120. doi:10.1111/j.1553-2712.2011.01160.x
7. Stephens RJ, Fairbanks RJ. Humans and multitask performance: let's give credit where credit is due. *Acad Emerg Med Off J Soc Acad Emerg Med.* 2012;19(2):232-234. doi:10.1111/j.1553-2712.2011.01264.x
8. Li SYW, Magrabi F, Coiera E. A systematic review of the psychological literature on interruption and its patient safety implications. *J Am Med Inform Assoc JAMIA.* 2012;19(1):6-12. doi:10.1136/amiajnl-2010-000024
9. Coiera E. The science of interruption. *BMJ Qual Saf.* 2012;21(5):357-360. doi:10.1136/bmjqs-2012-000783
10. Sweller J. CHAPTER TWO - Cognitive Load Theory. In: Mestre JP, Ross BH, eds. *Psychology of Learning and Motivation.* Vol 55. Academic Press; 2011:37-76. doi:10.1016/B978-0-12-387691-1.00002-8
11. Young JQ, Van Merrienboer J, Durning S, Ten Cate O. Cognitive Load Theory: implications for medical education: AMEE Guide No. 86. *Med Teach.* 2014;36(5):371-384. doi:10.3109/0142159X.2014.889290
12. Merkebu J, Veen M, Hosseini S, Varpio L. The case for metacognitive reflection: a theory integrative review with implications for medical education. *Adv Health Sci Educ Theory Pract.* 2024;29(4):1481-1500. doi:10.1007/s10459-023-10310-2
13. Walker S, Pham TN, Duong QH, Brock TP, Lyons KM. Cognitive and Metacognitive Processes Demonstrated by the Pharmacy Students When Making Therapeutic Decisions. *Am J Pharm Educ.* Published online March 10, 2022:8817. doi:10.5688/ajpe8817
14. Medina MS, Castleberry AN, Persky AM. Strategies for Improving Learner Metacognition in Health Professional Education. *Am J Pharm Educ.* 2017;81(4):78. doi:10.5688/ajpe81478
15. Kuiper RA, Pesut DJ. Promoting cognitive and metacognitive reflective reasoning skills in nursing practice: self-regulated learning theory. *J Adv Nurs.* 2004;45(4):381-391. doi:10.1046/j.1365-2648.2003.02921.x

16. Parsons AS, Wijesekera TP, Rencic JJ. The Management Script: A Practical Tool for Teaching Management Reasoning. *Acad Med.* 2020;95(8):1179-1185. doi:10.1097/ACM.0000000000003465

17. Cook DA, Stephenson CR, Gruppen LD, Durning SJ. Management Reasoning: Empirical Determination of Key Features and a Conceptual Model. *Acad Med.* 2023;98(1):80. doi:10.1097/ACM.0000000000004810

18. Daniel M, Durning SJ, Wilson E, Abdoler E, Torre D. Situated cognition: clinical reasoning and error are context dependent. *Diagnosis.* 2020;7(3):341-342. doi:10.1515/dx-2020-0011

19. Rencic J, Schuwirth LWT, Gruppen LD, Durning SJ. A situated cognition model for clinical reasoning performance assessment: a narrative review. *Diagn Berl Ger.* 2020;7(3):227-240. doi:10.1515/dx-2019-0106

20. Parsons AS, Wijesekera TP, Olson APJ, Torre D, Durning SJ, Daniel M. Beyond thinking fast and slow: Implications of a transtheoretical model of clinical reasoning and error on teaching, assessment, and research. *Med Teach.* Published online June 5, 2024:1-12. doi:10.1080/0142159X.2024.2359963

21. Guerrasio J. *Remediation of the Struggling Medical Learner.* 2nd Edition. Association for Hospital Medical Education; 2018.

22. DeKosky AS, Sedrak MS, Goren E, Dine CJ, Warburton KM. Simple Frameworks for Daily Work: Innovative Strategies to Coach Residents Struggling With Time Management, Organization, and Efficiency. *J Grad Med Educ.* 2018;10(3):325-330. doi:10.4300/JGME-D-17-00756.1

23. Gabbard GO. The role of compulsiveness in the normal physician. *JAMA.* 1985;254(20):2926-2929.

24. Kalet A, Chou CL, eds. *Remediation in Medical Education: A Mid-Course Correction.* Springer International Publishing; 2023. doi:10.1007/978-3-031-32404-8

25. Swets JA, Dawes RM, Monahan J. Psychological Science Can Improve Diagnostic Decisions. *Psychol Sci Public Interest J Am Psychol Soc.* 2000;1(1):1-26. doi:10.1111/1529-1006.001

26. Maniscalco B, Charles L, Peters MAK. Optimal metacognitive decision strategies in signal detection theory. *Psychon Bull Rev.* Published online November 18, 2024. doi:10.3758/s13423-024-02510-7

27. Boutis K, Pecaric M, Seeto B, Pusic M. Using signal detection theory to model changes in serial learning of radiological image interpretation. *Adv Health Sci Educ Theory Pract.* 2010;15(5):647-658. doi:10.1007/s10459-010-9225-8

28. Braun LT, Zottmann JM, Adolf C, et al. Representation scaffolds improve diagnostic efficiency in medical students. *Med Educ.* 2017;51(11):1118-1126. doi:10.1111/medu.13355

29. Small C, Land AM, Haist SA, Estrada CA, Snyder ED. Managing Cognitive Load to Uncover an Unusual Cause of Syncope: Exercises in Clinical Reasoning. *J Gen Intern Med.* 2016;31(2):247-251. doi:10.1007/s11606-015-3534-9

30. Gupta N, Feingold K, Dhaliwal G. Stressing Signal Versus Noise: An Exercise in Clinical Reasoning. *J Gen Intern Med.* 2017;32(1):122-126. doi:10.1007/s11606-016-3887-8

31. Custers EJFM. Thirty years of illness scripts: Theoretical origins and practical applications. *Med Teach.* 2015;37(5):457-462. doi:10.3109/0142159X.2014.956052

32. Bowen JL, ten Cate O. Prerequisites for Learning Clinical Reasoning. In: ten Cate O, Custers EJFM, Durning SJ, eds. *Principles and Practice of Case-Based Clinical Reasoning Education: A Method for Preclinical Students.* Springer; 2018. Accessed January 15, 2025. http://www.ncbi.nlm.nih.gov/books/NBK543761/

33. Pirolli P, Card S. Information foraging. *Psychol Rev.* 1999;106(4):643-675. doi:10.1037/0033-295X.106.4.643

34. Brown PJ, Marquard JL, Amster B, et al. What do Physicians Read (and Ignore) in Electronic Progress Notes? *Appl Clin Inform.* 2014;5(2):430-444. doi:10.4338/ACI-2014-01-RA-0003

35. Illingworth DA, Thomas RP. Strength of Belief Guides Information Foraging. *Psychol Sci.* 2022;33(3):450-462. doi:10.1177/09567976211043425

36. Mohan D, Fischhoff B, Angus DC, et al. Serious games may improve physician heuristics in trauma triage. *Proc Natl Acad Sci U S A.* 2018;115(37):9204-9209. doi:10.1073/pnas.1805450115

37. Kobayashi L, Shapiro MJ, Gutman DC, Jay G. Multiple encounter simulation for high-acuity multipatient environment training. *Acad Emerg Med Off J Soc Acad Emerg Med.* 2007;14(12):1141-1148. doi:10.1197/j.aem.2007.05.015

38. Fraser TN, Genuardi M, McCullough SA, Peloquin G, Currier PF, Miloslavsky EM. Observations: A Pilot Study of Multiple Simultaneous Critical Care Simulations. *J Grad Med Educ.* 2015;7(2):303. doi:10.4300/JGME-D-15-00074.1

39. Huang WC, Hsu SC, Yang CH, et al. A novel approach: Simulating multiple simultaneous encounters to assess multitasking ability in emergency medicine. *PloS One.* 2021;16(9):e0257887. doi:10.1371/journal.pone.0257887

40. Tsoy D, Sneath P, Rempel J, et al. Creating GridlockED: A Serious Game for Teaching About Multipatient Environments. *Acad Med.* 2019;94(1):66. doi:10.1097/ACM.0000000000002340

CHAPTER 14

Struggles in Urgent Situations

RESPONDING TO A CLINICAL EMERGENCY OR SUDDEN CHANGE IN CLINICAL STATUS

TO VARYING DEGREES, all clinicians face urgent situations in the context of patient care. In certain fields of medicine, the threat of crisis is more immediate than others. Most medical learners receive some version of scenario-based life support education aimed at preparing them to respond quickly in specific emergency settings.[1] Beyond basic skills training, the extent to which management of urgency and emergency is explicitly taught in medical education or training programs depends on the institution/program and the specialty. Caring for an acutely sick patient requires a unique and complex skillset that spans the competencies of medical knowledge, clinical reasoning, communication, professionalism, and technical skills. In this chapter, we focus on the clinical reasoning aspects of managing urgency.

In chapter 13, we introduced clinical task triage as a reasoning-based ability of the highest order, drawing upon basic intellectual, cognitive, metacognitive, and social-emotional capacities. Similarly, responding appropriately in urgent situations requires that the clinician: (a) recognizes the acuity and/or change in clinical status, (b) synthesizes information and generates early diagnostic hypotheses (diagnostic reasoning), (c) assesses clinical severity and immediate clinical trajectory (prognostic reasoning), and (d) formulates and enacts a plan for treatment and/or additional testing (management reasoning). Clinical reasoning in these settings is unique in that the emphasis is more immediately upon prognosis and management than diagnosis, and decisions must be made rapidly and without the full dataset. From the perspective of dual process theory (DPT), a clinician's ability to think on their feet largely reflects the recognition of patterns in the clinical picture (System 1) that facilitate diagnosis, prognosis, and management.[2–4] Pertinent knowledge is required to interpret data and proceed through the reasoning steps, but it is how the knowledge is organized in long-term memory that facilitates quick action.[5–7] Medical knowledge alone (e.g., memorizing guidelines and/or algorithms) does not predict the ability to recognize and/or stratify clinical urgency.[8] Faced with unfamiliar clinical problems early in training, learners must rely on educational frameworks (System 2) to reason in the face of urgency or emergency.[9] A well-known example is the "Hs and Ts" mnemonic taught as part of Advanced Cardiac Life Support Training.[1] The Hs and Ts represent the reversible causes of cardiac arrest characterized by pulseless electrical activity, and use of this mnemonic is meant to expedite diagnostic and management decisions in this situation. With practice, frameworks such as this one, even when medical care is not this algorithmic, can become intuitive and are internalized by the learner as schemas.[10] As introduced in chapter 3, educational frameworks based in System 2 thinking are not a singular strategy for improving clinical reasoning among novice or struggling learners; instead, they serve as a bridge while learners hone their pattern recognition.[2,11] Pattern recognition is honed by growing knowledge and experience as learners develop a mental library of scripts and schema tailored to specific urgent situations.[6,7]

Experts responding to an urgent situation rely not only on intuition but also on the ability to pause, reflect, and actively engage in System 2 thinking—particularly in the face of the unexpected. As discussed in chapter 11, this process also informs the ability to prognosticate. Trauma surgeons, for example, often take advantage of the representativeness heuristic (in which the correct assessment of severity depends on how well the specific case reflects a prototype) to triage their patients.[12] Reliance on this heuristic may lead to under- or over-triage if the typical severity clues are not present. Thus, it is important that the surgeon maintains the ability to shift in the moment to a more analytic reasoning process when circumstances demand. This interchange is also a critical part of management reasoning in urgent clinical situations. For example, when responding to a patient with acute hypoxia and tachycardia, an experienced clinician intuitively activates and enacts a management script that includes gathering laboratory data and performing a chest X-ray, electrocardiogram, arterial blood gas, and computed tomography pulmonary angiogram (CTPA) (System 1).[13] Prior to implementing all the items on the script, the clinician may shift to analytical thinking to consider the risk-benefit ratio of obtaining a CTPA in this patient who also has acute kidney injury (System 2).[14,15] Even in urgent situations, an expert's management script must consider contextual factors, uncertainty, high-value care, and shared decision-making as influencers of their testing and treatment threshold.[16–18] Over time, the process of toggling back and forth between System 1 and 2 thinking can lead to a deepening understanding of the material to which the clinician is exposed.[9,19]

Urgent and emergent clinical situations are characterized by their unpredictability. Information emerges in an irregular pattern, and the relationship between variables is often nonlinear. Effective clinical reasoning under pressure depends on working memory, processing speed, attentional capacity, ability to suppress distractions, and cognitive flexibility. The pressures and complexities of the clinical environment may expose bottlenecks in any of these areas that lead medical learners who might do well in a testing or simulation situation to struggle with managing urgency *in vivo*. As is the case for triaging tasks under time pressure, urgent situations may present a challenge for those who rely on a slower pace with less adrenaline to gather their thoughts and make decisions. Additionally, clinicians must manage their own emotional response—in the moment—to what is often an emotionally charged set of circumstances. Success in urgent situations is determined by an interplay between rational and emotional intelligence. In a crisis, the emotional mind (amygdala) is rapidly activated, allowing for quick action but without time for reflection and analysis.[20] The rational mind (prefrontal cortex) serves as a command center that governs the above functions and allows for effective clinical decision-making and emotion regulation. The ability to reflect on one's own thinking processes (metacognition) is critical to decision-making and avoidance of error. Finally, clinically urgent or emergent situations demand a certain degree of ownership in which the clinician takes initiative, makes decisions, leads a team, and holds themselves accountable for the process. The importance of situational awareness, assertive communication, and engagement in high-stakes clinical situations is discussed in more detail in chapter 15.

CHARACTERIZING LEARNER STRUGGLE IN URGENT SITUATIONS

Medical learners who underperform in the setting of clinical urgency or emergency typically exhibit one of the following behavioral patterns. Myriad overlapping factors potentially underlie these observed behaviors, including those intrinsic and extrinsic to the learner. For each behavioral sub-phenotype, we consider the subjective experience of the learner and potential root causes. Of note, this chapter focuses on urgent situations that occur in non-operative settings. Operative reasoning, including troubleshooting in the face of a procedural emergency, is covered in chapter 15.

1. Ignores, avoids, or adopts passive role

Case 1: *An intern is paged about a cross-cover patient who develops a fever following a blood transfusion. The intern orders acetaminophen without physically assessing the patient and misses a new oxygen requirement.*

Case 2: *An attending physician arrives to assist with a pediatric patient in cardiac arrest and finds the junior resident running the code alone. The senior resident enters the patient's room five minutes later with a fresh cup of coffee in hand.*

Case 3: *During a busy trauma response in the emergency department, a junior resident is called to help the rest of the team. Upon seeing the senior resident at the bedside, the junior resident leaves the room to place orders on a different patient, then returns. As the senior resident readies to place a chest tube, the junior resident steps away again to check in with the social worker and chaplain.*

What might be going on for the learner: Learner does not recognize the urgency, recognizes the urgency but is unsure what to do, recognizes the urgency but does not understand role and/or is uncomfortable in role, and/

or is emotionally detached from the clinical situation.

Discussion: Learners who appear to ignore or behave passively during urgent clinical situations are often labeled as unprofessional. This "failure to engage" phenotype of professionalism is often not a "primary" professionalism issue at all but rather an avoidant behavioral response that signals inadequate medical knowledge, faulty pattern recognition (e.g., limited or disorganized diagnostic, prognostic, and/or management script), performance anxiety, or neurodivergence (e.g., missing the social cue of urgency). Some learners struggle to understand their role or are intrinsically uncomfortable in urgent situations despite recognizing the urgency and wanting to help. Others appear uninvested in the care of acutely sick patients due to stress, fatigue, burnout, depression, substance use disorder, existential anxiety about their career, and/or feelings of inadequacy.

2. Moves slowly, hesitantly, or freezes

Case 4: *A medical student is paged about a cross-cover patient with sudden drop in oxygen saturation, increased respiratory rate, and altered mental status. Instead of immediately assessing the airway, breathing, and circulation, the student begins a systematic review of the patient's medical record, meticulously analyzing labs, imaging, and the medication administration records to identify a comprehensive list of potential causes for the deterioration.*

Case 5: *An OB/GYN resident is called to assist with a patient at 39 weeks' gestation. The patient has been laboring for several hours when sudden fetal bradycardia is detected, with fetal heart rate dropping to 80 bpm and not recovering with initial intrauterine resuscitation measures. The labor and delivery nurses look to the resident for direction, suggesting preparation for an emergent C-section. The resident hesitates and appears to freeze, unable to issue orders or initiate the necessary steps for the procedure.*

What might be going on for the learner: Learner recognizes the urgency but is unsure what to do, fears missing something, does not understand role and/or is uncomfortable in role, lacks cognitive flexibility, and/or is emotionally flooded.

Discussion: The tendency to move slowly or even freeze in the face of clinical urgency often reflects lack of germane knowledge or pattern recognition, as described above, and/or the inability to efficiently move to a more analytic reasoning approach when faced with the unexpected. Conversely, overreliance on System 2 thinking slows down the decision process and is not ideal in an emergency.[21] In chapter 12, we considered the learner whose discomfort with uncertainty and/or fear of missing something can lead them to overthink management decisions, leading to inaction. Additionally, some learners display inflexible patterns of thinking or behavior in their approach to patient care. For instance, we have worked with learners who have trouble moving forward with a management plan without first confirming the diagnosis and/or find it difficult to change course once they have started down a specific path. Significant rigidity in urgent situations may signal an underlying diagnosis (e.g., an anxiety disorder, ADHD, or autism spectrum disorder (ASD) or traits) in which the learner relies on routines to self-regulate and manage their symptoms. Deviating from routine, in this case, consistent patterns of thinking, can exacerbate feelings of being out of control or worries about missing something. For some learners, freezing reflects a physiological response to fear and perceived danger characterized by slowed thinking and inability to act.

3. Overconfident, over functions, or behaves aggressively

Case 6: *A resident is called to the bedside of a patient admitted for pneumonia who has suddenly developed hypotension and tachycardia. Upon entering the room, the resident immediately begins issuing orders, without pausing to fully assess the situation. She assumes the clinical deterioration represents septic shock and focuses on treating worsening pneumonia, ignoring the nurse who mentions that the patient complained of chest pain earlier. She does not listen to the chest or order an EKG. Within minutes, the patient goes into cardiac arrest, later determined to be a myocardial infarction.*

Case 7: *A resident assesses a neonate with worsening respiratory distress and hypoxia despite being on continuous positive airway pressure (CPAP). Without consulting the fellow, he requests an arterial blood gas and orders a full sepsis workup and broad-spectrum antibiotics. The fellow arrives at the bedside and notices a distended, tympanic abdomen, then reviews the* *history of feeding intolerance and correctly diagnoses necrotizing enterocolitis with secondary respiratory compromise and initiates the appropriate treatment plan.*

Case 8: *A general surgery resident evaluates a patient who recently had abdominal surgery and is suddenly tachycardic and hypotensive, with increasing abdominal pain. The resident immediately begins issuing orders with raised voice: "Get two units of blood, stat!" and "Call the OR now and book a room—this is a disaster!" and "Why didn't you call me earlier? Who is in charge here?" The nurse and intern, also at the bedside, hesitate, unsettled by the resident's tone, and suggest calling the attending. The resident snaps, "I don't need permission to manage a bleeding patient. Just move!"*

What might be going on for the learner: Learner is overly confident or lacks the ability to reflect, recognizes the urgency but is unsure what to do, fears missing something, does not understand role, and/or is emotionally flooded.

Discussion: The overconfident learner displays a misalignment between acknowledgement of clinical uncertainty and accurate pattern recognition. This pattern of behavior can lead to errors of commission (e.g., wrong diagnosis or wrong treatment) or omission (e.g., not fully appreciating the severity of the disease process). The over-functioning learner (defined here as overtesting, overtreating, acting prematurely, and/or failing to delegate) may also lack reflective ability. Case 7 highlights the importance of formulating an effective problem representation—in the moment—to activate the appropriate illness and management scripts. In this case, the resident was unable to activate a management script with consideration of patient and context-specific features, treating symptoms in isolation and leading to unnecessary, potentially harmful interventions and a missed diagnosis. Recognition of "a late preterm infant with respiratory distress and feeding tolerance who presents with worsening abdominal distension" should have prompted the appropriate differential diagnosis and targeted interventions. Overtesting and/or overtreating may reflect unfamiliarity with the principles of probabilistic or Bayesian reasoning.[22] Learners who act impulsively or fail to delegate may not understand their role or may be impervious to social cues. Alternatively, these behaviors may be driven by intense anxiety and/or feelings of inadequacy. For some, these observations indicate an underlying diagnosis such as an anxiety disorder, ADHD, or ASD or traits.

Aggressive behavior in a clinical emergency may be rooted in a lack of understanding of roles and/or triggered by emotional flooding. Goleman describes the *amygdala hijack* as an immediate, overwhelming emotional reaction that is initiated when the limbic system perceives a threat and triggers a fight-or-flight (or freeze, as discussed earlier) response before the cortical centers can enact a rational response.[20] The emotional reaction is typically out of proportion to the stimulus and, in the case of the resident in case 9, may lead to hostile or disrespectful communication that disrupts team cohesiveness and/or causes inappropriate clinical decision-making. While this can happen to anyone, common mitigating factors include stress, fatigue, and the impact of early-life experiences and/or concomitant mental or physical health conditions.

Table 14.1. Learner Factors That Contribute to Struggle in Urgent Situations

- Lacks relevant medical knowledge
- Related to above, lacks pattern recognition to guide diagnostic, prognostic, and management reasoning)
  - — May reflect inexperience, lack of dedicated clinical reasoning teaching, and/or ineffective knowledge acquisition and organization
- Does not appreciate principles of probabilistic or Bayesian reasoning
- Contextual factors (e.g., environmental noise and chaos, level of supervision, availability of resources, patient volume and acuity, time of day, competing clinical demands, interruptions and distractions, team dynamics and role ambiguity, institutional culture and expectations, familiarity with the clinical setting, presence of standardized protocols or lack thereof, pressure to perform, emotional intensity of the case, etc)
- Underlying mental health concern, leading to lack of engagement, missing urgency cue, and/or flawed clinical reasoning

(continued)

(Table 14.1 continued)

- — Stress, fatigue, burnout, feelings of inadequacy, existential anxiety about career
- — Anxiety disorder, including performance anxiety
- — Depressive disorder, substance use disorder
- — ADHD, other relative weakness in executive function (e.g., processing speed, cognitive flexibility)
- — Autism spectrum disorder or traits
- — Adverse childhood experiences
- Does not understand role

The role of context in urgent clinical encounters cannot be overstated, as it directly shapes the reasoning process and contributes to learner struggles.[23,24] As understood by situated cognition,[25,26] context encompasses the clinical environment, available resources, team dynamics, and competing demands—all of which can influence a learner's ability to recognize and respond to urgency. For example, a third-year medical student rotating in the ICU may struggle to identify early signs of sepsis in a decompensating patient, not because of a lack of knowledge, but because they are unaccustomed to interpreting subtle clinical changes in a high-acuity setting where multiple providers are managing concurrent crises. Similarly, a resident in the emergency department may hesitate to take ownership of a crashing patient when surrounded by senior clinicians, misinterpreting their role as purely supportive rather than active. Surrounding chaos and the degree to which clinical care is protocolized can impact learner performance in urgent situations. Many of these reflect the degree of demand on different components of executive functioning and/or threats to emotion regulation. For example, a learner may do fine when the timing and management of urgent situations are somewhat predictable but run into difficulty when a patient's clinical presentation is undifferentiated and/or unexpected. In contrast, a learner working in a resource-limited setting such as an overnight cross-cover shift with minimal backup may default to excessive testing or over-cautious management due to a lack of confidence in their ability to make high-stakes decisions independently. These contextual factors amplify existing cognitive load, heighten emotional reactivity, and can exacerbate struggles with pattern recognition and prioritization in urgent situations. As is true with all the phenotypes of clinical reasoning we have discussed, struggle may become more apparent with higher volume and/or acuity.

The prevalence of learner struggle with managing clinical emergencies varies depending on the level of training, medical specialty, and the scope of direct observation within the program. For instance, these issues may come to attention earlier in emergency medicine or critical care medicine than they would in a primarily outpatient-based specialty such as family medicine, in which emergencies are less frequent. Programs that routinely utilize simulated urgent encounters as a formative educational assessment tool may pick up an underlying issue earlier. Between the years of 2018 and 2025, nearly 40% of graduate medical learners in our program who were referred for clinical reasoning remediation were observed to struggle in urgent situations, either due to their inability to recognize urgency or to create an appropriate rapid management plan. Because appropriate response in urgent situations combines diagnostic, prognostic, and management reasoning, this phenotype of clinical reasoning struggle is never seen in isolation. Common coexisting behavioral concerns in our cohort included patient presentations, triaging tasks, and creating plans independently. The fact that issues with task triage and urgency management travel together makes sense, as they share many of the same underlying issues. If a learner cannot recognize urgency, it will be difficult to triage tasks effectively.

ASSESSMENT OF LEARNER BEHAVIOR IN URGENT CLINICAL SITUATIONS

Evaluating learner response to clinical urgency can be challenging, as urgent situations often occur on an unpredictable timeline, outside of typical workflow. In settings where management of unstable patients is the rule rather than the exception, factors like clinical pace, lack of privacy, and competing demands present barriers to meaningful direct observation and delivery of feedback *in situ*.[27] The likelihood that a supervising attending is present to observe the learner throughout the event varies depending on the clinical setting, and thus feedback is often fragmented and/or obtained from interdisciplinary team members. Simulation-based assessments afford educators the opportunity to observe a learner's behavior in urgent situations that are realistic and in which variables can be controlled and modified without risk to a patient. Thoughtfully designed simulation-based assessment has been shown to be reliable and valid for learners at various stages of training.[28]

Several methods have been developed to assess clinician performance during medical emergencies. Team Emergency Assessment Measure (TEAM) and Observational Skill-based Clinical Assessment tool for Resuscitation (OSCAR) are tools that employ behavioral scoring systems to evaluate teamwork and clinical decision-making in simulated resuscitation scenarios.[29,30] Another instrument rates clinicians on technical and nontechnical skills when managing septic shock in a simulated setting.[31] CERTAIN (Checklist for Early Recognition and Treatment of Acute Illness) is a video-based tool that relies on a checklist to assess performance in simulated pre-cardiac-arrest medical emergencies.[32] Checklists have been touted as an ideal way to translate clinical guidelines into structured tools that outline tasks for specific situations of clinical urgency, thereby increasing objectivity and standardization of assessments.[33,34] Ottestad and colleagues developed a scoring system to evaluate resident performance in simulated septic shock scenarios in the intensive care unit which highlights the importance of the "technical" (e.g., how well learners follow guidelines) and "nontechnical" (e.g., leadership, communication, contingency planning, and resource utilization) skills of managing clinical urgency.[31]

We have developed and have validity evidence for a structured approach to the formative assessment of the learner evaluating patients during urgent situations known as REACT (Rapid Evaluation Assessment of Clinical Reasoning) (Figure 14.1).[35] This tool provides behavioral anchors corresponding to five aspects of clinical performance: (1) hypothesis-driven data gathering and recognition of urgency (prognostic reasoning), (2) interpretation of data and formulation of a differential diagnosis (diagnostic reasoning), (3) initial and ongoing treatment (management reasoning), (4) communication, and (5) metacognition. Metacognitive reflection, in this case, encouraging the learner to reflect on their decision-making and their subjective experience during the event, is a critical part of honing clinical reasoning in general and can enhance the feedback process.[36] This tool was designed for use in the simulated setting to allow for easier isolation and measurement of variables of interest. While the tool is unlikely to capture all the variables that impact performance in real-life urgent scenarios, its framework serves as a reasonable starting point for feedback and coaching discussions.

Rapid Evaluation Assessment

Essential Tasks

Learner Function	Specified Task
Collecting • **Data gathering** *—recognition of urgent or emergent clinical scenario*	• **Collect/Report** history and exam data in hypothesis-directed manner • **Recognize** patient and disease specific factors as potential etiologies of decompensation • **Recognize** severity of clinical problem and contextual signs of urgency or emergency
Interpreting • **Diagnostic reasoning** *—differential diagnosis*	• **Generate** prioritized differential diagnosis of most likely, less likely, unlikely in urgent clinical situations
Management • **Management reasoning** *—initial management option selection* *—response to dynamic information*	• **Direct** evaluation and treatment towards high priority diagnoses • **Initiate** management in patient with urgent decompensation • **Recognize** need to escalate patient care
Communicating • **Patient-centered care** *—communicate care plan and goals of care* *—achieve a shared mental model*	• **Communicate** with health care team members according to role and responsibility to improve task efficiency • **Maintain** focus and two-way communication with patient or surrogate decision-maker in urgent clinical situations
Reflecting • **Metacognition** *—reflection of urgent or emergent clinical scenarios*	• **Demonstrate** the ability to think about one's own thinking (metacognition) in urgent clinical situations • **Mitigate** cognitive tendencies or emotional/situational factors influencing clinical decision making
	Overall score _____ /15

Figure 14.1. Rapid Evaluation Assessment of Clinical Reasoning Tool (REACT (Adapted with permission from the author.)[35]

f Clinical Reasoning Tool (REACT)

Assessment of Behaviors

Assessment		
❍ Non-focused history and exam ❍ Included extraneous information ❍ Missed key findings ❍ Did not recognize contextual clues of urgency	❍ History and exam reflect potential diagnoses ❍ Limited recognition of urgent contextual clues ❍ Included limited pertinent positive and negative findings	❍ Logical history and exam for potential diagnoses ❍ Questions assessed likelihood of specific diagnoses ❍ Full recognition of urgency contextual clues ❍ Prioritization on pertinent positive and negative findings
❍ Differential diagnosis missing likely or "can't miss" diagnoses in urgent situations ❍ Includes inappropriate diagnoses	❍ Differential diagnosis included likely and "can't miss" diagnoses in urgent situations but missed key diagnoses ❍ Inappropriate rank-order of diagnoses	❍ Accurately ranked differential diagnosis including key, likely, and "can't miss" diagnoses in urgent situations ❍ Prioritized urgent diagnoses appropriately
❍ Direct evaluation and treatment towards high priority diagnoses ❍ Initiate management in patient with urgent decompensation ❍ Recognize need to escalate patient care	❍ Major focus of evaluation and treatment on likely and urgent diagnoses ❍ Included non-essential testing ❍ Evaluated for response to initial management plan	❍ Efficiently directed management towards most likely and urgent diagnoses ❍ Deferred tests directed towards less likely or less important diagnoses ❍ Evaluated for response to initial interventions
❍ Did not engage health care team members ❍ Did not communicate care plan with patient/family ❍ Did not clarify patient's goals of care	❍ Limited engagement of health care team members to improve task efficiency ❍ Limited effort to communicate with patient/family but used medical jargon or failed to ensure understanding ❍ Limited clarification of patient's goals of care	❍ Fully engaged health care team members according to role and responsibility to improve task efficiency in urgent situation ❍ Effectively communicated care plan with patient/family and ensured understanding ❍ Effective clarification of patient's goals of care
❍ Unaware of cognitive tendencies or emotional/situational factors that may have influenced decision-making ❍ Unable to mitigate cognitive tendencies or emotional/ situational factors	❍ Limited awareness of cognitive tendencies or emotional/situational factors that may have influenced decision-making ❍ Limited mitigation of cognitive tendencies or emotional/ situational factors	❍ Full awareness of cognitive tendency or emotional/situational factors that may influence decision-making ❍ Effectively mitigates reactions to urgent clinical situations
1 point	2 points	3 points

An alternative framework for considering learner performance in urgent situations borrows from a familiar and trusted model of assessment in medical education known as RIME.[37]

Recognize — Does the learner recognize sick versus not sick? Once they recognize the urgency, can they initiate appropriate steps to seek help and stabilize the patient?

Interact — Does the learner communicate effectively as a leader? Can the learner participate in a collaborative and/or supporting role if necessary? Can the learner interact with the patient/family/multidisciplinary team?

Manage — Can the learner effectively manage the clinical situation? Can they anticipate what might happen and plan accordingly? Do they adjust their decision-making appropriately in the face of changing data?

Educate — Can the learner step aside and support and mentor a junior learner to take over as leader?

RIMEurgency does not yet have validity evidence for educational use, but anecdotally it provides a straightforward structure for focused feedback in real-time. Like the original RIME framework, *RIMEurgency* prompts educators to look for things that are familiar and intuitive in a learner's performance.

EXAMPLE: STRUCTURED DIRECT OBSERVATION TOOL TO ASSESS LEARNER RESPONSE TO URGENCY[38]

Mutter and colleagues have developed a repository of simulated clinical scenarios that evaluate a medical intern's response to urgent pages from the nursing team.[38] Their approach is highlighted as an exemplar of structured direct observation that is easily adaptable for use in the formative assessment of clinical reasoning and communication in a variety of simulated clinical situations. Here, the assessment of the learner's response is scaffolded by a checklist that is brief, straightforward, and requires little instructor training.

VIGNETTE

CC: Shortness of breath (SOB)

PAGE: Urgent need action: 3134 w SOB, O2 sat 83%. NAME OF CALLER

When student calls, evaluator should answer phone with:

"This is NAME."

If student does not exactly specify what they are calling about, evaluator should say: "What are you calling in reference to?"

If student does specify why they are calling, evaluator should state:

"Mr. Wallace started to c/o SOB when I was helping him get to his chair a few moments ago."

If asked about specifically, the following should be provided.

If student asks for information you do not have, state "I do not have that information."

Coach	Learner
Vitals:	• BP 138/86 • HR 120 • RR 40 • T 37.2/99.0 • O2 sats dropped to 83% on RA but came up to 96% with 3L of oxygen via nasal cannula.
Is the patient having chest pain?	• No
Assessment/How does he look?	• Alert and oriented, but appears uncomfortable • He is talking to me but having to stop to take breaths. • Lungs: CTAB. Breath sounds are present bilaterally. • CV: RRR, no MRG • Pulses normal
Access	• He has 2 peripheral IVs
Most recent CBC	• H/H 9.2/27
DVT prophylaxis	• He is not receiving any anticoagulation. He has not been wearing his SCDs.

Evaluation of phone call:

Communication:	
Student identified themselves	
Student identified reason for calling	
Student asked specific, goal-directed questions	
Student indicated they would call their senior resident	
Student initiated read-back (closed-loop communication)	
Student explained they were concerned about PE.	
Assessment and management:	
Student asked for vitals	
Student asked about chest pain	
Student asked for assessment of patient	
Student asked about DVT prophylaxis	
Student indicated they would come see the patient immediately	
Student asked for the following:	
— Portable CXR	
— EKG	
— Cardiac enzymes	
— ABG	
Student mentioned likely need for CTPA	
Student did not send patient off the floor for chest x-ray	

Comments:

COACHING THE LEARNER WHO STRUGGLES IN URGENT SITUATIONS

While behaviors tend to cluster in a limited number of patterns, the factors that underlie learner struggle in urgent situations are diverse. Therefore, we advocate for an individualized coaching approach that begins with understanding the subjective experience of the learner. Interventions should target the root of the behavior rather than the behavior itself. For example, lecturing a disengaged learner on the importance of patient ownership is unlikely to be effective unless the underlying causes of disengagement are addressed. This type of investigation requires a safe and neutral space and, ideally, a longitudinal relationship with a trusted and respected coach. Given the importance of separating summative assessment from coaching, we encourage institutional leaders and program directors to delegate this role to a different faculty member.

In the initial meeting(s), the coach can utilize the ADAPT (Ask, Discuss, Ask, Plan Together)[39] framework introduced in chapter 6 to share feedback, understand the learner's perspective, and begin to set goals for coaching.

A — The coach begins by asking questions that promote reflection on prior experiences in urgent situations: Can you recall a recent experience with a clinically unstable patient or clinical emergency? What went well? What did not go as well as you had hoped? Can you take me through the event, step by step? What feedback have you gotten about your performance in urgent situations? Inviting the learner to describe their decision-making and their subjective experience during the event should provide valuable information about learner insight and potential area(s) of deficiency (e.g., insufficient knowledge, lack of appreciation of urgency, lack of a management script). Because management of clinical emergencies is a multifaceted ability, the coach and learner should consider all aspects of performance including medical knowledge, clinical decision-making, and interpersonal communication.

D — Feedback about a recent event (or events) should be specific, behavior-based, and free of judgment. "I noticed [or "others noticed"] that you appeared hesitant" is preferable to "You looked really nervous." Similarly, "It seems like you're not invested" is a judgmental statement, while "When you leave the room during and emergency, one might conclude that you are not invested. I'm curious what was coming up for you when you left the room."

A — As the conversation continues, the coach encourages the learner to reflect on recent situations, exploring learner frameworks for managing unstable patients. The coach is encouraged to review common clinical scenarios to probe how the learner's knowledge is organized and apply the assessment framework introduced in chapter 6 to home in on the specific clinical reasoning concern(s). "Do you have a systematic way of approaching urgency in general?" It is important to query the learner about their performance in other settings as well as their understanding of, and comfort with, their role in an emergency. It can be helpful to have the learner reflect on role models. "What have you seen done well, or not so well, in similar situations?" While the coach should not take on the role of therapist, it is important to query the learner generally about level of fatigue, external stressors, and subjective feelings about anxiety during or in anticipation of urgent events.

PT — At the conclusion of the first meeting, the coach should have a good idea about learner insight and ability to reflect, as well as what underlying patterns of thinking or experience are contributing to the observed difficulties. Depending on the concerns raised, the coach and learner then co-create a coaching plan with specific, measurable, and time-bound goals. All coaching plans center on the principles of deliberate practice, which are discussed in more detail below. Given the challenges associated with direct observation of clinical emergencies, the plan must be learner-centered, with the learner taking on the responsibility of cueing the observations. If the initial meeting raises concern for an underlying mental health diagnosis, the learner should be referred for additional evaluation and/or treatment in accordance with institutional policy.

For all sub-phenotypes of struggle in clinically urgent situations, we advocate for coaching to begin in a simulated environment (e.g., coach's office, simulation center) where underlying issues can be explored and skills can be practiced without risk to the patient. In the examples that follow, we provide general guidance for the structuring of these meetings, recognizing that resources vary between programs. Depending on the specialty, it is often beneficial for learners to work with multiple coaches with different areas of content expertise.

RE-ENGAGING SYSTEM 2 WHEN NEEDED

All learners who underperform in the face of clinical acuity benefit from the development of frameworks to scaffold their approach to urgent situations. A coaching approach focused on analytical thinking might feel counterintuitive in clinical situations that require rapid management decisions. Yet this must be the starting point as pattern recognition is not effective for unrecognized problems. With practice and experience, these frameworks are internalized as schemas that foster intuitive reasoning.

Sub-phenotype 1: Lacks a systematic approach to urgent clinical situations in general

ABCDEF is a mnemonic that structures the approach to an acutely ill patient and segues into the exercises that follow. Initially, this framework can be introduced to guide deliberate practice across a range of clinical scenarios in a simulated environment (e.g., a coach's office, a simulation center) with a think-aloud approach in the presence of a coach.

A — Assess severity of illness and expected short-term course (prognostic reasoning)
B — Basic investigation, targeted management, and resuscitation (management reasoning)
C — Consider "can't miss" underlying etiologies (diagnostic reasoning)
D — Delegate/Discuss with the interprofessional team and/or consultants
E — Explain to the patient/family
F — Follow-up and contingency planning

The coach introduces the mnemonic and presents the learner with a case vignette. Together, they proceed through the steps. Depending on learner level and proficiency, the process facilitates both teaching and assessment of the clinical reasoning process by providing an exemplar.

VIGNETTE

A 75-year-old male with a past medical history of coronary artery disease status post stenting to the left anterior descending artery in 1995, ongoing tobacco use, and benign prostatic hypertrophy was admitted for observation following transurethral resection of a bladder tumor after recent diagnosis of bladder malignancy. The cross-covering resident receives the following page from nursing staff: URGENT: Medical Emergency Team (MET) call for new SOB, RR 30, 02 sat 87% on 2L NC.

A — In order to project the patient's immediate clinical course, the initial assessment begins with the vital signs—for this patient, looking specifically for fever, tachycardia, hypotension and/or decreased urine output. On the way to the bedside, the resident quickly scans the signout document and, once at the bedside, obtains relevant information from the nurse and confirms code status.

B — Initial management is aimed at stabilizing the vital signs. For this patient, based on what we know, this means providing supplemental oxygen. The resident performs a focused history and physical examination. In this case, history includes questions about onset of dyspnea and the coexistence of cough and chest pain. The physical examination concentrates on assessment of mental status, work of breathing, neck veins, lungs, heart, and extremities. Initial diagnostic testing may include an electrocardiogram, chest X-ray, CBC, CMP, urinalysis, blood and urine cultures, arterial or venous blood gas, lactate level, and cardiac biomarkers.

C — Considering common and "can't miss" diagnoses is a form of early hypothesis generation which, for experts, occurs almost immediately in the clinical reasoning process and generally informs "B," (focused history, physical examination, and initial diagnostic testing). The definition of "common" varies depending on the setting, time, and place. In emergency situations, the pre-test probability that the underlying diagnosis is on the "can't miss" list is high. Therefore, because of context, "common" becomes "can't miss." In this case, the learner initially considers pulmonary embolism (PE), acute coronary syndrome (ACS), pneumonia, and pneumothorax. In a simulated setting, the coach probes the learner's reasoning, asking why they included these diagnoses and excluded others? What fits and does not fit for each diagnosis on their list?

D — If team members are available, roles can be delegated. For example, the resident instructs the intern to interview and examine the patient while the resident reviews the data or talks to the nurse. The resident communicates the need for ongoing monitoring and shares their thought process with the interprofessional team. The team involves the attending physician if necessary. Consults to specialists are called if additional help is needed.

E — Once the patient is stabilized and an initial plan put in place, the resident and/or intern speaks with the family. At that time, they obtain and/or reconsider code status, gather additional history, and explain recent events and plan.

F — The patient is re-assessed, starting with vital signs and including data resulting from the initial assessment. The learner projects the clinical course based on any new data. Management typically becomes algorithmic at this point (e.g., if x, then y). In this case, if the oxygen requirement has increased and/or if the patient is hypotensive despite initial resuscitation, the resident should call the intensive care unit to initiate transfer and consider noninvasive ventilation and/or intubation with mechanical ventilation. If the chest X-ray and other initial work-up is unrevealing, the resident obtains a CTPA if the kidney function is normal or a V/Q scan. And so on. The coach encourages the learner to verbalize how they are making decisions and how management will change depending on pending results and proposed testing.

As the learner proceeds through the case, the coach poses "what if" questions to probe their knowledge and decision-making. For instance, the coach might ask, How would the management change if the patient developed an acute change in mental status? Since prognostic reasoning is an important part of response to clinical urgency, the learner should be encouraged to provide interval prediction of clinical course as data change throughout the exercise. The learner practices using the framework in the clinical environment and, in subsequent meetings with the coach, reflects on its utility. As the learner practices using ABCDEF in a variety of authentic and simulated encounters, the approach becomes more intuitive.

Sub-phenotype 2: Recognizes urgency, but struggles to act quickly

Learners with underdeveloped pattern recognition often appear hesitant or move slowly in an emergency. Conversely, they may appear to over function. For many, this reflects the fact that relevant knowledge is not stored in a way that facilitates rapid decision-making. Traditionally, clinical reasoning interventions have focused on diagnostic reasoning, providing learners with System 2-based frameworks that prioritize arrival at a diagnosis. In an urgent situation, retrieval of knowledge is more efficient if the knowledge is contextualized to specific clinical scenarios, which is analogous to the shift from topic-based to symptom-based learning discussed in chapter 9. Therefore, coaching in this situation centers on providing frameworks to help the learner develop a mental library of urgency schemas for commonly encountered high-acuity situations. These schemas would include elements of both illness and management scripts, reflecting that response in a clinical urgency is an amalgamation of diagnostic and management reasoning.

As with other scripts and schemas, they are idiosyncratic, and their use will vary by specialty and clinical setting. Effective response to clinical urgency begins with a problem representation that prompts hypothesis generation through illness script activation and a menu of management options through management script activation. Diagnostic reasoning is focused on identifying the conditions that are likely to kill the patient. Urgency schemas are unique in that the management in high-stakes situations is typically algorithmic (e.g., "if x, then y"). Probably the best-known and most well-accepted algorithms for managing urgency are those provided by the American Heart Association's Advanced Cardiac Life Support (ACLS) program. Clinical situations are often more nuanced. In interviewing experts about the use of schemas in urgent situations, representative sentiments included:

A lot of what we do is quite reactive and instinctive. This is why it is so hard with struggling learners to give them structure to go by.

We all do it "almost the same but never quite the same"—which is why there is no set protocol.

Table 14.2 outlines the components of an effective urgency schema, highlighting the unique blending of diagnostic, management, and prognostic reasoning in clinical decision-making. Coaches should provide frameworks to promote development of these schemas.

Table 14.2. Elements of an Urgency Framework to Promote Schema Formation

- Diagnostic reasoning
  - — Problem representation
  - — Early hypothesis generation
    - + "Can't miss" diagnoses
- Management reasoning
  - — Universal approach
    - + For all patients—initial labs, imaging, procedures, consultants, medications, monitoring
  - — Conditional approach
    - + Algorithmic approach to testing and treatment (if x, then y)
- Prognostic reasoning
  - — Contingency planning

Example: A medical student wishes to gain proficiency in identifying and managing hypertensive emergencies in the hospital, specifically in a non-operative setting. The coach encourages the student to review a textbook on pathophysiology as well as the American Heart Association (AHA) guidelines on blood pressure management[40,41] and schedules a follow-up meeting to begin to develop an urgency framework for this condition. In this case, the definition of hypertensive emergency, SBP > 180 or DBP > 110 mm Hg with new or worsening target organ damage, effectively serves as the problem representation, which is further characterized by the type and extent of target organ damage. In clinically urgent scenarios with a defined problem, all diagnoses are "can't miss" diagnoses. Treatment of hypertensive emergency is unique in that most decisions are dictated both by the underlying cause and the extent of target organ damage. After consulting the source material, the student decides to create a table that is organized by organ impacted, with additional categories for catecholamine excess and pregnancy. The table considers these cause-and-effect factors simultaneously, recognizing that differentiating between the two will not impact immediate management. For example, microangiopathic hemolytic anemia (MAHA) can be a cause as well as an effect of severe hypertension. For the purposes of immediate evaluation and management, whether MAHA is a cause or effect does not impact management or immediate contingency planning. In contrast, an illness script for an isolated condition would include enabling conditions and consequences.

The work-up of hypertensive emergency is generally guided by presenting signs and symptoms. With the coach's help, the learner also indicates in bold print the diagnostic testing that should be undertaken in all patients who meet the blood pressure criteria for this condition. The student learns from their reading that, in most cases, blood pressure must be lowered gradually to avoid ischemia to tissues accustomed to higher levels of blood pressure. However, in other clinical situations, for example, aortic dissection, the recommendation is to lower blood pressure quickly. These decisions, as well as those related to choice of antihypertensive agent, also relate to the underlying diagnosis and/or type of target organ damage which facilitates their inclusion in the same table. In the process of creating the schema, the coach (in this case, a content expert) helps fill in the gaps and areas of uncertainty, adding practical guidance.

EXAMPLE FRAMEWORK TO PROMOTE URGENCY SCHEMA FOR HYPERTENSIVE EMERGENCY

Heart/aorta

- **If**: chest pain, back pain, dyspnea, palpitations, recent use of cocaine or amphetamines, signs of volume overload on examination
- **Then consider**: acute coronary syndrome (ACS), decompensated heart failure, aortic dissection
- **Diagnostic testing**: EKG, CXR, cardiac biomarkers, urine drug screen (UDS), contrast-enhanced CT or MRI of chest or transesophageal echocardiogram

- **Blood pressure lowering**:
  - — Aortic dissection – SBP to < 120 mm Hg within 20 minutes
  - — Decompensated heart failure – SBP to < 180 mm Hg or MAP decline 25%
  - — ACS – depends on underlying BP, but typically rapid lower to SBP < 160 mm Hg
  - — Pulmonary edema not due to decompensated heart failure (hypertensive cardiogenic pulmonary edema) – depends on underlying BP, but typically rapid lower to SBP < 160 mm Hg
- **Choice of antihypertensive agent**:
  - — Aortic dissection
    - + Preferred initial management – beta blocker (e.g., esmolol, labetalol)
    - + Avoid vasodilator (e.g., hydralazine, sodium nitroprusside, nicardipine) unless already on beta blocker
  - — Acute coronary syndrome (without decompensated heart failure)
    - + Preferred initial management – beta blocker
    - + Avoid vasodilator unless already on beta blocker
  - — Cocaine chest pain with hypertension
    - + Preferred initial management – nitrates, benzodiazepines
    - + Avoid beta blocker
  - — Decompensated heart failure
    - + Preferred initial management – nitrates, calcium channel blocker (CCB)
    - + Avoid beta blocker
  - — Pulmonary edema not due to decompensated heart failure (hypertensive cardiogenic pulmonary edema) – nitrates, loop diuretic, morphine

Brain

- **If**: headache, nausea and vomiting, confusion, restlessness, focal neurologic symptoms, seizures, history of head trauma
- **Then consider**: acute hemorrhagic stroke, acute ischemic stroke, hypertensive encephalopathy (PRES [posterior reversible encephalopathy syndrome]), brain tumor
- **Diagnostic testing**: CT or MRI of the brain

(continued)

- **Blood pressure lowering:**
  - Acute hemorrhagic stroke – recommendations vary, requires close monitoring, treatment should be individualized
    - Avoid SBP < 140 mm Hg
    - If acute intracranial hypertension and SBP > 220 mm Hg, rapid lower to < 220 mm Hg, maintain > 140 mm Hg
  - Acute ischemic stroke –
    - If no thrombolysis planned
      - If SBP < 220 mm Hg, resume outpatient antihypertensive medications
      - If SBP > 220 mm Hg, or if other target organ damage, lower 15% in first 24 hours
    - If thrombolysis planned
      - Lower SBP to < 185 mm Hg before giving thrombolytics, and keep < 180 mm Hg over first 24 hours
  - Hypertensive encephalopathy (PRES) – immediate MAP decrease 10 to 25%, then gradual lowering of no more than 25% over next 24 hours
  - Head trauma - avoid aggressive lowering of BP
- **Choice of antihypertensive agent:**
  - Labetalol, CCB (clevidipine, nicardipine), enalaprilat
  - Avoid fenoldopam, nitroprusside, and nitroglycerine if high intracranial pressure or bleed

Eye

- **If:** visual changes
- **Then consider:** hypertensive retinopathy, increased intracranial pressure (see Brain)
- **Diagnostic testing:** fundoscopic examination
- **Blood pressure lowering:** SBP < 180, initial target MAP decline of 15%
- **Choice of antihypertensive agent:**
  - Avoid fenoldopam if high intra-ocular pressure

Kidney

- **If**: history of kidney disease, history of scleroderma, confusion, oliguria/anuria, signs and symptoms of volume overload, signs of scleroderma on exam
- **Then consider**: acute kidney injury, microangiopathic hemolytic anemia (MAHA), bilateral renal artery stenosis, scleroderma renal crisis (SRC)
- **Diagnostic testing**: urinalysis with microscopy, serum electrolytes, serum creatinine, complete blood count (CBC) with smear, haptoglobin, LDH, urine protein-to-creatinine ratio, renal ultrasound with Dopplers or MRA renal arteries
- **Blood pressure lowering**:
  - For all but SRC – MAP decline 20 to 25% over several hours
  - SRC (or other high renin disorder) – return to previous baseline BP within 72 hours
- **Choice of antihypertensive agent**:
  - If not SRC (or other high renin disorder)
    - Clevidipine, nicardipine, labetalol, fenoldopam
    - Avoid sodium nitroprusside, IV ACEI
  - If SRC (or other high renin disorder)
    - IV ACEI (enalaprilat)

Catecholamine excess

- **If**: headache, tachycardia, diaphoresis, recent use of cocaine or amphetamines, recently stopped taking clonidine or other short-acting antihypertensive agents, use of monoamine oxidase inhibitors and tyramine-containing foods
- **Then consider**: sympathetic overactivity due to ingestion or withdrawal of clonidine, catecholamine-secreting tumor
- **Diagnostic testing**: UDS, plasma free metanephrines
- **Blood pressure lowering**:
  - Depends on organ(s) involved and whether underlying BP was normal
- **Choice of antihypertensive agent**:
  - Clevidipine, nicardipine, phentolamine (first line if catecholamine-secreting tumor)
  - Avoid beta blocker (unless hypertension is due to beta blocker withdrawal)
  - Nitroprusside* can be used for intra-operative management of hypertension

Pregnancy

- **If**: pregnant + visual symptoms, dyspnea, headache
- **Then consider**: preeclampsia/eclampsia, HELLP
- **Diagnostic testing**: urine hcg, UPCR, CBC with smear, serum creatinine, liver function tests
- **Blood pressure lowering**:
  — Generally rapid lowering SBP < 160 mm Hg
- **Choice of antihypertensive agent**:
  — Labetalol, hydralazine, nicardipine, magnesium sulfate
  — Avoid ACEI, ARB, direct renin inhibitor, sodium nitroprusside

*requires intra-arterial blood pressure monitoring, monitoring for cyanide toxicity

---

An alternative framework depicts the management of hypertensive emergency as an algorithm with three branch points: (1) targeted diagnostic testing based on presenting signs and symptoms; (2) how quickly, and by how much, the blood pressure should be lowered; and (3) choice of antihypertensive agent.

We encourage struggling learners to begin by co-creating with their coach a list of commonly encountered urgent scenarios relevant to their clinical exposure. Early in the coaching process, the problem representation should be relatively undifferentiated (e.g., hypertensive emergency). Over time and with experience, the situations become more refined (e.g., hypertensive emergency in a 22-year-old patient undergoing an operative procedure). Development of these scripts occurs over time through an iterative process between coach and learner that involves considering variations in clinical presentation and course. Through the process of considering "what if" questions, the learner develops greater capacity for adaptability. Priming the learner to prepare for the unexpected, as we will discuss in more detail in chapter 15, improves their ability to troubleshoot in the moment. The learner then practices applying the framework in the clinical and/or simulated environment, continuing the process of refinement, and revisits their approach in subsequent meetings with the coach. Ultimately, the framework is internalized as a highly personalized schema, thus reorganizing the learner's thinking and minimizing cognitive load during complex decision-making.

Sub-phenotype 3: Over-reliant on intuition and makes errors, or struggles with the unexpected

Urgent situations are often passed from clinician to clinician with labels. For example, consider the patient with history of alcohol use disorder who presents to the emergency department with confusion, tachycardia, and fever. After initial triage, the emergency room physician treats the patient with benzodiazepines, documents the diagnosis of "alcohol withdrawal delirium," and transfers the patient to the medical intensive care unit (MICU). If the MICU team anchors on the label of "alcohol withdrawal" and continues the treatment approach without considering new evidence such as persistent fever, stiff neck, and recent history of a sinus infection, they may miss an alternative diagnosis such as bacterial meningitis. In all cases, learners who encounter clinically urgent situations should be encouraged to create their own problem representation, in the moment, to limit confirmation bias. When assuming care for a sick patient, it is important to consider the existing label and ask: What doesn't fit? What information might have been left out? What is another way to tie this together?[42]

This skill is mastered through deliberate practice in which the learner works through cases with the coach in a simulated setting (e.g., coach's office or simulation center). The coach provides a clinical scenario then walks the learner through decision points, inserting stops to help the learner practice slowing down consciously.

Example: The learner is called to the bedside of a 55-year-old woman admitted from the emergency department that morning with pyelonephritis. Vital signs are notable for temperature 39.4 C, BP 78/48 mm Hg, pulse of 132 bpm. Her urine output over the last six hours has been 10 mL.

The coach prompts the learner to verbalize their problem representation and an initial menu of management options. The learner rapidly recognizes this clinical picture as septic shock, and this pattern recognition triggers the following immediate interventions: bolus of isotonic intravenous fluid; broader antibiotic coverage; additional diagnostic testing including lactate level, blood cultures; and preparation for a central line for possible administration of vasopressor support. The coach relays that, despite fluid bolus, broadening of antibiotic coverage, and initiation of norepinephrine, the patient's blood pressure remains low at 88/52 mm Hg. Lactate level is 6.2 mmol/L, and she is now somnolent. The learner must now transition to analytic reasoning to more broadly assess potential etiologies and consider modifications in management. If the learner struggles with a place to start, the coach can pose questions such as: How would you assess adequacy of your fluid resuscitation? What might you be missing with the current antibiotic coverage? Are there situations in which antibiotics alone are not sufficient to treat infection? What are other causes of hypotension that you may have missed? The coach can take the learner down several hypothetical pathways with "what if" questioning, (e.g., What if the patient developed hypoxia and crackles on examination after the initial fluid bolus?). In one scenario, the learner orders a stat CT of the abdomen and pelvis to rule out urinary tract obstruction or abscess, which reveals a 6 cm obstructing ureteral stone with significant hydronephrosis, not appreciated on the initial ultrasound performed on admission. The learner toggles back to System 1 for rapid implementation of a plan, which includes urgent consultation of interventional radiology for likely placement of a percutaneous nephrostomy tube and possible MICU transfer. Once the nephrostomy tube is placed, the learner can return to analytical thinking to consider further management decisions (e.g., narrowing of antibiotics, preventive management of nephrolithiasis) and review the entire hospital course, reflecting on the progression of events and looking for areas of improvement in future patient encounters.

It may feel counterintuitive to slow down in situations that typically demand quick action, but we advocate that all learners enact a "medical timeout" when faced with a clinical emergency. Evidence points to the importance of the medical pause, which can be accomplished in as little as ten seconds, in disrupting negative momentum (e.g. failing to consider new information that is inconsistent with the initial diagnosis).[43–45] Pausing in this context is both a cognitive and, as we will discuss later in this chapter, physical exercise, that promotes reflection. Reflection allows integration of working memory and long-term memory, allowing learners to tap into more creative problem-solving.[45] There is a wide body of literature on the use of reflection for improving clinical reasoning.[44,46–49]

Table 14.3. Use of the Medical Timeout in Clinically Urgent Situations

- **Cognitive**
  - Triggers
    - Something doesn't feel right, something is atypical or unfamiliar
    - Uncertain diagnosis
    - Immediate management options require weighing of risks and benefits
    - Rapidly changing data or patient status
    - Unsure of next steps due to complexity
  - Action
    - Verbalize the need for a timeout
      - Can we take a moment to review?
      - I need a second to regroup.
    - Seek clarification, ask for help
    - Rename and reframe the problem[19]
      - Construct new problem representation
    - Think aloud
- **Physical**
  - Triggers
    - Feeling overwhelmed, anxious, flooded
    - Feeling stuck, frozen, trouble focusing
  - Action (internal dialogue)
    - Name the feeling
    - STOP exercise

In subsequent meetings with the coach, the learner reflects on the use of the medical timeout in the clinical environment. The coach asks about feasibility, impact on team dynamics, and learner's awareness of their feelings in general. The coach should also consider the length of the timeout and encourage reflection on the potential adverse events that can result from slowing down for too long or at the incorrect time.[21]

Sub-phenotype 4: Does not recognize urgency

It should be clear relatively quickly if the problem is that the learner fails to appreciate the cues, whether social or clinical, that indicate urgency. Prognostic reasoning, and specifically rapid assessment of illness severity, is discussed in detail in chapter 11. If the learner's performance does not improve with deliberate practice of newly developed frameworks, and/or if there are more global concerns about awareness or interpersonal interaction, referral for mental health evaluation and/or treatment should be considered in accordance with programmatic and institutional policy.

Sub-phenotype 5: Recognizes urgency but does not understand their role, is uncomfortable in their role, or appears uninvested in their role

Learners who do not understand their role, are uncomfortable in their role, or appear uninvested in their role in clinically urgent situations may appear hesitant or avoidant. Conversely, they may behave aggressively and compensate for their uncertainty or discomfort by over functioning. As we have discussed, coaching begins with understanding the learner's perspective and considering underlying contributors such as fatigue, stress, burnout, anxiety, depression, and/or feelings of inadequacy or fear of failure. Using the ADAPT framework,[39] the coach engages the learner in a series of reflective exercises tailored to the concern.

The following are example topics for reflective exercises, building on earlier recommendations for structuring the initial meeting with the coach:

- For all learners: Have you seen someone manage an emergency particularly well? What did you admire about how they handled the situation? Conversely, what behaviors have you observed to be ineffective in an urgent situation?
- If the learner appears hesitant, is overly deferential, or struggles to communicate or behave assertively: How do you see your role in emergencies? Why is assertive communication important during an emergency? Do you find yourself waiting for others to act, or waiting for permission, before stepping in? What holds you back? What does being "deferential" mean to you? Do you see it as a sign of respect, uncertainty, or something else?

- If the learner struggles to delegate: Why is teamwork important in managing an emergency? Do you trust your teammates to carry out delegated tasks? If not, what contributes to your hesitation? How do you feel about giving instructions to others in high-pressure situations? Do you worry about being perceived as bossy?

For all learners, it is important that the expectations for their role be clearly stated and that they understand these expectations. Part of reflection is helping the learner understand how they are perceived and how their behavior is or is not achieving their goals in the situation. Regardless of the underlying issue(s), most learners gain comfort and improve assertiveness through engaging in deliberate practice of managing urgent situations in a simulated setting (e.g., simulation center). If, during the process of reflection, concerns arise about underlying mental health conditions, referral for evaluation and/or treatment should be considered in accordance with programmatic and institutional policy.

Sub-phenotype 6: Becomes emotionally flooded in urgent situations

All clinicians experience a range of emotions when faced with a patient who is acutely ill. Without awareness of these emotions and their physical sensations in the body, it is possible to become flooded. Emotional flooding can impair decision-making and may lead to ineffective communication, either of which can negatively impact the ability to lead in a clinical emergency. Emotion regulation begins with self-awareness and recognizing feelings in the moment. Encouraging learners to name their feelings—"if you name it, you can tame it"[50]—can help them gain control in situations in which they tend to become emotionally hijacked. The learner should be encouraged to reflect on how they typically behave when emotionally triggered. Some learners will recognize that they tend to avoid, freeze, or become quiet. Others may notice that they raise their voice and/or exhibit nonverbal cues that are perceived as aggressive. The coach can ask how the learner's typical reactions have helped or hindered their ability to be effective in clinical emergencies. For learners who struggle to name their feelings, we encourage the use of a feelings wheel. Many wheels are available —common emotions experienced in urgent situations are excitement, fear, inadequacy, helplessness, guilt, compassion, and frustration.[51]

Austrian neurologist, psychologist, and Holocaust survivor Dr. Viktor Frankl is often quoted as having said, "Between stimulus and response there is a space. In that space is our power to choose our response. In our response lies our growth and freedom." The STOP exercise,[52] taught in many mindfulness courses, can be helpful to structure this pause when a learner notices themselves feeling flooded. This practice allows the learner to create that space in which they can choose an effective response rather than impulsively reacting to the situation. The pause also provides the opportunity for grounding to help the learner relax and calm themselves.

S top: pause for a moment
T ake a breath: to calm
O bserve your experience
    What am I feeling?
    What are my goals?
    What are my choices?
P roceed with awareness

In addition to applying these principles to their clinical work, the learner is encouraged to adopt the habit of naming emotions and using the STOP exercise in their day-to-day activities and to share their experience with the coach in subsequent meetings. Over time, this practice helps learners improve emotional regulation and resilience in challenging situations.

THE IMPORTANCE OF DEBRIEFING AFTER AN EVENT

Given the importance of situativity,[53–55] assessment and coaching must eventually take place *in situ*. Effective coaching of the learner who struggles in urgent situations is rooted in the principles of deliberate practice and therefore necessitates direct observation, which can be difficult given the unpredictability of these events. When possible, we recommend that all learners debrief with supervisors (e.g., faculty, peers, near peers) and/or members of the interprofessional team within 24 hours of an event. Debriefing has been promoted for health care workers to facilitate learning and to improve emotional processing and well-being after unanticipated, difficult, or adverse events. Multiple models exist to structure these discussions, though the literature suggests that debriefing does not happen often enough outside of the simulated environment.[56,57] Given the logistical constraints of most busy clinical environments, it generally works best if the debriefing process is learner-led. In fact, an early goal of coaching the learner who struggles in urgent situations is role playing and strategizing how to solicit feedback.

The power of the debrief is in reflection on what went well or did not go well, what was unexpected, what was difficult, and what came up for the learner during the event. The 3D model, rooted in the Kolb Experiential Learning Cycle, offers a structured approach to evaluate learner performance through inquiry and reflection.[58]

- **Defusing**—learner perspective (the "what")
  - Learner and observer recap event
  - Learner describes emotional experience

    Let's talk about how that went.

    What did you notice…?

    How did it feel to…?

- **Discover**—analyze performance (the "why")
  - Observer shares what they saw, probes rationale (mental model) behind decisions
  - Learner reflects on how this event relates to prior experience
  - Observer shares their mental model

    I noticed that…

    Can you tell me why…?

    If you had done x, how would that have changed y?

    How have you typically handled/seen this situation handled in the past?

    I typically…

- **Deepen**—connect learning to future practice (the "what next")
  - Observer prompts learner to consider how they will apply lessons learned to future practice
  - Summary of lessons learned

    The next time you encounter x, what will you do differently?

    Can you think of other situations where what you have learned today can be applied?

    What is one thing to take away from today?

SUMMARY

Clinically urgent situations present the ultimate opportunity for medical learners to apply clinical reasoning in context, and performance is influenced by a multitude of factors intrinsic and extrinsic to the learner. Simply knowing the guidelines or steps of an algorithm does not ensure success in vivo. Emergencies are unique in that the learner must combine elements of diagnostic, prognostic, and management reasoning to make decisions amid ambiguity and, invariably, commotion. Effective clinical reasoning relies both on pattern recognition and cognitive flexibility, as no two emergencies are the same. Most struggling learners benefit from an approach that combines the development of urgency-tailored frameworks with deliberate practice of skills in a simulated setting to promote adaptability. Coaching should be individualized, with careful consideration of the factors that underlie observed behaviors. For each phenotype of struggle, we have suggested how simulation can be incorporated to facilitate deliberate practice of skills. The exercises and approaches introduced in this chapter can inform the teaching of all medical learners.

References

1. Advanced Cardiovascular Life Support (ACLS). cpr.heart.org. Accessed February 5, 2025. https://cpr.heart.org/en/cpr-courses-and-kits/healthcare-professional/acls
2. Norman G, Pelaccia T, Wyer P, Sherbino J. Dual process models of clinical reasoning: The central role of knowledge in diagnostic expertise. *J Eval Clin Pract.* 2024;30(5):788-796. doi:10.1111/jep.13998
3. Smith ER, DeCoster J. Dual-Process Models in Social and Cognitive Psychology: Conceptual Integration and Links to Underlying Memory Systems. *Personal Soc Psychol Rev.* 2000;4(2):108-131. doi:10.1207/S15327957PSPR0402_01
4. Evans JStBT. Dual-Processing Accounts of Reasoning, Judgment, and Social Cognition. *Annu Rev Psychol.* 2008;59(1):255-278. doi:10.1146/annurev.psych.59.103006.093629
5. Custers EJFM. Thirty years of illness scripts: Theoretical origins and practical applications. *Med Teach.* 2015;37(5):457-462. doi:10.3109/0142159X.2014.956052
6. Charlin B, Tardif J, Boshuizen HPA. Scripts and Medical Diagnostic Knowledge: Theory and Applications for Clinical Reasoning Instruction and Research. *Acad Med.* 2000;75(2):182-190.
7. Charlin B, Boshuizen HPA, Custers EJ, Feltovich PJ. Scripts and clinical reasoning. *Med Educ.* 2007;41(12):1178-1184. doi:10.1111/j.1365-2923.2007.02924.x

8. Heidemann LA, McTaggart S, Monrad SU, Hartley S. Can Incoming Interns Be Entrusted to Recognize Medical Emergencies? Implementation of a Vignette-Based Cross-Cover Assessment. *J Grad Med Educ.* 2022;14(4):488-492. doi:10.4300/JGME-D-21-01193.1

9. Croskerry P. A Universal Model of Diagnostic Reasoning. *Acad Med.* 2009;84(8):1022. doi:10.1097/ACM.0b013e3181ace703

10. Cammarata M, Dhaliwal G. Diagnostic Schemas: Form and Function. *J Gen Intern Med.* 2023;38(2):513-516. doi:10.1007/s11606-022-07935-1

11. Norman G. Dual processing and diagnostic errors. *Adv Health Sci Educ Theory Pract.* 2009;14 Suppl 1:37-49. doi:10.1007/s10459-009-9179-x

12. Mohan D, Arnold RM, Fischhoff B, et al. Inside the Black Box of Deliberate Practice: How do Coaches Coach to Improve Trauma Triage. *J Surg Res.* 2024;302:669-678. doi:10.1016/j.jss.2024.07.114

13. Parsons AS, Wijesekera TP, Rencic JJ. The Management Script: A Practical Tool for Teaching Management Reasoning. *Acad Med.* 2020;95(8):1179-1185. doi:10.1097/ACM.0000000000003465

14. Cook DA, Stephenson CR, Gruppen LD, Durning SJ. Management Reasoning: Empirical Determination of Key Features and a Conceptual Model. *Acad Med J Assoc Am Med Coll.* 2023;98(1):80-87. doi:10.1097/ACM.0000000000004810

15. Cook DA, Stephenson CR, Gruppen LD, Durning SJ. Management reasoning scripts: Qualitative exploration using simulated physician-patient encounters. *Perspect Med Educ.* 2022;11(4):196-206. doi:10.1007/s40037-022-00714-y

16. Abdoler EA, Parsons AS, Wijesekera TP. The future of teaching management reasoning: important questions and potential solutions. *Diagn Berl Ger.* Published online November 23, 2022. doi:10.1515/dx-2022-0048

17. Wijesekera TP, Parsons AS, Abdoler EA, Trowbridge RL, Durning SJ, Rencic JJ. Management Reasoning: A Toolbox for Educators. *Acad Med.* 2022;97(11):1724. doi:10.1097/ACM.0000000000004796

18. Penner JC, Minter DJ, Abdoler EA, Parsons AS. Reasoning on Rounds Volume 2: a Framework for Teaching Management Reasoning in the Inpatient Setting. *J Gen Intern Med.* Published online December 20, 2024. doi:10.1007/s11606-024-09039-4

19. Moulton C anne E, Regehr G, Mylopoulos M, MacRae HM. Slowing Down When You Should: A New Model of Expert Judgment. *Acad Med.* 2007;82(10):S109. doi:10.1097/ACM.0b013e3181405a76

20. Goleman D. *Emotional Intelligence.* Bantam Books; 1995.

21. Monteiro S, Sherbino J, LoGiudice A, Lee M, Norman G, Sibbald M. The influence of viewing time on visual diagnostic accuracy: Less is more. *Med Educ.* 2024;58(7):858-868. doi:10.1111/medu.15380

22. Brush JE Jr, Lee M, Sherbino J, Taylor-Fishwick JC, Norman G. Effect of Teaching Bearman, MargaretBayesian Methods Using Learning by Concept vs Learning by Example on Medical Students' Ability to Estimate Probability of a Diagnosis: A Randomized Clinical Trial. *JAMA Netw Open.* 2019;2(12):e1918023. doi:10.1001/jamanetworkopen.2019.18023

23. Konopasky A, Artino AR, Battista A, et al. Understanding context specificity: the effect of contextual factors on clinical reasoning. *Diagnosis.* 2020;7(3):257-264. doi:10.1515/dx-2020-0016

24. Durning SJ, Artino AR, Boulet JR, Dorrance K, van der Vleuten C, Schuwirth L. The impact of selected contextual factors on experts' clinical reasoning performance (does context impact clinical reasoning performance in experts?). *Adv Health Sci Educ Theory Pract.* 2012;17(1):65-79. doi:10.1007/s10459-011-9294-3

25. Daniel M, Durning SJ, Wilson E, Abdoler E, Torre D. Situated cognition: clinical reasoning and error are context dependent. *Diagnosis.* 2020;7(3):341-342. doi:10.1515/dx-2020-0011

26. Rencic J, Schuwirth LWT, Gruppen LD, Durning SJ. A situated cognition model for clinical reasoning performance assessment: a narrative review. *Diagn Berl Ger.* 2020;7(3):227-240. doi:10.1515/dx-2019-0106

27. Natesan S, Jordan J, Sheng A, et al. Feedback in Medical Education: An Evidence-based Guide to Best Practices from the Council of Residency Directors in Emergency Medicine. *West J Emerg Med.* 2023;24(3):479-494. doi:10.5811/westjem.56544

28. Boulet JR, Murray D, Kras J, Woodhouse J, McAllister J, Ziv A. Reliability and validity of a simulation-based acute care skills assessment for medical students and residents. *Anesthesiology.* 2003;99(6):1270-1280. doi:10.1097/00000542-200312000-00007

29. Walker S, Brett S, McKay A, Lambden S, Vincent C, Sevdalis N. Observational Skill-based Clinical Assessment tool for Resuscitation (OSCAR): development and validation. *Resuscitation.* 2011;82(7):835-844. doi:10.1016/j.resuscitation.2011.03.009

30. Cooper S, Cant R, Porter J, et al. Rating medical emergency teamwork performance: development of the Team Emergency Assessment Measure (TEAM). Resuscitation. 2010;81(4):446-452. doi:10.1016/j.*resuscitation.*2009.11.027

31. Ottestad E, Boulet JR, Lighthall GK. Evaluating the management of septic shock using patient simulation. *Crit Care Med.* 2007;35(3):769-775. doi:10.1097/01.CCM.0000256849.75799.20

32. Erdogan A, Dong Y, Chen X, et al. Development and validation of clinical performance assessment in simulated medical emergencies: an observational study. *BMC Emerg Med.* 2016;16:4. doi:10.1186/s12873-015-0066-x

33. Schmutz J, Eppich WJ, Hoffmann F, Heimberg E, Manser T. Five Steps to Develop Checklists for Evaluating Clinical Performance: An Integrative Approach. *Acad Med.* 2014;89(7):996. doi:10.1097/ACM.0000000000000289

34. Rosen MA, Pronovost PJ. Advancing the Use of Checklists for Evaluating Performance in Health Care. *Acad Med.* 2014;89(7):963. doi:10.1097/ACM.0000000000000285

35. Peterson BD, Magee CD, Martindale JR, et al. REACT: Rapid Evaluation Assessment of Clinical Reasoning Tool. *J Gen Intern Med.* 2022;37(9):2224-2229. doi:10.1007/s11606-022-07513-5

36. Marcum JA. An integrated model of clinical reasoning: dual-process theory of cognition and metacognition. *J Eval Clin Pract.* 2012;18(5):954-961. doi:https://doi.org/10.1111/j.1365-2753.2012.01900.x

37. Pangaro L. A new vocabulary and other innovations for improving descriptive in-training evaluations. *Acad Med.* 1999;74(11):1203.

38. Cetrone E, Mutter K, Pedersen K, Shah N, Martindale J. A Paging Training Program for a Fourth-Year Internship Readiness Course. *MedEdPORTAL J Teach Learn Resour.* 16:11021. doi:10.15766/mep_2374-8265.11021

39. Kogan J. The Adapt Model for Feedback. ACGME Remediation Toolkit. Learn at ACGME. August 31, 2024. Accessed February 4, 2025. https://dl.acgme.org/courses/acgme-remediation-toolkit

40. Whelton PK, Carey RM, Aronow WS, et al. 2017 ACC/AHA/AAPA/ABC/ACPM/AGS/APhA/ASH/ASPC/NMA/PCNA Guideline for the Prevention, Detection, Evaluation, and Management of High Blood Pressure in Adults: Executive Summary: A Report of the American College of Cardiology/American Heart Association Task Force on Clinical Practice Guidelines. *Hypertens Dallas Tex 1979.* 2018;71(6):1269-1324. doi:10.1161/HYP.0000000000000066

41. Bress AP, Anderson TS, Flack JM, et al. The Management of Elevated Blood Pressure in the Acute Care Setting: A Scientific Statement From the American Heart Association. *Hypertens Dallas Tex 1979.* 2024;81(8):e94-e106. doi:10.1161/HYP.0000000000000238

42. Lighthall GK, Vazquez-Guillamet C. Understanding Decision Making in Critical Care. *Clin Med Res.* 2015;13(3-4):156-168. doi:10.3121/cmr.2015.1289

43. Yale S, Cohen S, Bordini BJ. Diagnostic Time-Outs to Improve Diagnosis. *Crit Care Clin.* 2022;38(2):185-194. doi:10.1016/j.ccc.2021.11.008

44. Mamede S, Hautz WE, Berendonk C, et al. Think Twice: Effects on Diagnostic Accuracy of Returning to the Case to Reflect Upon the Initial Diagnosis. *Acad Med.* 2020;95(8):1223. doi:10.1097/ACM.0000000000003153

45. Lee JY, Szulewski A, Young JQ, Donkers J, Jarodzka H, van Merriënboer JJG. The medical pause: Importance, processes and training. *Med Educ.* 2021;55(10):1152-1160. doi:10.1111/medu.14529

46. Mamede S, Schmidt HG. Deliberate reflection and clinical reasoning: Founding ideas and empirical findings. *Med Educ.* 2023;57(1):76-85. doi:10.1111/medu.14863

47. Mamede S, Schmidt HG. The structure of reflective practice in medicine. *Med Educ.* 2004;38(12):1302-1308. doi:10.1111/j.1365-2929.2004.01917.x

48. Mamede S, Schmidt H. Reflection in Diagnostic Reasoning: What Really Matters? *Acad Med.* 2014;89(7):959-960. doi:10.1097/ACM.0000000000000306

49. Mamede S, van Gog T, van den Berge K, et al. Effect of availability bias and reflective reasoning on diagnostic accuracy among internal medicine residents. *JAMA.* 2010;304(11):1198-1203. doi:10.1001/jama.2010.1276

50. The Whole-Brain Child. Dr. Dan Siegel. Accessed February 5, 2025. https://drdansiegel.com/book/the-whole-brain-child/

51. Feelings Wheel. Accessed February 5, 2025. https://feelingswheel.com/

52. *Fully Present.*; 2017. Accessed February 5, 2025. https://www.hachettebookgroup.com/titles/susan-l-smalley-phd/fully-present/9780738214221/

53. Durning SJ, Artino AR. Situativity theory: a perspective on how participants and the environment can interact: AMEE Guide no. 52. *Med Teach.* 2011;33(3):188-199. doi:10.3109/0142159X.2011.550965

54. Merkebu J, Battistone M, McMains K, et al. Situativity: a family of social cognitive theories for understanding clinical reasoning and diagnostic error. *Diagn Berl Ger.* 2020;7(3):169-176. doi:10.1515/dx-2019-0100

55. Parsons AS, Wijesekera TP, Olson APJ, Torre D, Durning SJ, Daniel M. Beyond thinking fast and slow: Implications of a transtheoretical model of clinical reasoning and error on teaching, assessment, and research. *Med Teach.* Published online June 5, 2024:1-12. doi:10.1080/0142159X.2024.2359963

56. Sweeney RE, Clapp JT, Arriaga AF, et al. Understanding Debriefing: A Qualitative Study of Event Reconstruction at an Academic Medical Center. *Acad Med.* 2020;95(7):1089. doi:10.1097/ACM.0000000000002999

57. Evans TR, Burns C, Essex R, et al. A systematic scoping review on the evidence behind debriefing practices for the wellbeing/emotional outcomes of healthcare workers. *Front Psychiatry.* 2023;14:1078797. doi:10.3389/fpsyt.2023.1078797

58. Zigmont JJ, Kappus LJ, Sudikoff SN. The 3D Model of Debriefing: Defusing, Discovering, and Deepening. *Semin Perinatol.* 2011;35(2):52-58. doi:10.1053/j.semperi.2011.01.003

CHAPTER 15

Struggles in the Operating Room

As one of my professors once explained, doing surgery is no more physically difficult than writing in cursive. Surgical mastery is about familiarity and judgment. You learn the problems that can occur during a particular procedure or with a particular condition, and you learn how to either prevent or respond to those problems.

—Atul Gawande, MD, "Personal Best," *Annals of Medicine*, *The New Yorker*, Sept 26, 2011

CASE 1

Dr. Li is 8 months into his clinical PGY4 year of surgery residency. In the operating room (OR), he struggles to anticipate the steps in the case. His technical skills are average. He can provide assistance but is unable to take over as the primary technician during portions of the case. He requires constant cues and corrections to perform a task. As a result, he is provided less autonomy in the OR as compared to his peers. Additionally, he lacks the confidence to make critical decisions in the OR. For example, he is unable to determine if he has successfully obtained the critical view of safety during a laparoscopic cholecystectomy. He is becoming more self-conscious and, as a result, his nervousness is apparent while performing technical tasks. When given the opportunity to perform parts of a case, he rushes in fear of having the opportunity taken away from him. Multiple attending surgeons have lamented that he requires close supervision as they fear he may cause a complication during the case. Dr. Li's medical knowledge is average, and there have been no significant concerns regarding his management of patients on the inpatient floor or intensive care unit services. However, his performance in the OR is below the required standard. Program leadership is concerned that he may not be able to assist in PGY5 or chief-level cases. Furthermore, fellowship applications are approaching, and many faculty are uncomfortable providing letters of support for Dr. Li's application to fellowship.

DEFINING OPERATIVE REASONING

The operating room is a unique environment in which medical learners are faced with high-stakes clinical situations where the risk of patient harm is always immediate. Complexity is magnified by time pressures, the potential for interruptions and unexpected events, and the need to interact with a multidisciplinary team. In contrast to most other clinical settings, direct observation of the learner in the operating room is a constant, whether by the trainee's supervisor or by other members of the team. Operative performance spans the competencies of medical knowledge, patient care, professionalism, interpersonal and communication skills, systems-based practice, and problem-based learning and improvement.[1,2] Historically, studies describing remediation of surgical trainees have focused on technical skill (defined as using instruments effectively and efficiently) or medical knowledge.[3] Much has been written about the conceptualization and remediation of technical skill.[3–5] However, technical skill deficiency is the primary problem in only a small minority of struggling procedural learners.[6,7] Literature in the last twenty years reflects an increasing appreciation of the nontechnical elements of operative performance and their association with error and adverse events.

Leaders in surgical education have defined common themes of struggle among learners in the operating room that go beyond medical knowledge and technical skill, suggesting that operative performance is fundamentally a clinical reasoning ability.[3,8–14] In chapter 4, we presented a hierarchy of skills, visualized as a pyramid, that are related to clinical reasoning. At the bottom of the pyramid are basic intellectual, cognitive, and social-emotional capacities. Higher order abilities include metacognition and self-regulation.

At the highest level, learners integrate these skills to think critically and manage patients in the busy clinical environment. As discussed, the cognitive processes of clinical reasoning can be coached as micro skills with explicit consideration of context. Clinical reasoning *in vivo* considers the interface between the learner and the clinical environment. This relationship is best understood using the theory of *embodied cognition* in which the mind, body, and environment are interconnected and interdependent for both making diagnoses and enacting management plans.[15] This is particularly true for learners in procedural fields. Effective clinical reasoning in the operating room requires the learner to link their knowledge with their perceptions and motor capabilities. While basic knowledge and technical skill are necessary, simply knowing the facts or being facile with hands and instruments is not sufficient.

Operative clinical reasoning comprises three interrelated components, each of which are teachable, assessable, and remediable through coaching (Table 15.1). These concepts are applicable to learners in any procedural field, including general surgery, surgical subspecialties, anesthesiology, obstetrics and gynecology, interventional radiology, and medical subspecialties that involve procedures (e.g., cardiology, gastroenterology).

Table 15.1. The Components of Operative Reasoning

1. **Forward planning**
    a. Physical preparation
    b. Cognitive preparation
2. **Troubleshooting**
3. **Situational awareness**
    a. Self (role, emotions, limits of knowledge and skill)
    b. Others (roles, perspectives, emotions, limits of knowledge and skill)
    c. Clinical circumstances (time pressures, changes in clinical data or clinical status)
        i. Perception, integration, and projection

FORWARD PLANNING

As defined by Sanfey and colleagues, forward planning refers to the clinician's ability to anticipate needs, to think ahead, and to prepare the operative field in an appropriate manner.[3] Physical preparation involves room set up (positioning, draping, lighting) and choice of instruments and sutures.[14] Depending on the clinical setting and type of training program, medical learners may or may not play an active role in the physical set up of the operative environment. In contrast, cognitive preparation is a fundamental ability required for all procedurally based learners and includes conceptualization of the procedure in distinct steps, recognition of potential points of error, and identification of strategies to mitigate risk. Also called mental rehearsal, cognitive preparation requires focused review of the relevant anatomy and pathophysiology, consideration of the indications for and potential complications of the procedure, and choice of incision, instrument positioning, and dissection.

Effective forward planning considers the expected as well as the unexpected. This complex skill relies on intact foundational knowledge (e.g., of the indications and risks of the procedure, anatomical landmarks, and pathological abnormalities),[16] an understanding of the base rates of common surgical complications, and basic cognitive and executive capacities including attention, working memory, and the ability to visualize a sequence of events and anticipate potential outcomes. Forward planning incorporates principles of prognostic reasoning (discussed in chapter 11), specifically, an assessment of the current clinical severity and future clinical trajectory. Prior research suggests that explicit teaching of operative planning is not universal in surgical training programs.[17]

Learners who struggle with forward planning are often described in the operating room as "hesitant" or "slow." They tend to "get stuck" on early procedural steps and require a great deal of direction to make forward progress in the case. They may appear flustered when asked to demonstrate their thinking during Socratic questioning or when clinical circumstances require them to troubleshoot.

TROUBLESHOOTING

Part of forward planning is anticipating unforeseen events and avoiding error. Troubleshooting refers to an in-the-moment ability to handle the unexpected or, in Sanfey's words, "to improvise."[3] The *unexpected* comprises a spectrum, from a slightly atypical unfolding of events to a true emergency. Responding in these situations requires rapid task shifting ("multitasking") and triage. Like task triage and response in urgent situations (examined in chapters 13 and 14, respectively) troubleshooting is a higher-order ability that relies on relevant medical knowledge, intact foundational executive functions, metacognitive awareness, and self-regulation.

For example, when faced with unexpected bleeding during a surgical procedure, the learner must (1) recognize in the moment that something is wrong (situational awareness), (2) synthesize clinical information to generate diagnostic hypotheses (diagnostic reasoning), (3) assess clinical severity and immediate clinical trajectory (prognostic reasoning), and (4) act (management reasoning). To further complicate matters, decisions must be made without full information. As discussed in chapter 12, management reasoning in the face of uncertainty can be difficult for some medical learners. Experienced clinicians develop a mental library of organized knowledge[18]—in this case, schemas of what is normal and what might go wrong in each procedure—that enable them to recognize instability and make quick decisions in the face of emergency.[19] Troubleshooting occurs by toggling back and forth between System 1 (rapid assessment by pattern recognition) and System 2 (slowing down to think more analytically when necessary) thinking when reasoning through an acute problem.[20] This is analogous to what Schon describes as transitioning from knowing-in-action to reflection-in-action.[21]

Example: *An orthopaedic surgeon is performing a total hip replacement on an elderly patient. Near the end of the procedure, as she is impacting the femoral stem into the femoral canal, the surgeon notes that the implant fits more loosely than expected within the bone. She recognizes that this may be due to a crack in the femur, necessitating an urgent change in operative plan. She quickly reviews her options for further investigation and ultimate repair, articulating her thought process aloud. While often largely intuitive, an expert's reasoning during the troubleshooting process can be broken down into steps:*

- *Assessment of the situation, understanding what has happened—this step often involves unplanned testing and/or intervention [imaging, exposure to determine site of fracture]*

To test her hypothesis that the loose fit of the implant is due to a fracture, she exposes and examines the proximal end of the femur. She also calls radiology to obtain an intraoperative X-ray, which confirms her suspicion. The radiograph demonstrates the extent of the fracture, which propagates approximately 10 cm distally, so the surgeon extends the incision distally to directly visualize the entire fracture.

- *Weighing available options for intervention [do I have to revise the femoral component/take it out and redo, or cable or plate it out?]*

With this information, the surgeon then considers her options for addressing the fracture. She knows that these could include exchanging the current implant for a longer femoral stem to bypass the fracture, placing cables around the bone to reduce the fracture, and/or adding a plate and screw construct to stabilize the fracture.

- *Selecting an intervention*

Because she determined that the current implant is loose, the surgeon knows that it must be exchanged. She then removes the current stem to better assess the condition of the bone and form her plan. The fracture pattern appears straightforward, and the bone is otherwise in good condition, so she decides to address it using cables.

- *Gathering available resources to enact the intervention [ask device representative what stems they have available, please bring plates, cables]*

While making each of these assessments and decisions, the surgeon communicates them to everyone in the room, mobilizing the team to address the situation as efficiently as possible.

- *Communication with the team to ensure appropriate and efficient response*

In reality, many of these steps are occurring simultaneously. Communication with the team is an ongoing process. As soon as the surgeon recognizes the possibility of a fracture, she voices her concerns to everyone in the room (We may have fractured the femur, so we will need an X-ray and additional equipment). This focuses the attention of the team on the new development. While the surgeon is waiting for the X-ray to confirm the fracture, she asks the circulating nurse to send for the cable set and discusses other available stem options with the implant rep. She also notifies the anesthesia team that there may be additional operative time and blood loss. By the time she has fully formed her plan, the necessary instruments are open and available for her to move forward.

Effective troubleshooting in the operating room requires basic executive function such as attention, processing speed, working memory, mental flexibility, and inhibitory control. Metacognition and self-regulation are also essential components of troubleshooting, as the learner must be able to reflect upon their own thinking and emotions in the moment—as well as those of their team members—and assertively communicate any changes in plan while remaining calm and centered.

Learners who struggle with troubleshooting may appear to freeze, hesitate, or seem stuck in the face of an unexpected procedural complication. This may reflect limited capability for pattern recognition due to lack of experience or limited/disorganized knowledge (i.e., management script)[22–24] for the problem in front of them. In chapter 14, we discussed the learner who appears "paralyzed" in the face of uncertainty, often due to overthinking (excessive reliance on System 2 reasoning), anxiety and/or rigidity. Some learners inherently have trouble deviating from a planned course. Because it is impossible to anticipate every untoward clinical event, cognitive flexibility is critical for the learner to apply knowledge and previous experience to the current situation. Conversely, inexperience, anxiety, and/or rigidity may cause the learner to overcompensate or react in an inappropriately aggressive manner in the face of a complication. In chapters 13 and 14, we review the mental health conditions that may underlie difficulties handling interruptions and responding to clinical urgency, respectively.

SITUATIONAL AWARENESS AND KNOWING WHEN TO SLOW DOWN

Situational awareness is central to clinical reasoning, especially in environments where decision-making occurs amid changing data and circumstances. In the operating room, learners must simultaneously pay attention to self, others, and the clinical environment around them. Self-awareness includes cognizance of one's role, one's own emotions, one's level of fatigue and physical condition, the limits of one's own knowledge and skill, and one's emotional and physical impact on others. Humans have limited capacity for attention,[25,26] and this level of vigilance can result in significant cognitive load.[27,28] Errors may occur when attention is divided or misdirected.[29]

Multiple paradigms of situational awareness exist. The Endsley model has been widely applied in health care and describes situational awareness in three hierarchical levels: perception, comprehension, and projection.[30] Initially developed for use in military aviation in the 1980s, this model has informed the conceptualization of operative reasoning in surgery and anesthesiology.[25,26,29,31,32] Errors can occur at each level.[21] Level I (perception) errors involve a failure to collect the relevant information or appreciate the relevant change in clinical circumstances. Difficulties at Level II (comprehension) occur when the clinician perceives the information but is unable to integrate it with the overall clinical picture, often due to ineffective pattern recognition. Level III (projection), the most sophisticated level of situational awareness, is essentially prognostic reasoning and relies on both perception and comprehension. Errors of projection occur when the clinician understands what is happening but incorrectly anticipates the next steps. Situational awareness as defined in this model underlies the ability to effectively troubleshoot in the operating room.

A key aspect of operative judgment is the surgeon's ability to *slow down when [they] should*, as described in a series of seminal articles by Moulton and colleagues.[21,25,33–35] Slowing down, in their conceptualization, represents a deliberate shift from automatic to effortful thinking and comprises a spectrum of behavior from a physical pause (e.g., stopping to refocus, consulting a colleague, reviewing data, or eliminating distractions) to a nearly imperceptible fine-tuning of attentional focus.[33] It is intuitive for a surgeon to pause when called upon to troubleshoot in an intraoperative emergency. However, these investigators observed that expert surgeons also routinely engage in a more proactive form of slowing down (e.g., at critical points of a case).[34] They point to numerous factors that might impede the practice of slowing down proactively, including fatigue, physical or mental health conditions, personality characteristics, and situational influences such as time pressure or availability of resources. In our characterization of operative reasoning, ineffective forward planning would also negatively impact this process. We emphasize the importance of *when [they] should* because, in fact, slowing down simply for the sake of slowing down may actually increase error rates due to overthinking.[36]

More broadly, we consider situational awareness in the operating room to mean reading the room. Used both literally and figuratively, reading the room in this context means monitoring the patient's condition, interpreting the nonverbal cues of team members, and maintaining cognizance of others' moods and stress levels. Experts know when to check in with colleagues, when to acknowledge that things are or are not going well, and when to pause and explain their reasoning. Struggles with interpersonal awareness may reflect social anxiety, neurodiversity, lack of experience with social interactions, early life challenges, or other mental or physical health conditions.

Some learners struggle to adapt to the unspoken rules of social behavior in the operating room and/or do not intuitively understand their role and/or the roles of other team members. They may fail to appreciate the hierarchy, appearing overly eager, arrogant, or unwilling to delegate. Conversely, they may be excessively deferential and reluctant to take ownership during a case. The operating room is an emotionally charged environment, and learners describe feeling exhilarated, anxious, rushed, and inadequate, sometimes all at once. All team members experience a range of emotions during a procedure. These emotions are often associated with physical sensations in the body such as increased heart rate, sweating, or tremor. Without awareness, it is possible to become emotionally flooded in situations of high acuity or conflict or in response to stress. Flooding is a situation in which the rational mind (neocortex) is hijacked by the emotional mind (amygdala and limbic system). Some people are more prone to emotional flooding than others, and one's tendency to flood can be measured.[37,38] When a clinician is caught up in emotions, they tend to react without thinking, they may not communicate effectively, and they often feel out of control. Flooding impairs working memory and concentration[39] and thus may make it difficult to adhere to a predetermined plan, to appreciate changes in clinical circumstance, and/or to troubleshoot. The ability to self-regulate is commonly negatively impacted by sleep deprivation. Additional contributors include stress, concomitant mental or physical health conditions, substance abuse, and early childhood experiences.

THE IMPORTANCE OF ASSERTIVE COMMUNICATION AND TAKING INITIATIVE IN THE OPERATING ROOM

Clinicians engage in multiple types of communication in the operating room, from providing direction, to alerting of a change in clinical status, to teaching, to engaging others in problem-solving. The ability to speak clearly, directly, respectfully, and calmly, especially in times of stress or changing clinical circumstance, is a critical part of operative performance. Assertive communication is likely to promote collaboration and effective team dynamics. In contrast, aggressive communication, characterized by hostility and/or disrespect, may adversely impact the team's ability to work together to care for the patient and respond appropriately to adverse events. Because these skills are often not explicitly taught, trainees frequently rely on role modeling by observing and unconsciously imitating the conduct of supervising faculty. In the high-stakes, often high-stress environment of the operating room, it is not uncommon for behaviors such as yelling or condescension to be perpetuated unintentionally.

In addition, learners are expected to take initiative and provide technical assistance in a procedure without being prompted. Common descriptors of those who struggle with assertiveness include "timid," "functions as a bystander," and "doesn't take ownership." Early on, these observations often reflect the learner's uncertainty about their role in the OR, which often dissipates with time and positive role modeling. Persistence of these behaviors may limit the progression toward autonomy in the operating room, as trust is gained through these verbal and nonverbal cues of engagement. Anecdotally, women are more likely to appear hesitant, lack confidence, or display discomfort with uncertainty in procedural settings. Hesitancy or lack of ownership in the operating room is often blamed on deficient medical knowledge or technical skills and/or unpreparedness (e.g., lack of forward planning). As we will discuss, deliberate practice of forward planning and troubleshooting can improve confidence and bolster assertiveness in the procedural setting. However, even with appropriate knowledge, mastery of basic technical skills, and adequate preparedness, some learners struggle to be assertive—especially in the face of uncertainty or complexity. Timidity as a character trait may signal different neurochemistry, with a lower threshold for activation of the limbic system.[39] Hesitancy can reflect perfectionistic traits, performance anxiety, and/or imposter syndrome. Discomfort with uncertainty may stem from prior experience such as an adverse event. The challenge for educators is to differentiate the learner who is hesitant due to lack of capability from the learner who is hesitant due to imposter syndrome, anxiety, or the processing of a traumatic event(s).

Most surgical educators that we interviewed are more comfortable working with the overconfident trainee than the underconfident trainee, which in part reflects the value placed on confidence and decisiveness in the operating room. Much is written about reining in the "cowboy" who moves too fast, fails to appreciate nuance, overestimates their ability, or is resistant to supervision or feedback.[11] Coaching the overconfident trainee is most successful if it begins with identifying the cause the behavior, which is often rooted in insecurity or a misunderstanding of expectations. Surgical trainees may work to project an image of confidence based on perceived expectations of how a surgeon is supposed to behave,[40] and sometimes they go overboard. Coaching continues with the setting of clear expectations for appropriate and inappropriate behavior followed by role modeling and frequent, direct, real-time feedback. Learners should be encouraged to reflect on how their behavior is and is not helping them reach their goals.

Similarly, coaching the learner who struggles with assertiveness or lack of engagement begins with understanding their experience and raising awareness of what comes up for them emotionally and physically in the operating room. Many learners describe feeling flooded with anxiety, uncertainty, or feelings of inadequacy and, whether or not they realize it, respond by shutting down, getting stuck, or pulling back. Often this is an unconscious, learned response that has developed early in life to protect the individual from feeling these difficult feelings. The process is initially adaptive but becomes maladaptive later in life. Most medical learners set very high standards for themselves, and some may become fixated on how they fall short of these standards, including perseverating on past mistakes. Many individuals with whom we have worked describe a harsh inner critic and/or the tendency to fixate on criticism. Encouraging them to name these feelings and normalizing that everyone feels this way from time to time can be validating. A coach can help the learner to reflect on how the inner critic is both adaptive and maladaptive. A coach or therapist can work with the learner to explore the origins of the inner critic. Evidence supports that humans disproportionately notice and give weight to negative experiences over neutral or positive experiences.[41] This negativity bias leads many learners to ruminate on what they perceive as negative feedback or mistakes.

Evidence-based strategies to help struggling learners cope with these negative feelings and disrupt this type of automatic reaction include mindfulness, self-compassion, and positive practices. For example, the learner can be encouraged to write down three positive work-related experiences at the end of each day (e.g., something they did to help a patient, a piece of positive feedback they received, something they did today that they could not do six months ago). Intentionally drawing attention to the positive events in our lives can train us to do this more naturally. Negative feedback will always sting. And yet real-time feedback is, by necessity, a constant in the operating room. There is an art to giving corrective feedback to the hesitant learner, and it begins with setting expectations. We advocate for a direct approach. Ideally one on one, and not in the operating room itself, acknowledge that you have noticed the learner is hesitant. Explore and validate this hesitancy. Talk to them about how they are being perceived and the positive and negative consequences of hesitancy in an operative setting. Sanford's challenge and support model posits that learners thrive and grow when mentors strike a balance between challenge and support.[42] Often, supervisors will shy away from the timid learner for fear of making them feel more self-conscious. Unfortunately, this often only exacerbates the hesitancy.

Even with clear expectations and positive role modeling, some learners demonstrate persistent uncertainty or discomfort with their role and default to a passive stance, appearing disengaged in the operating room. Anecdotally, many individuals who trained during the COVID-19 pandemic describe feeling generally detached from their patients and in their learning experience. Other learners walk into a case without knowing the patient's full history or having considered the steps of the surgery being performed and yet expect to be given autonomy and responsibility in the operating room just by virtue of being there. It can be challenging to cultivate a sense of ownership with some learners. As is true with earlier examples, working with the disengaged learner begins with understanding the root of the disengagement. How do they understand their role? Often helping these learners to reconnect with whatever drew them to their field of training can be helpful. Setting clear and specific expectations around engagement in the operating room is important, as is role modeling. When feasible, structuring rotations to maximize patient continuity to facilitate more meaningful learner-patient relationships can be helpful. We discuss how to give feedback on operative performance in more detail later in the chapter.

IDENTIFICATION AND ASSESSMENT OF OPERATIVE REASONING DEFICITS

Early identification of operative reasoning deficiency is critical because coaching takes time and requires considerable practice. Several factors contribute to delays in recognition. That a learner will struggle in the operating room is sometimes, but not always, predictable based on their performance in the non-operative setting (e.g., on the consult service, in the intensive care unit). Demonstration of operative reasoning requires a certain degree of autonomy which most surgical learners are not granted until later in their training. Additionally, the surgical training paradigm has changed, most notably by the adoption of the 80-hour work week over the last 20 years. Studies have documented a reduction in quality and quantity of operative experience for general surgery trainees,[14] leading to concerns about preparedness for independent practice. In addition, with a move away from the traditional apprenticeship model,[10] learners spend less time with supervising attendings. This shift impacts the consistency of direct observation, lessens the effect of role modeling on the development of reasoning, and often means that the learner is receiving less meaningful feedback. Concurrently, learners are exposed to sicker and more complex patients in a systems culture that often prioritizes operating room efficiency over time for teaching.[4]

Unlike technical skills, operative reasoning is not universally taught or assessed in surgical training programs.[12] Morbidity and mortality conferences have historically served as a tool to teach clinical reasoning by encouraging learners to discuss their decision-making process and learn from peers and experts.[43–45] Some programs have created interactive teaching conferences centered around complex clinical reasoning scenarios that allow interactive learning in a lower-stakes environment.[46] Creative technology has been developed and employed to assess the technical aspects of operative performance (e.g., high-fidelity simulation, virtual reality), but widespread use of standardized tools to assess clinical reasoning in the operating room is lacking. Direct observation forms the cornerstone of assessment of any type of clinical reasoning. Given the discontinuity that exists in many training programs, it is critical that someone—a program leader, mentor, or coach—is connecting the dots when concerns arise.

In 2023, the American Board of Surgery developed entrustable professional activities (EPAs) that incorporate elements of operative reasoning for commonly encountered clinical scenarios.[47] Some surgical programs have reported improvements in quantity and quality of feedback in the operating room using a smartphone application known as SIMPL.[48] While these provide a variety of workplace-based frameworks for assessment of operative reasoning, implementation has been variable. For programs with the technology, video-based coaching in which a surgeon's operative performance is recorded and reviewed with a coach offers a workplace-based assessment tool that allows for individualized feedback and instruction in both technical and nontechnical skills.[14] Finally, many procedurally based specialties still require oral board examinations for certification. The structure and content of these exams vary by specialty, with some questions focusing on intraoperative reasoning. In theory, the real-time interaction between tester and learner provides the opportunity to gain a more nuanced understanding of the learner's reasoning process that is not readily captured through written multiple-choice questions. As we will discuss, our coaching approach borrows from the oral boards format, with particular focus on exploring and developing cognitive flexibility.

The literature on assessment of the nontechnical components of operative performance has primarily focused on team dynamics and communication and/or situational awareness of the individual.[13] In most of these studies, situational awareness is defined using the Endsley model and thus reflects components of diagnostic, management, and prognostic clinical reasoning. Indirect measures of situational awareness rely on behavioral rating scales to approximate clinicians' internal cognitive processes.[13,32] Examples of tools adapted from the aviation industry and validated for use in anesthesiology and surgery include, respectively, ANTS (Anaesthetists' Non-Technical Skills)[26,32] and NOTSS (Non-Technical Skills for Surgeons).[12,32,49] The NOTSS system, developed in the UK nearly 20 years ago,[31] provides a framework to structure direct observation of the nontechnical aspects of surgery including preparation, awareness, teamwork, and effective communication in the operating room. Inter-rater reliability of both ANTS and NOTSS is variable, and both require expertise and training to administer.[13,26,32] As a surrogate for situational awareness, gaze behavior has been studied via eye tracking devices in simulated settings as a means of measuring distribution of visual attention.[26] Similarly, sensors that measure physiological and behavioral responses have been suggested as a means of approximating cognitive variables such as cognitive load.[13,28]

In contrast, direct measures of situational awareness allow the evaluator to probe the clinician's thought process during or immediately after an operative procedure.[13,32] SAGAT (Situational Awareness Global Assessment Technique) measures perception, integration, and projection via scenario-specific questionnaires that require frequent stops in the clinical action. Initially developed by Endsley and colleagues for use in the aviation industry, SAGAT has been validated in a variety of health care settings.[29,50] Because the tool relies on scheduled pauses to ask questions, its practical use is restricted to simulated settings. SART (Situational Awareness Rating Technique)[26] and S-SART[51] (Surgical Situational Awareness Rating Technique) employ a self-rating questionnaire administered post hoc to assess understanding, attentional demand, and attentional supply. Direct comparison of SART and SAGAT have shown little correlation, and widespread implementation has been limited by concerns about content validity.[26]

Script concordance testing, introduced in chapter 5, has been explored in many procedural fields as a means of assessing clinical reasoning in training and practicing clinicians.[52–57] Two studies have demonstrated the efficacy of script concordance testing as a means of evaluating intraoperative decision-making[55,56] and airway management[57] in anesthesiology residents, respectively. In a third study, investigators from five programs in obstetrics and gynecology created approximately 100 clinical scenarios to assess judgement in gynecologic surgery cases and designed a reliable and valid instrument for assessing intraoperative decision-making.[55] While concerns about feasibility have limited the more widespread use of script concordance testing as an assessment method, we draw upon its fundamental principles when creating coaching plans for learners who struggle with troubleshooting.

COACHING THE LEARNER WHO STRUGGLES WITH OPERATIVE REASONING

While small studies offer evidence-based methods to help trainees evaluate or improve their operative performance, best practices in coaching operative reasoning remain undefined.[14] Learners are often told to "read more" or "practice more." *Practice*, which typically implies repetition of an action to develop a skill and is often performed unaccompanied, is helpful in developing and improving basic technical expertise. However, both the technical and nontechnical aspects of operative performance eventually require *deliberate practice*, which refers to a more reflective process involving acknowledgement of areas of weakness and the setting of specific goals for improvement.[58,59] Effective deliberate practice relies on structured direct observation and real-time feedback around a defined task and can best be conceptualized as a collaborative process that is undertaken by the learner and a coach together.[16] Remediating operative reasoning can appear daunting due to the nature of schedules and the importance of skill-building in a realistic environment, and often requires some creativity. The process frequently begins in a simulated setting such as a coach or supervisor's office or, for those with these resources, a simulation center. This graded approach works particularly well for troubleshooting and/or adapting flight plans to changing or unexpected circumstances in which variables can be controlled in a risk-free, low-stakes environment. Deliberate practice of these fundamental operative reasoning abilities is most effective when there is some adrenaline present. As an example, educators in the UK have developed a simulation-based coaching program that focuses on the nontechnical aspects of operative performance using the NOTSS framework.[12]

Some surgical educators have expressed concern about the patient safety implications associated with remediating technical skills in the operating room. The operating room, however, offers an ideal setting for deliberate practice of operative reasoning, provided there is time for planning and goal setting (i.e., the night before, or just before, the case) and debrief (i.e., at the end of, or right after, the case). To promote self-regulated learning, we recommend tasking the learner with initiating and structuring these pre- and post-procedure meetings. Because many struggling learners are initially uncomfortable with receiving feedback, it is important to set expectations ahead of time, specifying where, when, and how the feedback will be provided. Setting the stage is critical to ensure the learner views the feedback as credible and trustworthy.[60] Given the nature of surgical training, it is likely that the struggling learner will be observed by many different people in many different settings. This underscores the importance of a learner-directed coaching approach in which the learner may have to cue the direct observation and solicit the feedback.

Surgical coaching interventions, occurring in simulated settings and in the operating room, have demonstrated a positive impact on both technical and nontechnical skills. Evidence supports that the quality of coaching is an important determinant of learner expertise in procedural settings.[10,16,61] Effective coaching of operative reasoning typically necessitates a longitudinal relationship between learner and coach during which trust and self-awareness can be cultivated. Ideally, the coach observes the learner some of the time and, when not available to observe, can communicate with other supervising faculty and oversee the skill development from a higher level. In earlier chapters, we have discussed the importance of separating summative assessment from coaching, and thus we recommend that institutional or program directors not assume the role of coach. We recognize that not all institutions or programs have the resources to provide this infrastructure. The good news is that the principles of deliberate practice can be applied in any setting in which the learner is working with a supervisor. Just 1 to 5 minutes of direct observation is enough to provide clear and specific feedback—provided the correct structure is in place.[62] When resources permit, the coach's role is to raise the bar on each cycle of deliberate practice to ensure that the learner is constantly being challenged and improving.

CASE 1, CONTINUED

Dr. Li is not inspiring confidence in the operating room. Despite average medical knowledge and technical skills, he appears to lack assertiveness and self-direction and requires considerable assistance. Perhaps as a consequence of recognizing his own limitations, he seems nervous and tends to rush.

Because there are so many potential explanations for these observations, in this and all cases, effective coaching requires an individualized approach that begins with understanding the learner's perspective and, ultimately, the issues that underlie the behavior. It is important to remember that timidity does not necessarily signify incompetence, just as confidence does not always reflect competence. Dr. Li's difficulties may stem from inadequate forward planning either from lack of preparation (e.g., did not review the relevant anatomy beforehand) or ineffective preparation (e.g., has the relevant knowledge but did not create an effective mental rehearsal). As we have discussed with other phenotypes of clinical reasoning struggle, some learners rely more heavily on frameworks than others to reliably think on their feet in the clinical context. Perhaps Dr. Li feels prepared, but when he gets into the operating room and things are different than he expected, the problem is a lack of cognitive flexibility to allow him to adapt. This struggle to apply knowledge learned from "situation A" to "situation A prime" is more challenging to remediate. Dr. Li may lack situational awareness and, specifically, an understanding of his role and/or how things work in the OR. Some learners pick up on these cues more readily than others. He may struggle with assertiveness or taking initiative in general, and these traits are often magnified in conditions of clinical uncertainty. There may be an underlying mental or physical health condition such as anxiety or depression, or he may be experiencing fatigue or burnout.

Table 15.2 outlines a structured approach to working with the learner with operative reasoning deficiency that makes the following two assumptions: (1) that a coach is available to oversee the process, and (2) that most of the deliberate practice is occurring in or near the operating room itself during scheduled cases. Based on a model proposed 15 years ago by surgical educators at Southern Illinois University, steps 2 through 4 comprise a deliberate practice cycle characterized by direct observation with real-time feedback and time for reflection that occurs immediately before, during, and after an operative procedure.[17] While these steps eventually can and should be learner-directed and incorporate multiple observers, it is ideal in the beginning to pair the learner with a faculty member who can approach the situation more holistically.

In our proposed model, the initial meeting is centered around building rapport, assessing learner perspective, and laying the groundwork for skill development during the coaching process. Using the ADAPT model (Ask, Discuss, Ask, Plan Together),[63] the coach begins by posing questions that promote reflection on prior performance. Questions such as, What are you working on? What has/has not been going well? and What type of feedback have you received from other faculty members? provide a reasonable, if generic, place to start. If the coach has recently observed the learner in the operating room, they can encourage the learner to think back on that experience. The coach continues to ask clarifying questions to probe the learner's insight, subjective experience when being observed in the OR, and overall well-being before sharing their own (or others') observations about the learner's performance. The learner is doing at least half of the talking during the "ask" phase. In Dr. Li's case, the coach should resist the temptation to interject statements such as, "Yes, it looked like you were struggling in there," or "It sounds like you are not taking initiative in the OR, and that is really creating a lot of concern about your ability to progress." When delivering the corrective feedback during the "discuss" phase, it is preferable to describe the behaviors observed (e.g., hesitancy) rather than what they might signify (e.g., lack of knowledge, lack of preparation). Statements beginning with "I saw..." or "Others noticed..." maintain this focus on the behavior and avoid personal judgments that may trigger defensiveness or lead to the learner shutting down. The coach need not take on the role of therapist but should be aware of underlying mental health conditions as potential contributory factors in operative performance concerns. If these initial conversations raise concern for an underlying issue, the learner should be referred for additional evaluation and/or treatment as dictated by programmatic policy.

The initial meeting continues with an effort to identify the clinical reasoning in need of development. We have hypothesized that Dr. Li's difficulties stem in part from lack of effective forward planning and/or situational awareness. Thus, the coach should explore and provide feedback on his preparation process and his understanding of roles and how he is being perceived in the clinical setting. Depending on the underlying issue, the coach and learner move into a collaborative plan, identify specific goals of coaching, and tee up steps 2 through 4 (the deliberate practice cycle). The plan may involve additional meetings to promote development (e.g., how to prepare effectively for a case). For most learners, preparation builds confidence in high-stakes situations. If the learner lacks a system for preparation, the coach can share theirs and/or encourage the learner to observe them preparing for a case. Table 15.2 lists the components of the flight plan. Some learners benefit from using templates or checklists to guide their forward planning. It can be helpful to review and/or role play recent or hypothetical cases, either assigned ahead of time or presented in real time, to assess and provide feedback on learner preparation, knowledge of relevant anatomy and pathophysiology, insight and ability to reflect, and mental flexibility (by reviewing "what if" scenarios). For programs with these resources, the simulation center can provide an excellent setting for these types of exercises.

Situational awareness, as we have defined it, is a coachable skill, though individuals have differing capacities to develop emotional intelligence in general. Some learners benefit from scaffolding to improve their awareness in the OR setting. The STEPPS checklist acknowledges the status of the patient, status of team members, environment (resources, equipment), and progress toward goal (e.g., Are we making progress? Do we need to change course?).[3] In this case, the coach is encouraged to explore Dr Li's understanding of roles in the operating room. As discussed earlier in this chapter, assertiveness is likely to improve once the learner is provided with support, clear expectations, and frameworks to promote effective clinical reasoning. The learner should leave the initial meeting(s) with a clear idea of expectations and areas on which to focus their attention during the upcoming deliberate practice cycle. The coach should clarify learner understanding by asking them to reflect the plan and to identify any areas of uncertainty or confusion.

For all learners in procedural specialties, meeting with the supervising faculty member immediately prior to the case is crucial to identify skills within the zone of development on which to focus the teaching and observation in the OR. Depending on the learner and the type of procedure, this meeting might occur anywhere between the day before to minutes before the case is to begin. The learner should be encouraged to prepare for the case as outlined in Table 15.2, using templates or checklists if helpful to structure their preparation. For many struggling learners, coaching centers around making the planning process itself more explicit. Reflection on their methods of preparation before, during, and after the case serves as a means of identifying areas for further development and/or content areas in which further study is needed. Taking the time to touch base and review/assign roles, set time limits (when applicable), and anticipate events should facilitate a smoother, more efficient experience for both learner and observer and may allow the learner more autonomy. In anticipation of patient- or procedure-specific potential difficulties, the learner should be encouraged to identify points in the case that warrant slowing down. Because the observer may not be aware of Dr. Li's situation, it is important that Dr. Li assume a proactive role in both ensuring these meetings occur and in setting expectations for the observation.

CASE 1, CONTINUED

Dr. Reynolds, an attending surgeon, has posted an elective robotic low anterior resection for rectal cancer. Dr. Li will be assisting her. In preparation for the case, Dr. Reynolds meets with Dr. Li the morning prior to surgery. Dr. Reynolds reviews the patient's history with Dr. Li, explaining her reasoning for neoadjuvant treatments and the final decision for surgery. They then review the details of the operation, including the expected port placements and robotic instruments that are needed to accomplish the surgery. Dr. Reynolds outlines the critical steps of the surgery, including the high ligation of the critical vessels, identification and preservation of the left ureter, obtaining the appropriate planes for the total mesorectal excision, and, most importantly, plan for achieving a successful anastomosis. Dr. Reynolds then queries Dr. Li's comfort level with each critical step of the case. Dr. Li expresses that he would like to be able to identify and perform the high ligation of the inferior mesenteric vessel and most of the rectal dissection. With this information Dr. Reynolds goes through various scenarios with Dr. Li: For example: What if, after transecting the major vessel, you experience rapid pulsatile bleeding? What if you find that you have in fact transected the left ureter? What are your landmarks and steps to identifying the correct vessel?

Dr. Reynolds then discusses with Dr. Li that the rectal dissection involves careful tumor manipulation, and any error to this dissection could compromise the patient's oncologic outcome. If she decides that the tumor is too risky, she will likely perform this step herself. This reassurance will help Dr. Li with his confidence level during the case—specifically, that it hasn't been "taken away" from him because of his technical capabilities. Rather, it is the patient-specific anatomy that forbids this.

During the case, the direct observation and feedback is centered around the goals and objectives defined in the pre-brief. This is an opportunity for the coach to both role model and probe the learner's reasoning process. Statements like "Talk me through your decision-making," or "What if…?" can be helpful.

Dr. Reynolds and Dr. Li proceed with the case. They have completed the left colon mobilization and identified the left ureter. They are now ready to transect the inferior mesenteric artery. Dr. Reynolds queries Dr. Li regarding his approach to ligating this major artery. Dr. Li verbalizes that he would like to utilize the vessel sealer device to ligate the artery. Dr. Reynolds then asks him to consider what he would do if, after transecting the vessel, he encounters mild bleeding? Moderate bleeding? Significant bleeding that occludes his view? They then run through each scenario and ensure that all necessary equipment for these contingency plans is available.

If circumstances permit, the struggling learner can be encouraged to talk a more junior learner through the case. For the learner who is working to improve assertiveness, drawing attention to examples of your own assertive communication during the case can be helpful. Over time, this practice builds self-awareness and encourages the learner to be more deliberate about why and how they are performing the steps of the case and/or making certain decisions. Role modeling can be an effective way to teach learners how and when to *slow down* during a procedure. Because the processes of shifting attention and responding to changing clinical circumstances are typically so automatic for experts, educators must practice their own situational awareness, becoming more deliberate about articulating their thought process in key moments.

The post-case debrief can be quick (< 5 minutes) and may take place at the end of the case (e.g., while the learner is closing, if the room has cleared out) or immediately after the case. The purpose of this meeting is to promote reflection on what worked/did not work, what came up for the learner as they were practicing the skill(s), and how they did or did not meet the previously outlined expectations. The debrief is also the time to address any unexpected events that occurred during the procedure. The ADAPT framework works well for structuring the debrief. In Dr Li's case, the coach might begin by asking questions such as, What went well? How did your preparation strategy work today? Is there anything that you missed in preparation? How did it feel to behave more assertively?

The case proceeds smoothly, and Drs. Reynolds and Li are performing the anastomosis. At this critical step, it is clear that Dr. Li is not familiar with the technical aspects of firing the anastomotic stapler. His struggles result in a tear in the bowel. They re-do the anastomosis and complete the surgery. Later in the day, Dr. Reynolds meets with Dr. Li. Dr. Li admits that he has only used that particular stapler a handful of times, and each time he struggles with the mechanics of manipulating the instrument. Drs. Reynolds and Li then formulate a clear action plan to have Dr. Li meet with the stapler device representative for hands-on training. Additionally, Dr. Reynolds reinforces the need for open and clear communication and self-awareness surrounding his comfort level going forward.

In other scenarios, feedback for the learner working on situational awareness might center around whether the learner demonstrated awareness of others' points of view, appropriately delegated, or sought help when reaching their limits of confidence. In this model, the conversation continues with the observer providing feedback on the skills being observed, ensuring the learner understood the feedback. At the conclusion of the feedback and reflection, learner and coach co-create goals for future study and direct observation. Pendleton's rules[64] provide a related, alternative structure for providing post-procedure feedback, as follows: (1) Observer asks learner to identify 3 things that went well, (2) Observer provides 3 things that went well, (3) Observer asks for 3 things that could be improved, (4) Learner identifies 3 things that could be improved and offers strategies for improvement, and (5) Together, observer and learner summarize important points. Both feedback approaches encourage metacognitive reflection which is a critical component of operative reasoning. If insight is limited, the observer may need to lead the conversations early in the coaching processes. With practice, the process should become more learner-directed.[64] The debrief builds self-awareness and improves the learner's ability to estimate their procedural competency, identifying specific areas of strength and weakness.

If the coach is not performing the direct observation as the learner cycles through these deliberate practice activities, the learner should be encouraged to check in regularly with the coach to process feedback, hone skill development, and assess the progress of the coaching intervention.

Table 15.2. A Practical Approach to Coaching Operative Reasoning

1. **Initial Meeting(s)**—*learner and coach meet in a private setting outside of the OR*
   — Review feedback and concerns
   — Explore learner's perspective, assess for underlying factors

(continued)

(Table 15.2 continued)

- "Diagnose" clinical reasoning issue(s), introduce frameworks
  + Forward planning: explore and role model preparation strategies
  + Troubleshooting: mock oral board cases, probe mental flexibility
  + Situational awareness: explore understanding of roles, STEPPS
- Set expectations for coaching process, develop a plan to ensure direct observation with real-time feedback
- Refer for additional evaluation and/or treatment if concern about underlying mental or physical health condition

2. Immediately prior to case—*learner and coach (or observer, if different than coach) meet the day before, or day of, the surgery*

- Ask learner to prepare/review, in advance, for verbal discussion or in writing
  + Indications for the procedure
  + Clinical picture, key imaging,
  + Physical set up
  + Operative steps
  + Points of potential risk, with contingency planning
  + Points of uncertainty, with contingency planning
  + Operative notes from related cases
- Review learner's plan, explore reasoning behind the plan, provide feedback, identify additional areas for preparation and/or study
- Assign roles
- Set time limits for certain steps
- Identify potential points of *slowing down*
- Anticipate events, contingency planning
- Set 2 to 3 specific goals for the case with measurable outcomes and expectations for feedback

(Table 15.2 continued)

3. **During case**—*coach either directly observes learner during case or provides tips to supervising faculty to guide structured direct observation*
   - Provide specific feedback on skills being practiced
   - Ask questions to prompt reflection
   - Encourage learner to articulate thought process during key steps or when troubleshooting
   - Draw attention to points of slowing down
   - Instruct learner to talk a more junior learner through the case/decisions
   - Ask "what if?" or "what is your next step?" questions to probe learner's knowledge and mental flexibility
   - Provide emotional support if learner appears distressed, practice grounding exercises (i.e., breathing)
4. **Immediately after case**—*learner and coach (or observer) meet to debrief day of, or day after case*
   - Provide specific feedback on performance aligned with previously set expectations
   - Encourage learner to reflect on performance (e.g., preparation process, situational awareness, progression through steps as planned, ability to adapt in the moment, emotional regulation)
   - Identify areas for continued practice and goals for the next direct observation
5. **Ongoing meetings**—*learner and coach may continue meeting to review cases, feedback*

COACHING TROUBLESHOOTING IN THE OPERATING ROOM

As discussed, problem solving when things go awry in the operating room is a multifaceted ability that incorporates elements of forward planning, situational awareness, and assertiveness. There is considerable overlap between intraoperative troubleshooting and other reasoning-related abilities discussed in this book, including designing a management plan (chapter 12), triaging tasks (chapter 13), and responding to clinical urgency (chapter 14). The coaching approach for learners who struggle when faced with the unexpected during a procedure, either by freezing, hesitating, appearing stuck, or over functioning, follows the structure outlined in Table 15.2. By encouraging reflection on prior events, the coach explores the learner's experience—cognitively, emotionally, and physically—during prior events and provides feedback on how the learner is perceived in these situations. It can be helpful to review prior or hypothetical cases in a mock oral boards format to better understand the clinical reasoning issue that underlies the struggle with troubleshooting. For instance, does the learner lack frameworks for recognizing (or management scripts for managing) common intraoperative complications? Do they struggle with rapid task shifting? Are they overcome with fear or flooded with uncertainty which prevents the ability to access knowledge and/or respond appropriately to the change in clinical status? These questions can usually be answered relatively quickly in one meeting. From there, the coaching plan is developed, targeting the specific area of concern.

All learners can benefit from restructuring knowledge to facilitate script activation and pattern recognition in situations that require rapid decision-making. In chapter 14, we introduced the *urgency framework* as a coaching tool to promote contextualization of knowledge and more efficient retrieval and application of knowledge in the moment. We adopt a similar approach for the learner who "draws a blank" when expected to troubleshoot in the operating room. The learner is encouraged to create a list of commonly encountered intraoperative urgencies or emergencies relevant to their scope of practice and to develop frameworks for managing these situations that combine elements of diagnostic, management, and prognostic reasoning. A simplified framework for unexpected intraoperative bleeding, with clinical example, is presented below as an example:

1. **Problem representation**
   60-year-old woman undergoing a routine laparoscopic cholecystectomy develops sudden and unexpected bleeding during dissection, and the surgical field is obscured

2. **Statement of immediate goal(s)**
   Control the bleeding; stabilize patient's hemodynamics; maintain visualization of the field
3. **Diagnostic reasoning**
   Where is the bleeding originating? What are the contributing circumstances (e.g., coagulopathy, technical factors)? What are the worst-case scenarios?
4. **Management reasoning**
   a. Immediate actions
      Gain control of the surgical field (e.g., apply suction, pack the area); ensure patient stability (e.g., communicate with anesthesia team; prepare for resuscitation with fluids and/or blood products)
   b. More definitive management
      Restore hemostasis (combination of techniques depending on source/location of bleeding)
5. **Prognostic reasoning**
   Is the bleeding controlled or uncontrolled? Evaluate impact of initial attempts at hemostasis. Assess hemodynamic stability. Adjust approach as necessary (e.g., convert to open procedure).

The learner discusses these scenarios and/or reviews hypothetical or recently encountered scenarios with a coach in the office or in a simulation center. During the exercise(s), the coach probes the learner's knowledge and reasoning by changing key features of the case and asking "what if" questions. The learner receives in the moment feedback about their decision-making and is encouraged to reflect on the experience. Through an iterative process that occurs longitudinally, the frameworks are internalized as schemas.[19,65] Because the spectrum of the unexpected in the operating room is so broad, it is impossible to anticipate and plan for all untoward events. The strength of this approach, then, lies in its ability to promote adaptability, or the ability to apply lessons learned from "situation A" to "situation A prime." It is through repetition of the deliberate practice cycle, occurring initially in a simulated setting (e.g., a coach's office, the simulation center) and ultimately in the operating room, that cognitive flexibility is developed—which is ultimately what will determine the learner's ability to troubleshoot *in vivo*.

This approach borrows from the literature on script concordance testing, an assessment method designed to evaluate clinical reasoning in conditions of uncertainty. As an example, the following case vignette was designed to assess intraoperative reasoning in gynecologic surgery.

55 y/o female undergoing abdominal hysterectomy for menorrhagia. She has a 16-week size uterus with multiple fibroids on physical exam. During the hysterectomy you encounter bleeding from one uterine pedicle. The learner is asked: *a) if you were considering treating the bleeding by cauterizing the bleeding vessels, and then you find the ureter immediately adjacent to the bleeding vessel, that treatment becomes (check one): -2 (almost contraindicated), -1 (less appropriate or less useful), 0 (neither more nor less appropriate, +1 (more appropriate or even helpful), +2 (indicated or absolutely indicated).*[55] Though script concordance testing as a clinical reasoning assessment method is often impractical, the underlying concepts greatly inform the coaching of intraoperative reasoning. The case vignettes and "what if" questions, focusing on clinical situations for which there is no one "right" answer, provide a means of promoting cognitive flexibility and stimulating meaningful interaction between learner and expert during coaching sessions.

Drawing from the work of Moulton and colleagues, we encourage all learners to be deliberate about *slowing down* when (*when is key*) faced with the unexpected during a procedure.[33,34] Lee and colleagues integrate theories from education and psychology to characterize the "medical pause," the most extreme form of slowing down, citing its importance in promoting both patient safety and learning.[27] The pause allows the learner to engage their awareness, to notice what they are feeling, to scan the room for others' nonverbal cues, and to communicate with the team. For learners who experience performance anxiety, grounding tools such as box breathing (inhale 4 counts, hold breath for 4 counts, exhale 4 counts, hold exhalation for 4 counts) can help to relieve the physiologic symptoms of anxiety.[66] Diaphragmatic breathing has been shown to reduce self-doubt and enhance both working memory and motor skills in the operating room.[67] Moreover, we advocate for a "cognitive time-out" in which the learner articulates the problem representation as the first step of enacting their troubleshooting script. This process promotes shared recognition by the team of the situation and prioritizes immediate goals. Using the above example, the learner recognizes the problem and states, "We have brisk bleeding from a branch of the cystic artery. The surgical fields are obscured." This practice is important for situations less obvious than bleeding and is recommended anytime the learner is aware of a sense of discomfort, or that things aren't quite right.

For all the other issues, including becoming more facile with task shifting, managing emotions, and communicating assertively when under stress, our recommended approach is deliberate practice in a setting in which some adrenaline is present. Troubleshooting is an ideal skill to hone in a simulation center. Beginning in an area of content familiarity and employing cases where variables are limited and the pathway for decision-making is more well-defined, the learner can work through cases that require troubleshooting. Eventually the deliberate practice must continue in the clinical environment. As we have discussed, direct observation of this skill in the operating room should focus on the learner's thought process as they make decisions. The coach can serve as a role model by articulating their thought process as they themselves approach unforeseen events and by drawing attention to their own process of *slowing down* (emphasizing how and when) to regroup. Feedback should focus on how quickly the learner was able to adapt, their comfort with intervening or not intervening when appropriate, their facility with toggling back and forth between strategies or hypotheses, and their ability to articulate their decision-making processes.

APPLYING THESE LESSONS TO COACH LEARNERS IN ANESTHESIOLOGY

CASE 2

Dr. Carter is an anesthesiology resident who works hard and never complains, is always proactive about giving breaks to her colleagues, and performs thorough preoperative patient evaluations. However, concerns have arisen early in the second year about appropriate preparation and problem solving in the intraoperative environment. Evaluations note as areas for improvement that she often appears unprepared for potential emergencies and struggles to consider a comprehensive differential diagnosis when urgent situations occur.

An example of the insufficient preparation occurred when a patient experienced laryngospasm, and it was identified that there was no succinylcholine (emergency medication to treat laryngospasm) in the automated medication dispensing system, as that was not checked during the setup for her case. An illustration of ineffective troubleshooting involved a patient who developed hypotension during a multilevel spine surgery, and she increased vasopressors without recognizing that the patient was hypovolemic and should have been treated with fluids instead. Similarly, her patient's blood pressure cuff cycled without giving a read shortly after abdominal insufflation during a laparoscopic cholecystectomy. Dr. Carter persistently focused on fixing the blood pressure cuff itself by changing the cuff size and location of the cuff without recognizing true hypotension causing the cuff to not give a reading.

Dr. Carter has never had any difficulty with learning or performance in school. Her medical school performance reveals a ranking in the middle 50% of her graduating class and average standardized test scores. She acknowledges that she does feel overwhelmed sometimes in the operating room when things happen urgently and notes that her anxiety at these times makes it difficult to think clearly.

Trainee intraoperative reasoning issues in anesthesiology overlap with those observed in other procedural specialties and may include difficulties with forward planning, troubleshooting, and/or situational awareness. A learner who is struggling in one or more of these realms may demonstrate adequate or even above-average medical knowledge or technical skills. In fact, often these learners come to attention later than ideal because they have been putting in the effort, often with a good attitude, but fail to progress in their ability to anticipate and manage urgent clinical events.

As vigilance serves as the cornerstone of anesthesiology, early recognition of learner struggles with situational awareness is critical. Coaching the learner who struggles with situational awareness begins with considering the impact of factors that impair attention, such as distractors (e.g., loud music, internet browsers) and interruptions. The learner is encouraged to practice being mindful of where attention is directed during a case and employ visual tools or mnemonics to promote more methodical scanning of the environment.[29] Drawing from Endsley's model, tools like SAGAT provide a framework for coaching situational awareness, from perception (e.g., How is the patient's blood pressure?) to comprehension (e.g., Why is the patient hypotensive despite a fluid bolus?) to projection (e.g., Is the patient nearing cardiac arrest? Does the patient need a blood transfusion or vasopressor support?).[26]

The process for coaching anesthesiology learners who struggle with forward planning centers around the principles of deliberate practice that we have discussed earlier in this chapter. Employment of a checklist provides a structured approach to case preparation and can help ensure that nothing is forgotten. For example, MS MAIDS is an acronym that outlines the steps involved in preparing the OR prior to each case (M: machine check, S: suction, M: monitors, A: airway, I: intravenous kit, D: drugs, S: special equipment).[68] Direct observation of the learner attempting room setup using this tool may identify areas in need of more rigorous preparation and additionally presents the opportunity to assess and provide feedback about contingency planning. For example, if remembering D (drugs) is not enough, the coach can help the learner to create a detailed checklist including specific drugs expected to be immediately available in case of an emergency.

When issues with troubleshooting and situational awareness are identified, coaching in a simulated environment (either the coach's office or a simulation center) can be helpful. In either setting, simulation allows the learner to think aloud and debrief with a coach after each scenario and provides a safe learning space to develop and practice these skills. Talking through differential diagnoses of common perioperative adverse events (e.g., hypotension and hypoxia) facilitates the development of illness and management scripts that will be activated in context when they encounter these events in the OR. Because cognitive flexibility is so important for troubleshooting, as discussed earlier in this chapter with other procedurally based learners, we draw upon the principles of the script concordance test as learners develop and refine these scripts. It is critical that learners develop management scripts through growing knowledge and experience for commonly encountered operative adverse events, much like the development of urgency schemas as discussed in chapter 14.

In the simulated environment, learners can gain comfort adapting to changing circumstances without risk of harming a patient. Also, having an emergency manual readily available as an app on their phone can serve as a surrogate for a checklist as they work through emergency situations.[69] An example is a laminated algorithm for emergencies in anesthesia such as LAST syndrome or malignant hyperthermia.

When working with struggling learners, we typically employ an approach with multiple simulations of progressively increasing complexity followed by debriefing sessions. For the anesthesiology learner who is struggling with troubleshooting, a typical initial clinical scenario involves a standard induction in the operating room. In this case, the debriefing allows instructors to ensure the learner understands the logic and reasoning for the clinical decisions made during a normal clinical encounter. The second scenario presents a "curve ball" such as bronchospasm, an urgent but common problem, that develops after induction. This debriefing focuses on creating a differential diagnosis and talking through the reasoning behind treatment decisions in common intraoperative emergencies, as well as preparation for these events. Subsequent scenarios introduce rarer, yet life-threatening, scenarios such as a malignant hyperthermia crisis. The coach can thus differentiate between learner struggle with the basics, anticipating common emergencies, or recognizing uncommon emergencies.

A commonly used framework for structuring the debriefing sessions includes the following components: introduction, advocacy/inquiry, application to real settings, and summary.[70] Example introduction: "You just finished taking care of Mrs. Smith. There were some challenging moments. How are you feeling about it?" The advocacy/inquiry component allows the instructor to explore the learner's perspective and, if necessary, help move the learner to a new perspective. Example advocacy/inquiry question: "I saw that you hesitated to treat when the patient's heart rate increased. Could you walk me through what you were thinking at the time?" It is helpful to generalize and apply these lessons learned to the real clinical setting in which they will return. Example application to real settings: "How do you see this playing out with your future clinical practice?" Each debriefing should also end with a summary of take-away points for the learner to consider in between coaching sessions.

Direct observation is one of the most critical assessments that can be used to provide meaningful feedback to learners when coaching moves from the simulated environment to the clinical environment. Direct observation tools help provide standardized ways to structure feedback discussions. These may come in the form of checklists, the Structured Direct Observation Assessment Tool (SDOT),[71] ACGME milestone evaluations,[1] or mini-clinical evaluation exercise (Mini-CEX).[72] These tools provide means to observe, assess, and give feedback in a standardized format and should be succinct to minimize the burden and stress on the coach educator in a busy clinical environment. One of these direct observation tools should be used as the daily feedback form for all learners referred for coaching in the clinical environment within a training program. This standardization may help relieve the stigma of being referred for coaching.

Finally, if the resident identifies that anxiety is hindering their ability to perform to the best of their ability during urgent situations, referral to a mental health professional in accordance with programmatic and institutional policy may be warranted.

Dr. Carter is confidentially referred to a therapist for evaluation and treatment of performance anxiety. Simultaneously, she begins work with a clinical reasoning coach with whom she can engage in simulation scenarios, utilize checklists, and develop illness scripts and management scripts to address common adverse perioperative events.

SUMMARY

The window to coach the learner who struggles in procedural settings is narrow, and the stakes are high. Effective coaching must transcend reading plans and technical skills repetition. The components of operative reasoning and the related skills of assertive communication and engagement can be taught and honed through the process of deliberate practice. Evidence supports that coaching improves operative performance. Given the many logistical challenges that disrupt continuity between learner and educator in the current model of surgical training, coupled with the importance of self-regulated learning, coaching works best when it is learner centered. In fact, a critical aspect of coaching is empowering the learner to become an active participant in their own learning. In this chapter, we offer a practical approach to coaching the learner struggling with operative performance that takes advantage of existing points of interface between the learner and supervising faculty member. With minimal faculty development, this approach can be applied to all medical learners in procedural fields as part of their educational development.

Acknowledgement: Thank you to Katherine Fedder, MD, head and neck oncologic and microvascular surgeon and medical educator, for her input and guidance throughout the development of this chapter.

References

1. ACGME Home. Accessed January 22, 2025. https://www.acgme.org/
2. UME Competencies AAMC | AACOM | ACGME. Accessed January 22, 2025. https://engage.aamc.org/UME-Competencies-AAMC-ACGME-AACOM
3. Sanfey H, Williams R, Dunnington G. Recognizing residents with a deficiency in operative performance as a step closer to effective remediation. *J Am Coll Surg.* 2013;216(1):114-122. doi:10.1016/j.jamcollsurg.2012.09.008
4. Reznick RK, MacRae H. Teaching surgical skills—changes in the wind. *N Engl J Med.* 2006;355(25):2664-2669. doi:10.1056/NEJMra054785
5. Kalet A, Chou CL, eds. *Remediation in Medical Education: A Mid-Course Correction.* Springer International Publishing; 2023. doi:10.1007/978-3-031-32404-8
6. Williams RG, Roberts NK, Schwind CJ, Dunnington GL. The nature of general surgery resident performance problems. *Surgery.* 2009;145(6):651-658. doi:10.1016/j.surg.2009.01.019
7. Parsons AS, Dreicer JJ, Martindale JR, Young G, Warburton KM. A Targeted Clinical Reasoning Remediation Program for Residents and Fellows in Need. *J Grad Med Educ.* 2024;16(4):469. doi:10.4300/JGME-D-23-00822.1
8. Crannell WC, Brasel KJ. Dealing with the struggling learner. *Surgery.* 2020;167(3):523-527. doi:10.1016/j.surg.2019.06.013
9. Yule S, Flin R, Paterson-Brown S, Maran N. Non-technical skills for surgeons in the operating room: a review of the literature. *Surgery.* 2006;139(2):140-149. doi:10.1016/j.surg.2005.06.017
10. Min H, Morales DR, Orgill D, Smink DS, Yule S. Systematic review of coaching to enhance surgeons' operative performance. *Surgery.* 2015;158(5):1168-1191. doi:10.1016/j.surg.2015.03.007
11. Minter RM, Dunnington GL, Sudan R, Terhune KP, Dent DL, Lentz AK. Can this resident be saved? Identification and early intervention for struggling residents. *J Am Coll Surg.* 2014;219(5):1088-1095. doi:10.1016/j.jamcollsurg.2014.06.013
12. Yule S, Parker SH, Wilkinson J, et al. Coaching Non-technical Skills Improves Surgical Residents' Performance in a Simulated Operating Room. *J Surg Educ.* 2015;72(6):1124-1130. doi:10.1016/j.jsurg.2015.06.012
13. Cha JS, Yu D. Objective Measures of Surgeon Non-Technical Skills in Surgery: A Scoping Review. *Hum Factors.* 2022;64(1):42-73. doi:10.1177/0018720821995319
14. Hu YY, Mazer LM, Yule SJ, et al. Complementing Operating Room Teaching With Video-Based Coaching. *JAMA Surg.* 2017;152(4):318-325. doi:10.1001/jamasurg.2016.4619

15. Daniel M, Wilson E, Torre D, Durning SJ, Lang V. Embodied cognition: knowing in the head is not enough. *Diagn Berl Ger.* 2020;7(3):337-338. doi:10.1515/dx-2020-0004

16. Sauer CG, Newman LR, Leichtner AM. Training in Endoscopy: Coaching, Deliberate Practice, and Reflection. *J Pediatr Gastroenterol Nutr.* 2019;68(3):298-300. doi:10.1097/MPG.0000000000002231

17. Roberts NK, Williams RG, Kim MJ, Dunnington GL. The briefing, intraoperative teaching, debriefing model for teaching in the operating room. *J Am Coll Surg.* 2009;208(2):299-303. doi:10.1016/j.jamcollsurg.2008.10.024

18. Custers EJFM. Thirty years of illness scripts: Theoretical origins and practical applications. *Med Teach.* 2015;37(5):457-462. doi:10.3109/0142159X.2014.956052

19. Cammarata M, Dhaliwal G. Diagnostic Schemas: Form and Function. *J Gen Intern Med.* 2023;38(2):513-516. doi:10.1007/s11606-022-07935-1

20. Croskerry P. A Universal Model of Diagnostic Reasoning. *Acad Med.* 2009;84(8):1022. doi:10.1097/ACM.0b013e3181ace703

21. Moulton C anne E, Regehr G, Mylopoulos M, MacRae HM. Slowing Down When You Should: A New Model of Expert Judgment. *Acad Med.* 2007;82(10):S109. doi:10.1097/ACM.0b013e3181405a76

22. Parsons AS, Wijesekera TP, Rencic JJ. The Management Script: A Practical Tool for Teaching Management Reasoning. *Acad Med.* 2020;95(8):1179-1185. doi:10.1097/ACM.0000000000003465

23. Cook DA, Stephenson CR, Gruppen LD, Durning SJ. Management reasoning scripts: Qualitative exploration using simulated physician-patient encounters. *Perspect Med Educ.* 2022;11(4):196-206. doi:10.1007/s40037-022-00714-y

24. Abdoler EA, O'Brien BC, Schwartz BS. Following the Script: An Exploratory Study of the Therapeutic Reasoning Underlying Physicians' Choice of Antimicrobial Therapy. *Acad Med.* 2020;95(8):1238. doi:10.1097/ACM.0000000000003498

25. St-Martin L, Patel P, Gallinger J, Moulton C anne. Teaching the slowing-down moments of operative judgment. *Surg Clin North Am.* 2012;92(1):125-135. doi:10.1016/j.suc.2011.12.001

26. Schulz CM, Endsley MR, Kochs EF, Gelb AW, Wagner KJ. Situation awareness in anesthesia: concept and research. *Anesthesiology.* 2013;118(3):729-742. doi:10.1097/ALN.0b013e318280a40f

27. Lee JY, Szulewski A, Young JQ, Donkers J, Jarodzka H, van Merriënboer JJG. The medical pause: Importance, processes and training. *Med Educ.* 2021;55(10):1152-1160. doi:10.1111/medu.14529

28. Young JQ, Van Merrienboer J, Durning S, Ten Cate O. Cognitive Load Theory: implications for medical education: AMEE Guide No. 86. *Med Teach.* 2014;36(5):371-384. doi:10.3109/0142159X.2014.889290

29. Margolis RD, Ku CM. The "Difficult Learner" in anesthesiology: Challenges, pitfalls, and recommendations. *Pediatr Anesth.* 2021;31(1):92-102. doi:10.1111/pan.14059

30. Endsley MR. TOWARD A THEORY OF SITUATION AWARENESS IN DYNAMIC SYSTEMS. *Hum Factors.* 1995;37(1). Accessed February 4, 2025. https://trid.trb.org/View/426377

31. Yule S, Flin R, Paterson-Brown S, Maran N, Rowley D. Development of a rating system for surgeons' non-technical skills. *Med Educ.* 2006;40(11):1098-1104. doi:10.1111/j.1365-2929.2006.02610.x

32. Cooper S, Porter J, Peach L. Measuring situation awareness in emergency settings: a systematic review of tools and outcomes. *Open Access Emerg Med OAEM.* 2013;6:1-7. doi:10.2147/OAEM.S53679

33. Moulton C anne, Regehr G, Lingard L, Merritt C, MacRae H. Slowing Down to Stay Out of Trouble in the Operating Room: Remaining Attentive in Automaticity. *Acad Med.* 2010;85(10):1571. doi:10.1097/ACM.0b013e3181f073dd

34. Moulton C anne, Regehr G, Lingard L, Merritt C, Macrae H. "Slowing down when you should": initiators and influences of the transition from the routine to the effortful. *J Gastrointest Surg Off J Soc Surg Aliment Tract.* 2010;14(6):1019-1026. doi:10.1007/s11605-010-1178-y

35. Merritt C. Operating from the other side of the table: control dynamics and the surgeon educator. *J Am ….* Published online January 1, 2010. Accessed February 4, 2025. https://www.academia.edu/586713/Operating_from_the_other_side_of_the_table_control_dynamics_and_the_surgeon_educator

36. Monteiro S, Sherbino J, LoGiudice A, Lee M, Norman G, Sibbald M. The influence of viewing time on visual diagnostic accuracy: Less is more. *Med Educ.* 2024;58(7):858-868. doi:10.1111/medu.15380

37. Gottman JM. A theory of marital dissolution and stability. *J Fam Psychol.* 1993;7(1):57-75. doi:10.1037/0893-3200.7.1.57

38. Penberthy JK, Chhabra D, Ducar DM, et al. Impact of Coping and Communication Skills Program on Physician Burnout, Quality of Life, and Emotional Flooding. *Saf Health Work.* 2018;9(4):381-387. doi:10.1016/j.shaw.2018.02.005

39. Goleman D. *Emotional Intelligence.* Bantam Books; 1995.

40. Patel P, Martimianakis MA, Zilbert NR, et al. Fake It 'Til You Make It: Pressures to Measure Up in Surgical Training. *Acad Med.* 2018;93(5):769. doi:10.1097/ACM.0000000000002113

41. Vaish A, Grossmann T, Woodward A. Not all emotions are created equal: the negativity bias in social-emotional development. *Psychol Bull.* 2008;134(3):383-403. doi:10.1037/0033-2909.134.3.383

42. Sanford N. *Self and Society: Social Change and Individual Development.* Atherton Press; 1966:xvii, 381.

43. Beaulieu-Jones BR, Wilson S, Howard DS, et al. Defining a High-Quality and Effective Morbidity and Mortality Conference: A Systematic Review. *JAMA Surg.* 2023;158(12):1336-1343. doi:10.1001/jamasurg.2023.4672

44. Abraham S, Parsons A, Uthlaut B, Plews-Ogan P. Re-thinking morbidity and mortality. *Diagnosis.* 2020;1(ahead-of-print). doi:10.1515/dx-2020-0040

45. Fiorentino AR, Kieffer KA. Learning Outcomes from an Academic Internal Medicine Morbidity and Mortality Conference. *J Gen Intern Med.* 2022;37(9):2239-2245. doi:10.1007/s11606-022-07499-0

46. Minter DJ, Parsons AS, Abdoler E. Reasoning Report: Engineering Case Conferences to Maximize Clinical Reasoning Education for All Learners. *J Gen Intern Med.* 2024;39(15):3073-3076. doi:10.1007/s11606-024-08778-8

47. Montgomery KB, Mellinger JD, Lindeman B. Entrustable Professional Activities in Surgery: A Review. *JAMA Surg.* 2024;159(5):571-577. doi:10.1001/jamasurg.2023.8107

48. Abdou H, Kidd-Romero S, Brown RF, Kavic SM, Kubicki NS. Keep it SIMPL: Improved Feedback After Implementation of an App-Based Feedback Tool. *Am Surg.* 2022;88(7):1475-1478. doi:10.1177/00031348221082279

49. Wood TC, Raison N, Haldar S, et al. Training Tools for Nontechnical Skills for Surgeons-A Systematic Review. *J Surg Educ.* 2017;74(4):548-578. doi:10.1016/j.jsurg.2016.11.017

50. Hogan MP, Pace DE, Hapgood J, Boone DC. Use of human patient simulation and the situation awareness global assessment technique in practical trauma skills assessment. *J Trauma.* 2006;61(5):1047-1052. doi:10.1097/01.ta.0000238687.23622.89

51. Chen JJ, Gompers A, Evenson A, James BC, Royce C. Surgical Adaptation of the Situation Awareness Rating Technique (S-SART): Assessing Situational Awareness Among Medical Students. *J Surg Educ.* 2023;80(2):216-227. doi:10.1016/j.jsurg.2022.09.015

52. Meterissian SH. A novel method of assessing clinical reasoning in surgical residents. *Surg Innov.* 2006;13(2):115-119. doi:10.1177/1553350606291042

53. Kania RE, Verillaud B, Tran H, et al. Online script concordance test for clinical reasoning assessment in otorhinolaryngology: the association between performance and clinical experience. *Arch Otolaryngol Head Neck Surg.* 2011;137(8):751-755. doi:10.1001/archoto.2011.106

54. Sibert L, Darmoni SJ, Dahamna B, Hellot MF, Weber J, Charlin B. On line clinical reasoning assessment with Script Concordance test in urology: results of a French pilot study. *BMC Med Educ.* 2006;6:45. doi:10.1186/1472-6920-6-45

55. Park AJ, Barber MD, Bent AE, et al. Assessment of intraoperative judgment during gynecologic surgery using the Script Concordance Test. *Am J Obstet Gynecol.* 2010;203(3):240.e1-6. doi:10.1016/j.ajog.2010.04.010

56. Ducos G, Lejus C, Sztark F, et al. The Script Concordance Test in anesthesiology: Validation of a new tool for assessing clinical reasoning. *Anaesth Crit Care Pain Med.* 2015;34(1):11-15. doi:10.1016/j.accpm.2014.11.001

57. Omega A, Wijaya Ramlan AA, Soenarto RF, Heriwardito A, Sugiarto A. Assessing clinical reasoning in airway related cases among anesthesiology fellow residents using Script Concordance Test (SCT). *Med Educ Online.* 2022;27(1):2135421. doi:10.1080/10872981.2022.2135421

58. Ericsson KA. Deliberate Practice and the Acquisition and Maintenance of Expert Performance in Medicine and Related Domains. *Acad Med.* 2004;79(10):S70.

59. Abdulnour REE, Parsons AS, Muller D, Drazen J, Rubin EJ, Rencic J. Deliberate Practice at the Virtual Bedside to Improve Clinical Reasoning. *N Engl J Med.* 2022;386(20):1946-1947. doi:10.1056/NEJMe2204540

60. Kogan J. The Adapt Model for Feedback. ACGME Remediation Toolkit. Learn at ACGME. August 31, 2024. Accessed February 4, 2025. https://dl.acgme.org/courses/acgme-remediation-toolkit

61. Padia R, Wang C, Henry L, Ishman SL, Jamal N. How to be a Better Surgeon: The Evidence for Surgical Coaching. *Otolaryngol—Head Neck Surg Off J Am Acad Otolaryngol-Head Neck Surg.* Published online December 15, 2024. doi:10.1002/ohn.1091

62. Feedback for Coaches. Accessed February 4, 2025. https://depts.washington.edu/lgateway/elearning/fbc/story.html

63. Andolsek K, Padmore J, Hauer KE, Holmboe E. Clinical Competency Committees.

64. Ridder JMM van de, Wijnen-Meijer M. Pendleton's Rules: A Mini Review of a Feedback Method. *Am J Biomed Sci Res.* 2023;19(1):19.

65. Minter DJ, Manesh R, Cornett P, Geha RM. Putting Schemas to the Test: An Exercise in Clinical Reasoning. *J Gen Intern Med.* 2018;33(11):2010-2014. doi:10.1007/s11606-018-4599-z

66. Balban MY, Neri E, Kogon MM, et al. Brief structured respiration practices enhance mood and reduce physiological arousal. *Cell Rep Med.* 2023;4(1):100895. doi:10.1016/j.xcrm.2022.100895

67. Hopper SI, Murray SL, Ferrara LR, Singleton JK. Effectiveness of diaphragmatic breathing for reducing physiological and psychological stress in adults: a quantitative systematic review. *JBI Database Syst Rev Implement Rep.* 2019;17(9):1855-1876. doi:10.11124/JBISRIR-2017-003848

68. MSMAID. Accessed February 4, 2025. https://prolongedfieldcare.org/wp-content/uploads/2015/04/msmaid-show-notes.pdf

69. Home. Stanford Emergency Manual. Accessed February 27, 2025. https://emergencymanual.stanford.edu/

70. Rudolph JW, Simon R, Rivard P, Dufresne RL, Raemer DB. Debriefing with good judgment: combining rigorous feedback with genuine inquiry. *Anesthesiol Clin.* 2007;25(2):361-376. doi:10.1016/j.anclin.2007.03.007

71. CORD Standardized Direct Observational Assessment Tools. Accessed February 4, 2025. https://www.cordem.org/resources/residency-management/cord-standardized-assessment-methods

72. Norcini JJ, Blank LL, Duffy FD, Fortna GS. The mini-CEX: a method for assessing clinical skills. *Ann Intern Med.* 2003;138(6):476-481. doi:10.7326/0003-4819-138-6-200303180-00012

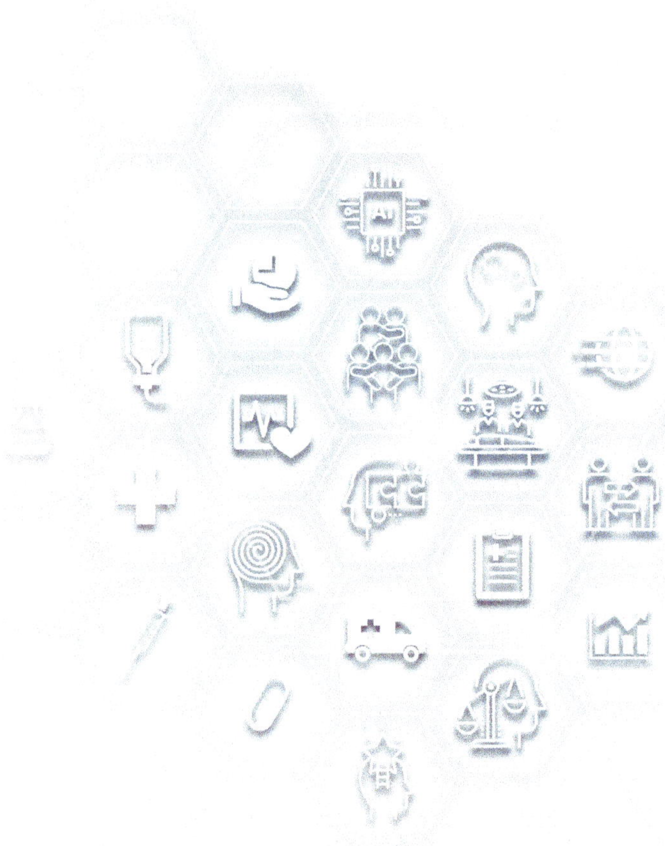

APPENDIX

Clinical Reasoning in the Workplace: A Blueprint for Direct Observation

Consistent with the principles of deliberate practice and self-regulated learning, direct observation is central to all aspects of the clinical reasoning coaching process. Experts uphold the importance of direct observation in the workplace, during actual clinical encounters, and using existing tools with validity evidence.[1–3] While the optimal duration of each direct observation session is unknown, meaningful work can be accomplished in a matter of minutes if goals and objectives are clearly determined ahead of time. With every subtype of clinical reasoning struggle presented in this book, we have provided deficit-specific and setting-specific guidance on structuring direct observation. However, as we have acknowledged throughout, addressing the significant barriers to more widespread use of direct observation in the workplace requires its intentional integration into clinical practice and dedicated faculty development.

Below, we present a framework for structuring direct observation of clinical reasoning in different workplace settings, outlining what to observe and linking observable activities to the clinical reasoning discussed in this book, referenced by chapter. Learners are encouraged to think aloud and explain their thought process as they are observed. Each encounter should begin with a brief discussion of goals and objectives and conclude with immediate, structured feedback. Feedback must be specific, timely, and behavior based. While designed to promote formative assessment of learners engaged in clinical reasoning coaching, this framework can be applied to all learners.

INPATIENT SETTING

- **Pre-rounding process:** observer spends 5 to 30 minutes with the learner as they prepare for attending rounds, at the bedside and/or away from the bedside
  - — Early hypothesis generation [chapters 7, 8]
  - — Hypothesis-driven data gathering, focused history/physical exam/ use of EHR [chapters 7, 8]
  - — Hypothesis refinement, synthesis of data, cognitive flexibility [chapters 7, 8]
  - — Effective diagnostic scripts and schemas [chapter 9]
  - — Prioritization of tasks within fixed time interval, contingency planning [chapters 11, 13]
- **Patient presentations on interdisciplinary rounds:** observer evaluates the presentation in entirety or chooses components (below) on which to focus the direct observation, including the learner's response to questions asked during the presentation
  - — Reflects all aspects of the pre-rounding process (as above)
  - — Problem representation, differential diagnosis with justification [chapters 7, 8, 10]
  - — Hypothesis refinement, synthesis of data, cognitive flexibility [chapters 7, 8]
  - — Prioritization of the problem list [chapters 9, 10, 11]
  - — Independent plan with justification, use of management script template [chapters 7, 8, 12]
  - — Effective diagnostic and/or management scripts and schemas [chapters 8, 9]
  - — Prognostic reasoning [chapter 11]
- **Encounter with patient at the bedside:** observer spends 5 to 30 minutes observing a patient encounter (new patient encounter, change in clinical status, counseling/explaining to patient) or specific elements of an encounter
  - — Early hypothesis generation [chapters 7, 8]
  - — Hypothesis-driven data gathering, focused history/physical exam/ use of EHR [chapters 7, 8]
  - — Hypothesis refinement, synthesis of data, cognitive flexibility [chapters 7, 8]
  - — Problem representation [chapters 7, 8, 10]

— Management with justification [chapters 7, 8, 12] if observe post-encounter decision-making and/or if decision-making is part of the encounter

— Effective diagnostic and/or management scripts and schemas [chapters 8, 9]

— Prognostic reasoning [chapters 10, 11]

— Triaging tasks: prioritization and integration of data, avoiding rabbit holes [chapter 13]

- **Written notes, discharge summaries**

— Hypothesis refinement, synthesis of data, cognitive flexibility [chapters 7, 8]

— Problem representation, differential diagnosis with justification [chapters 7, 8, 10]

— Prioritization of problem list [chapters 10, 11]

— Management with justification [chapters 7, 8, 12]

— Lack of effective diagnostic and/or management scripts and schemas [chapters 8, 9]

— Prognostic reasoning [chapters 10, 11]

- **Handoffs of care**

— Problem representation [chapters 7, 8, 10]

— Prognostic reasoning [chapters 10, 11]

— Prioritization of problem list [chapters 10, 11]

- **Calling consultants:** observer pays attention to framing of the clinical question and integration of the consultant's recommendations

— Problem representation [chapters 7, 8, 10]

- **Triaging a task list:** observer checks in during the workday and reviews the learner's task list with them

— Triaging tasks: managing interruptions, task shifting, prioritization of tasks, cognitive flexibility [chapter 13]

— Problem representation [chapters 7, 8, 10]

— Management reasoning [chapters 7, 8, 12]

— Hypothesis refinement, synthesis of data, cognitive flexibility [chapters 7, 8]

— Lack of effective diagnostic and/or management scripts and schemas [chapters 8, 9]

- **Response to clinically urgent or emergent situations:** observer debriefs with the learner within 24 hours of the event
  - — Response to urgency or emergency [chapter 14]
  - — Early hypothesis generation [chapters 7, 8]
  - — Problem representation [chapters 7, 8, 10]
  - — Prognostic reasoning [chapter 11]
  - — Management reasoning, management amid uncertainty [chapters 7, 8, 12]
  - — Hypothesis refinement, synthesis of data, cognitive flexibility [chapters 7, 8]
  - — Effective diagnostic and/or management scripts and schemas [chapters 8, 9]

OUTPATIENT SETTING

- **Preparation for clinic, precharting**
  - — Early hypothesis generation [chapters 7, 8]
  - — Hypothesis-driven data gathering: focused history/physical exam/ use of EHR [chapters 7, 8]
  - — Hypothesis refinement, synthesis of data, cognitive flexibility [chapters 7, 8]
  - — Triaging tasks: managing interruptions, task shifting, prioritization of tasks, cognitive flexibility [chapter 13]
  - — Effective diagnostic scripts and schemas [chapters 8, 9]
  - — Prioritization of tasks within fixed time interval, contingency planning [chapters 11, 13]
- **Encounter with patient**
  - — Early hypothesis generation [chapters 7, 8]
  - — Hypothesis-driven data gathering: focused history/physical exam/ use of EHR [chapters 7, 8]
  - — Hypothesis refinement, synthesis of data, cognitive flexibility [chapters 7, 8]
  - — Problem representation [chapters 7, 8, 10]
  - — Management with justification [chapters 7, 8, 12] if observe post-encounter decision-making and/or if decision-making is part of the encounter
  - — Effective diagnostic and/or management scripts and schemas [chapters 8, 9]

— Prognostic reasoning [chapter 11]
— Triaging tasks: prioritization and integration of data, avoiding rabbit holes [chapter 13]

- **Post-encounter decision-making**
  — Entering orders, selecting plan [chapter 12]
  — Problem representation, differential diagnosis with justification [chapters 7, 8, 10]
  — Hypothesis refinement, synthesis of data, cognitive flexibility [chapters 7, 8]
  — Prioritization of problem list [chapters 10, 11]
  — Management with justification [chapters 7, 8, 12]
  — Effective diagnostic and/or management scripts and schemas [chapters 8, 9]

- **Written notes**
  — Hypothesis refinement, synthesis of data, cognitive flexibility [chapters 7, 8]
  — Problem representation, differential diagnosis with justification [chapters 7, 8, 10]
  — Prioritization of problem list [chapters 10, 11]
  — Management with justification [chapters 7, 8, 12]
  — Effective diagnostic and/or management scripts and schemas [chapters 8, 9]
  — Prognostic reasoning [chapters 10, 11]

OPERATIVE SETTING

- **Before the procedure:** observer meets with the learner within 24 hours of the procedure to review the learner's physical and cognitive preparation
  — Forward planning [chapters 11, 15], anticipating:
    + Room setup
    + Flight plan/steps of the case
    + Points of potential risk or uncertainty, with contingency planning
    + Procedural risk assessment, critical anatomical or patient-specific considerations
    + Indications for the case
    + Optimization pre-operatively (e.g., anticoagulation, antibiotics, fluids, blood products)

- **During or immediately after the procedure:** observer debriefs with the learner within 24 hours of the procedure
  - Troubleshooting [chapters 11, 15]: responding to the urgent and/or unexpected
    - Problem representation [chapters 7, 8, 10]
    - Effective diagnostic and/or management scripts and schemas [chapters 8, 9]
    - Hypothesis refinement, synthesis of data, cognitive flexibility [chapters 7, 8]
    - Prognostic reasoning [chapters 10, 11]
    - Management reasoning, management amid uncertainty [chapters 7, 8, 12]
  - Situational awareness [chapter 15]

References

1. Kogan JR, Hatala R, Hauer KE, Holmboe E. Guidelines: The do's, don'ts and don't knows of direct observation of clinical skills in medical education. *Perspect Med Educ.* 2017;6(5):286-305. doi:10.1007/s40037-017-0376-7

2. Kogan JR, Holmboe ES, Hauer KE. Tools for direct observation and assessment of clinical skills of medical trainees: a systematic review. *JAMA.* 2009;302(12):1316-1326. doi:10.1001/jama.2009.1365

3. Hauer KE, Holmboe ES, Kogan JR. Twelve tips for implementing tools for direct observation of medical trainees' clinical skills during patient encounters. *Med Teach.* 2011;33(1):27-33. doi:10.3109/0142159X.2010.507710

ABOUT THE AUTHORS

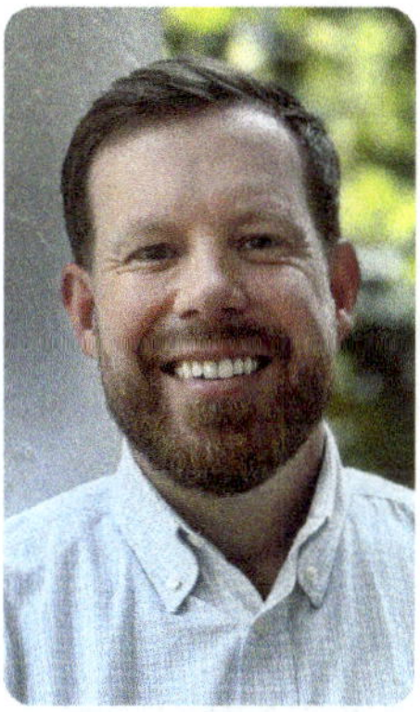

Used by permission

Andrew S. Parsons, MD, MPH is an associate professor of medicine at the University of Virginia School of Medicine where he serves as the Associate Dean for Clinical Competency. He is also the Director of Research and Academic Advancement for the Division of Hospital Medicine.

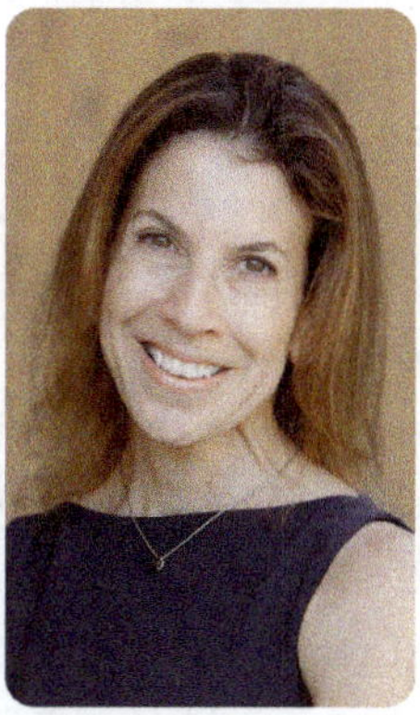

Photo by Jen Fariello

Karen M. Warburton, MD is a professor of medicine at the University of Virginia School of Medicine where she serves as Associate Designated Institutional Official for Trainee Advancement and Director of the Clinician Wellness Program.

ABOUT THE ASSOCIATION FOR HOSPITAL MEDICAL EDUCATION (AHME)

The Association for Hospital Medical Education, founded in 1956, is a national, non-profit organization involved in the continuum of hospital-based medical education. AHME's members represent several hundred teaching hospitals, academic medical centers, and consortia which are involved in the delivery of undergraduate, graduate, and continuing medical education. The mission of AHME is to promote improvement in medical education to meet health care needs, serve as a forum and resource for medical education information, develop professionals in the field of medical education, and advocate the value of medical education in health care.

To fulfill its mission, the Association annually provides a three-day educational conference (AHME Institute), one-day educational sessions (AHME Academy), and a series of six webinars. AHME publishes the *Guide to Medical Education in the Teaching Hospital* (a practical resource for medical education professionals), *Remediation of the Struggling Medical Learner* (a structured approach to identifying and supporting residents and students who aren't progressing at an expected pace), *Remediation Case Studies: Helping Struggling Medical Learners*, and two issues of *AHME News* annually. Additional resources are also made available on the AHME website (www.ahme.org). AHME has secured external funding to support clinical performance-improvement activities, solicited and reviewed proposals from member institutions, and awarded grants to support these projects. AHME also publishes the *Journal for Continuing Education in the Health Professions*, a peer-reviewed publication, in collaboration with the Alliance for Continuing Education in the Health Professions (ACEHP) and the Society of Academic Continuing Medical Education (SACME).

AHME supports four interest groups, which include the Council of Institutional Leaders, the Council of Program Administrators and Coordinators, the Council on Professional and Faculty Development, and the Council of Transitional Year Program Directors. The Association is a member organization of the Accreditation Council for Continuing Medical Education, an associate member organization of the Council of Medical Specialty Societies, as well as a liaison organization of the National Resident Matching Program. It also enjoys collaborative relationships with a number of other accreditation, regulatory, and professional organizations with an interest in medical education.

AHME | ASSOCIATION FOR HOSPITAL MEDICAL EDUCATION

INDEX

D

V

W

Y

www.ingramcontent.com/pod-product-compliance
Lightning Source LLC
LaVergne TN
LVHW052020200926
848481LV00005B/1542
9798218701697